IN HER LIFETIME

Female Morbidity and Mortali
in Sub-Saharan Africa

Committee to Study Female Morbidity and Mortality in Sub-Saharan Africa

Christopher P. Howson, Polly F. Harrison, Dana Hotra, and Maureen Law, *Editors*

Board on International Health

INSTITUTE OF MEDICINE

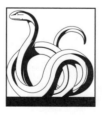

NATIONAL ACADEMY PRESS
Washington, D.C. 1996

NATIONAL ACADEMY PRESS • 2101 Constitution Avenue., N.W. • Washington, D.C.   20418

NOTICE: The project that is the subject of this report was approved by the Governing Board of the National Research Council, whose members are drawn from the councils of the National Academy of Sciences, the National Academy of Engineering, and the Institute of Medicine. The members of the committee responsible for the report were chosen for their special competences and with regard for appropriate balance.

This report has been reviewed by a group other than the authors according to procedures approved by a Report Review Committee consisting of members of the National Academy of Sciences, the National Academy of Engineering, and the Institute of Medicine.

The Institute of Medicine was chartered in 1970 by the National Academy of Sciences to enlist distinguished members of the appropriate professions in the examination of policy matters pertaining to the health of the public. In this the Institute acts under the Academy's 1863 congressional charter responsibility to be an adviser to the federal government and, upon its own initiative, to identify issues of medical care, research, and education. Dr. Kenneth I. Shine is President of the Institute of Medicine.

The project was supported by funds from the Carnegie Corporation (contract nos. B-5269 and D-93065). Additional project support was provided by the Special Programme of Research, Development, and Research Training in Human Reproduction, World Health Organization (contract no. HQ/93/043301); the Kellogg Endowment Fund; and the National Research Council's NAS/NAE independent funds and IOM independent funds.

Library of Congress Catalog Card Number: 95-72800

International Standard Book Number: 0-309-05430-3

Additional copies of this report are available from:

National Academy Press
Box 285
2101 Constitution Avenue, N.W.
Washington, DC 20418

Call 800-624-6242 or 202-334-3313 (in the Washington Metropolitan Area)

COVER: Oil painting by Ablade Glover. Reprinted, with permission, from the Carnegie Corporation of New York. Ablade Glover is a Ghanaian artist who has exhibited widely in the United States, Switzerland, Zimbabwe, England, Germany, and his home country. He is represented in collections in many countries. He studied art in the United Kingdom and at Kent State University and Ohio State University in the United States. Currently he is associate professor, Department of Art Education, University of Science and Technology, Kumasi, Ghana, on sabbatical in Accra, where he is directing a cooperative gallery called Artists Alliance.

Printed in the United States of America

The serpent has been a symbol of long life, healing, and knowledge among almost all cultures and religions since the beginning of recorded history. The image adopted as a logotype by the Institute of Medicine is based on a relief carving from ancient Greece, now held by the Staatlichemuseen in Berlin.

COMMITTEE TO STUDY FEMALE MORBIDITY AND MORTALITY IN SUB-SAHARAN AFRICA

MAUREEN LAW (*Chair*), Director General, Health Sciences Division, International Development Research Centre, Ottawa, Ontario, Canada

UCHE AMAZIGO, Visiting Professor, Department of Zoology, University of Nigeria, Nsukka, Enugu State

JUDITH FORTNEY, Corporate Director, Scientific Affairs, and Director, Division of Reproductive Epidemiology and Sexually Transmitted Diseases, Family Health International, Research Triangle Park, North Carolina

PHILIP L. GRAITCER, Associate Professor, Center for Injury Control, Rollings School of Public Health, Atlanta, Georgia

FRANCOISE F. HAMERS, EIS Officer, Division of STD/HIV Prevention, Centers for Disease Control and Prevention, Atlanta, Georgia

H. KRISTIAN HEGGENHOUGEN, Associate Professor, Department of Social Medicine, Harvard School of Medicine, Boston, Massachusetts

KARUNGARI KIRAGU, Research and Evaluation Officer, Center for Communication Programs, Johns Hopkins School of Hygiene and Public Health, Baltimore, Maryland

JOANNE LESLIE, Adjunct Assistant Professor, University of California at Los Angeles, School of Public Health, and Co-Director, Pacific Institute for Women's Health, Los Angeles, California

WALINJOM F. T. MUNA, Director, General Hospital of Yaounde, Yaounde, Republic of Cameroon

JONATHAN E. MYERS, Director, Occupational Health Research Unit, Department of Community Health, School of Medicine, University of Cape Town, South Africa

BENJAMIN O. OSUNTOKUN, Professor, Neurology Unit, Department of Medicine, University of Ibadan, Ibadan, Nigeria (Deceased)

PATIENCE W. STEPHENS, Demographer, the World Bank, Resident Mission, Accra, Ghana

JUDITH N. WASSERHEIT, Director, Division of STD/HIV Prevention, Centers for Disease Control and Prevention, Atlanta, Georgia

BELMONT E. O. WILLIAMS, Professor, Clark Atlanta University, and Assistant Clinical Professor, Department of Obstetrics and Gynecology, Morehouse School of Medicine, Atlanta, Georgia

Project Staff

CHRISTOPHER P. HOWSON, Project Director
POLLY F. HARRISON, Senior Program Officer
DANA HOTRA, Research Associate
DELORES SUTTON, Project Assistant
JAMAINE TINKER, Financial Associate
CAROLINE MCEUEN, Contract Editor
BERYL BENDERLY, Contract Writer

iii

Dedication

The Committee to Study Female Morbidity and Mortality in Sub-Saharan Africa dedicates this report to Patricia Rosenfield and Rosalee Karefa-Smart of The Carnegie Corporation. Their vision, hard work, and strong commitment to the life span perspective and female health made this project possible.

Acknowledgments

Although this book is cited as a report of the Committee to Study Female Morbidity and Mortality in Sub-Saharan Africa, the committee chair and Institute of Medicine wish to acknowledge the following committee members, IOM staff, and outside experts as primary authors: Chapter 1 (Beryl Benderly, consultant science writer; Polly Harrison; Christopher Howson); Chapter 2 (Kristian Heggenhougen; Polly Harrison; Dana Hotra); Chapter 3 (Joanne Leslie; Bibi Essama, University of California at Los Angeles); Chapter 4 (Judith Fortney; Karungari Kiragu); Chapter 5 (Benjamin Osuntokun); Chapter 6 (John Orley and Giovanni de Girolamo, World Health Organization); Chapter 7 (Walinjom Muna); Chapter 8 (Philip Graitcer); Chapter 9 (Jonathan Myers); Chapter 10 (Uche Amazigo); Chapter 11 (Judith Wasserheit; Francoise Hamers); and Appendix A (Christine Costello, National Academy of Sciences; Douglas Ewbank, University of Pennsylvania; Christopher Howson; Patience Stephens). For their part, the committee gratefully acknowledges the valuable contributions of the following people to their report: F. C. Okafor, Maureen Obi, and N. Ivoke, University of Nigeria, for their help with Chapter 10; Richard Rothenberg and Sevgi Aral, Centers for Disease Control and Prevention, for their insightful comments and suggestions regarding Chapter 11; and Susan Scrimshaw, University of Illinois at Chicago, for her sage editorial advice on the report as a whole. The committee owes a special debt of gratitude to Caroline McEuen, contract editor, for her substantive and creative editing of the final document.

The committee also thanks those individuals whose vision and hard work contributed to the early development of this project in 1986, including Polly Harrison, Jill Gay, April Powers, and Belkis Giorgis, Institute of Medicine; Susan Scrimshaw, University of Illinois at Chicago; Judith Bruce, the Population Council; Elayne Clift, Academy for Educational Development; Carol Corillon, National Academy of Sciences; Joan Dunlop, International Women's Health Coalition; Patrice Engle, Institute of Nutrition of Central America and Panama; Ruth Bamela Engo-Tjega, Labor Ministry-Cameroon; Benjamin Gyepi-Garbah, Barbara Hertz, and Althea Hill, the World Bank; Don Hopkins, the Carter Center; Sandra Huffman, Center to Prevent Childhood Malnutrition; Angela Kamara, Columbia University; Marjorie Koblinsky, the Ford Foundation; Michael Latham, Cornell University; Haydee Lopez, Chilean Medical Association; Cathie Lyons, The United Methodist Church; Ken McIntosh, Harvard Medical School; Henry Mosely, The Johns Hopkins University; Isabel Nieves, the Institute of Nutrition of Central America and Panama; Judy Norsigian and Norma Svenson, Boston Women's Health Book Collective; Adhiambo Odaga, Oxford University; Chloe O'Gara, U.S. Agency for International Development; Freda Paltiel, Canadian Ministry of Health; Barbara Pillsbury, University of California at Los Angeles; Barry Popkin, University of North Carolina; Eva Rathgeber, International Development Research Centre; Allan

Rosenfield, Columbia University; Nawal El Saadawi and Irene Santiago, Oxfam; Judith Timyan, International Center for Research on Women; and Ann Tinker, the World Bank.

The committee also thanks the many people who provided information, critical analysis, advice, and informal review in the last two years of the project, including Margaret R. Becklake, McGill University; Mark Belsey, World Health Organization; Ronald Blanton, Case Western Reserve University; Barry Bloom, Albert Einstein College of Medicine; Lita Curtis, Institute of Medicine; Aleya El-Bindari Hammad, World Health Organization; Lori Heise, Pacific Institute for Women's Health; Kenneth Hill, Johns Hopkins School of Hygiene and Public Health; King Holmes, University of Washington; Niki Jazdowska; Eileen Kennedy, International Food Policy Research Institute; Mere Kisekka, Ahmadu Bello University, Nigeria; Claude Lenfant, National Heart, Lung, and Blood Institute; Adetokunbo Lucas, Harvard School of Public Health; Deborah Maine, Columbia School of Public Health; Violaine Mitchell, Institute of Medicine; Jane Mutambirwa, University of Zimbabwe; Elena Nightingale, Carnegie Corporation of New York; Obioma Nnaemeka, University of Minnesota; Frederick Robbins, Case Western Reserve University; Jeanne Stellman, International Labor Organization; and Tomris Turmen and Carol Vlassoff, World Health Organization.

The committee would also like to thank individuals within the Institute of Medicine whose support was instrumental to the project. These include Christopher P. Howson, Study Director; Polly F. Harrison, Senior Program Officer; Dana Hotra, Research Associate, and Dee Sutton, Project Assistant, who typed volumes, arranged travel, and organized and assisted at meetings. Others within the Institute of Medicine and National Academy of Sciences who were instrumental in seeing the project to completion were Kenneth I. Shine, IOM President, who provided invaluable editorial advice at a key juncture in report preparation; Enriqueta C. Bond and Karen Hein, IOM Executive Officers; Susan M. Wyatt and Jamaine Tinker, Financial Associates; Mary Pat Nowack, Contract Specialist; Sharon Scott-Brown, Administrative Assistant; Michael Edington, Editor; and Betsy Turvene, Consultant. The commmittee is especially grateful to Claudia Carl, Administrative Associate, for her expert help in coordinating the outside review of this manuscript.

In particular, the committee would like to thank Timothy Rothermel of the United Nations Development Programme, and Paul Van Look, Einar Roed, and Guiseppe Benagiano of the Human Reproduction Programme, World Health Organization, for their help in securing additional funds for this project.

Finally, it is with great sadness that committee and staff note the death of Benjamin O. Osuntokun, Professor of Neurology, University of Ibadan, Nigeria, on 23 September 1995. His expertise, hard work, and graciousness as a physician and member of this committee were key to the success of this project. We will miss you, Ben.

Contents

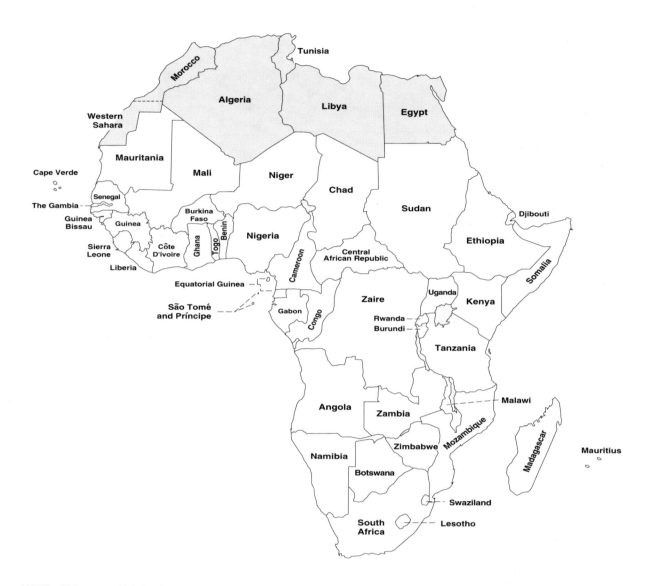

NOTE: This map, which has been prepared solely for the convenience of readers, does not purport to express political boundaries or relationships. The scale is a composite of several forms of projection. SOURCE: Reprinted, with permission, from National Research Council, *Social Dynamics of Adolescent Fertility in Sub-Saharan Africa*. Copyright 1993 by the National Academy of Sciences.

1

Summary

PREAMBLE

As mothers, as workers, as citizens, as members of families and communities, women play a central and increasingly complex role in the life of Sub-Saharan Africa. That reality, however, has been reflected in only a patchy, disjointed, and erratic way in the worlds of medicine and public health. Scientific attention and preventive health efforts have almost single-mindedly focused on women's health as it affects their offspring, and on women's lives as centered on reproduction alone. In essence, women have been treated as mothers or wives, rather than as individual female human beings living whole lives.

There are powerful reasons why this has been so; perhaps the most compelling of these has been demographic. Anxiety about population growth, and consequent concern about the high fertility rates in developing countries, drove the expansion of family planning services that began in the 1960s in much of the developing world. The emphasis, therefore, was on reproduction, not on reproductive health. These attempts to give women at least some control over the number and timing of births in their lives were eminently worthwhile, but they were incomplete.

The second reason has also involved numbers. The emphasis placed on the survival of infants and very young children during the past 15 years responded to the dictates of mortality statistics. To a degree, this was appropriate. Throughout the developing world, death rates in infants and children were higher than in any other age group, in many cases stunningly high. A large proportion of these deaths were seen to be—and, indeed, proved to be— avoidable, as relatively low-cost technologies and program interventions became increasingly available. Efforts to reduce mortality in this vulnerable population were essential but, again, were incomplete: the survival, health, and nutritional status of females seemed to matter—both physiologically and programmatically—only because they influenced child survival and well-being.

There are other reasons as well for the neglect of women's health issues. In virtually all countries, both developing and developed, government administration is categorical and disarticulated. Ministries of agriculture, health, education, infrastructure, labor, commerce, and industry do their work separately, unified only by the annual budgeting efforts of central finance ministries. Gender or age categories are almost never a target for public investment; when they are, such efforts are usually internal to a single sector. From a bureaucratic standpoint, this is logical, but such a disjointed approach rarely responds very well to the special needs of particular populations or to the resolution of wide-ranging national problems.

Finally, efforts over the past 25 years toward women's fuller participation in the life and development of nations have stressed their legal and political rights—to vote, to hold office, to work, to inherit. Yet, as necessary and urgent as this emphasis has been, it too is incomplete. Current directions are much more expansive; "women's *human* rights" include protection from political persecution and gender violence; property rights and fair compensation for work in a safe workplace; the ability to practice free and responsible parenthood; and the setting of reproductive rights in the context of overall health.

Every one of these initiatives has been crucial for large numbers of individuals and families. Had they not been undertaken, it would be more difficult now to think more expansively. At the same time, these partial approaches create a special dilemma for females because their responsibilities are so complex. The female role is at least a double one: women have the primary charge for reproduction and the care of their own offspring, and often care for the parental or grandchild generation as well. At the same time, in most of the developing world, and increasingly in the developed world, women play a major role in the production of goods and services. In Sub-Saharan Africa, female children are quite young when they are first called to share in family labor, first births come early, and life expectancy has been short; thus, females are bearing children, caring for them, and working throughout their lives.

As overall life expectancy in the region continues to lengthen, however, the span of those years widens, so that a model of health care in which females are statistically and medically important only in their ability to survive infancy and bear children is proving increasingly inadequate. The challenge that confronts us now is how to maintain female health and well-being across that widening and ever more complex span, and adjust to the new needs that will arise.

THE "LIFE SPAN" APPROACH

In 1988, when the Institute of Medicine began to conceptualize this study and held the first planning meeting, its articulation of a "life cycle" approach to thinking about female health was novel and innovative. There was virtually no published literature dedicated to the methodological potential of this approach, nor were there any case applications.

The basic premise of the approach is that human health and illness are not invariably haphazard, but an accumulation of conditions that begin earlier in life, in some respects before birth. A second premise holds that the factors that favor health and precipitate ill-health are not purely genetic or biological, but can be social, economic, cultural, and psychological, and that these elements can work together or against one another across the span of an individual's life in ways that we are only beginning to understand. The third premise is that any reasonable public health strategy must recognize these dynamics and the resulting continuity of risk over the entire course of the female lifetime.

Since that first meeting in 1988, momentum in domestic and international thinking has grown around the need for a more inclusive and integrative model of women's health and well-being, and "life cycle" as a term of art has acquired a certain currency. In 1994 the World Bank published two documents[1] with the life cycle as a central theme, and the United Nations International Conference on Population and Development enlarged the perspective on family planning beyond provision of contraceptives to the assurance of women's total health and economic well-being.[2] The Institute of Medicine and this committee are gratified to have contributed to the thought processes underlying these works and excited to see the concept taking hold.

Early in their deliberations, the authors of this report considered whether or not to stay with the term "life cycle." On the one hand, the concept had been the organizing device for the study and surely conveyed the desired elements of continuity and inheritance. On the other hand, the term has a procreative connotation that, in effect, excludes women who either produce no offspring or are past childbearing, and thus can be seen as reducing health to its reproductive value alone. From this perspective, for example, the health of a female adolescent is of interest only as a preface to the onset of her reproductive life, not as helping to make her whole life safer, better, and more productive. In addition, the emphasis on the healthy survival of the fetus makes it the prime beneficiary of health interventions; the mother is the target of those interventions only as the conduit of their beneficial effects, so that the benefit she derives is secondary. Reproduction is a central and uniquely valuable role of women and must be accounted for, but it is not all they do, and that must be accounted for as well.

In contrast, the term "life span" is neither ambiguous nor limiting. It clearly refers to an individual's entire life experience from birth to death, whether or not that includes reproduction. The term applies equally to analysis of male health. That the focus of this study is on female health should not be seen to imply a lack of concern for males. The health and well-being of males over the life span is of rightful and necessary concern in itself, as well as in its many implications for family health and well-being.

Finally, the term "life span" is becoming more widely applicable as more countries go through the demographic and epidemiologic transitions that will profoundly transform their health profiles. Although the communicable diseases still dominate national health profiles in Sub-Saharan Africa, the dimensions of the noncommunicable, social, and environmental diseases are growing. Overall life expectancy has increased, and infant-child mortality has fallen, so that growing numbers of individuals are surviving to experience the chronic effects of earlier·disease exposures and the "newer" diseases of the later years. Health systems throughout Sub-Saharan Africa, already greatly stressed, will have to find ways to respond, sooner rather than later. In many cases, that time has already arrived.

THE STUDY PROCESS

Background

As part of its continuing concern for the Sub-Saharan African region, The Carnegie Corporation of New York has had abiding interest in the present and future role of women in the development of the region, as well as in their ability to play that role. Given the breadth of that interest, the Corporation found the concept of a holistic approach to the health dimensions of women's role appealing. In consequence, the Corporation provided funds to the Institute of Medicine (IOM) for a planning meeting, held in 1991, to define the design, determine the scope, and develop a detailed plan for implementation of a study on female morbidity and mortality in Africa south of the Sahara. Subsequently, the Carnegie Corporation, the United Nations Development Programme, the World Health Organization, and the National Research Council provided additional funds in support of the study, the two committee meetings that followed, and publication of the final report.

The Committee and Its Process

The 14-member interdisciplinary committee appointed to conduct the study included experts in anthropology, chronic diseases, demography, epidemiology, infectious diseases, injury and violence, mental health, nutrition, obstetric health, occupational and environmental health, and sexually transmitted diseases and HIV. Half of the committee members were from Sub-Saharan Africa, and principal authorship for the chapters to be included in the report was evenly distributed among the committee members.

In evaluating the evidence on female health in Sub-Saharan Africa, the committee examined a wide range of information sources, including demographic and health surveys; epidemiologic studies; case series and individual case reports available both from peer-reviewed journals and the often rich, unpublished literature available locally in Africa; conference and symposium proceedings; newsletters from professional health organizations and women's groups; academic dissertations and theses; and the body of analysis carried out in conjunction with the World Bank's work on the global burden of disease. Whenever possible, the committee examined the primary data sources.

The committee anticipated that it would be hampered in its task by paucity of data, especially age-specific and sex-specific data. That issue surfaces throughout this document in different contexts, and is the subject of the Appendix to this volume. As is often the case, however, the "no data" concern was partially unfounded: there is a substantial body of information about Africa, women in Africa, and health in Africa. Nonetheless, gaining a solid, longitudinal understanding across the life span was impeded by incomplete data; unevenness in data quality, consistency, and reliability; and a lack of the kinds of disaggregation by age and sex that are absolutely essential to that understanding.

Study Objectives

The committee set out to accomplish two objectives. First, it wished to elaborate and test the life span model and its utility for thinking about health and illness as cumulative products of the synergy among different diseases and conditions. Sub-Saharan Africa was taken as the case in point, but the committee also hoped to demonstrate the general utility of the life span model. Second, it wished to provide a unified documentary base for use in developing a systematic agenda for research and health policy formulation around female health in Sub-Saharan Africa.

The committee expects that the audience for the report will include African and non-African researchers, policymakers in African ministries of health, international donor agencies, and indigenous and international nongovernmental organizations.

Dilemmas and Strategies

The committee faced two major challenges: selection of the topic areas, individual diseases, and disease clusters for its analysis, and how to organize its work and the final report, given that its subject matter was multifactorial in etiology, cumulative in manifestation, not always clearly linear or transparent, and sometimes biomedical and sometimes not. For example:

- Should malnutrition be considered as disease, predisposing condition, or sequela?
- Should the diseases selected be just those that are exclusive to, or more prevalent in, females, implying that all other diseases have the same ramifications for both males and females?
- Should the tropical infectious diseases be viewed as vector-borne or poverty-borne? More broadly, is poverty simply the largest health problem, and the problem from which all others derive?
- Should the study focus be solely biomedical? If so, did that mean that socioeconomic, cultural, and political dimensions were to be ignored? If not, were those dimensions to be taken up specifically in each chapter, or generically, as applicable to all health problems?
- Should the report be organized according to the phases of the life span, or by health problem?

The committee first decided that the study would emphasize the biomedical aspects of women's health, but would also establish at the outset the social, economic, and cultural factors that interact most powerfully with human biological processes. The committee recognized that this decision might be controversial, because it would appear to go against the current interest in more inclusive models of health in general, and women's health in particular. The biomedical focus might also appear to ignore the current sentiment in developing countries that Western medical models are rigid, mechanistic, narrow, and insensitive to cultural and gender realities.[3]

At the same time, disease cannot be understood without reference to biology. There is no question that the burden of disease on Sub-Saharan African women is very, very large, but in the committee's view it had not yet been "unpacked" and laid out systematically in a way that would reveal all its features. As a consequence, modern medical systems—not just in Africa, but worldwide—are not well informed about gender differences. This is partly the result of the general exclusion of women from clinical studies of the treatments being prescribed for them; the general belief that, in most situations, women and men will not differ significantly in their responses to treatment; and the notion that much of what women present as illness is psychosomatic.

This disregard of gender is a mistake. There are gender differences, and they are relevant. Differences between men and women in size, fat ratios, and metabolic rates are associated with differences in drug concentration, metabolism, and response. Psychosocial differences are associated with differences in exposures to all manner of risk. In addition, intergender differences change over time, in females in conjunction with menarche, menstruation, pregnancy, lactation, menopause, and aging. Finally, there is the possibility that genetic, physiologic, or morphologic traits associated with sex may either exacerbate or attenuate infection in males and females, and may even affect the incidence of disease and the processes of co-infection in ways that are not a function of exposure alone (see Chapters 4 and 10 in this volume).

In sum, examination of the biomedical component of the burden of morbidity and mortality is necessary and useful in any effort to understand the strategic points of vulnerability and the complex interplay of disease determinants, manifestations, and sequelae across an individual lifetime. Scrutiny of the possible earlier determinants of disease will suggest a very different research and intervention agenda than would be produced through traditional cross-sectional analysis. Such a perspective, and the knowledge it produces, will also be more likely to foster prevention and the idea of medicine as "a culturally tailored continuum of care."[4]

The committee also noted that the compilation of information about women's health in Sub-Saharan Africa would in itself be a useful service, and it would assist scholars and policymakers involved in the larger contextual issues influencing health. Indeed, statements of the scientific and statistical facts can be compelling in themselves, reaching beyond their more specific epidemiologic and program uses to raise consciousness or command policy attention. The examples of AIDS and female genital mutilation are particularly instructive in this regard.

Given the biomedical orientation of the report, the chapters are organized around discrete sets of health problems. Factors that influence or contribute to female health—education, income, availability of health services, and civil rights—are addressed in a separate, overarching chapter at the beginning of the report. Because individual chapters might be used independently, however, chapter authors were encouraged to highlight the socioeconomic and cultural factors that were particularly salient to the topic under discussion. The internal organization of each chapter follows the life span sequence: infancy, childhood, adolescence, adulthood, and older age, with information about demographic subgroups included as data permitted. The committee considered organizing the entire report according to the life span sequence. From a public health standpoint, this approach might be desirable. From a practical standpoint, however, that strategy would have introduced significant constraints and redundancies.

In selecting the focus of individual chapters, the committee concentrated on health problems that: (1) are exclusive to females; (2) place a greater absolute burden of morbidity, mortality, or disability on females than they place on males; and (3) produce burdens of comparable magnitude for both sexes, but have unique implications for females. The committee also discussed the merits of using a measure being developed by the World Health Organization and the World Bank in their work on the global burden of disease, the disability-adjusted life year, or DALY.[5] The measure proved useful in Chapter 10, which examines eight tropical infectious diseases and their relative burdens; the data bases for DALY computation in these instances were reasonably robust.

Definitions

Sub-Saharan Africa

This report considers the 39 mainland countries of the continent south of the Sahara, with the addition of the island nations, as Sub-Saharan Africa. That term is used throughout this report interchangeably with the terms "Africa" and "the region." The countries north of the Sahara are understood to constitute North Africa and to be oriented more toward the Middle Eastern Crescent than toward the rest of the continent to their south. The committee was fully aware of the subcontinent's great heterogeneity, and it accounts for this by providing individual country data and pointing to significant differences where they exist, as well as to zones of commonality.

Sex and Gender

Throughout this report, the term "sex" is used when the reference is to the fundamental biological distinctions between males and females; survey data, for example, are disaggregated by sex. Although formal lexicons equate the two terms, current usage of the term "gender" is more expansive. As applied in this report, "gender" includes not only biological or sex differences between males and females, but also subsumes the context of their behavior in society, the different roles they perform, the range of social and cultural expectations and the constraints placed on them by virtue of their sex, and the ways they cope with those expectations and constraints.[6]

Report Organization

In Her Lifetime is divided into 11 chapters. This segment, Chapter 1, introduces the study and presents its rationale, objectives, strategy, processes, definitions, and organization and summarizes its conclusions and recommendations. Chapter 2 describes socioeconomic and sociocultural contexts and influences. Chapters 3 through 11 present the evidence on female morbidity and mortality for specific diseases and conditions: nutrition; obstetric and gynecologic health; nervous system disorders; mental health problems; selected chronic diseases; injury; occupational and environmental health; tropical infectious diseases; and sexually transmitted diseases, including HIV infection. The Appendix describes the nature and extent of the evidentiary base on female health in Sub-Saharan Africa.

Each chapter starts with a brief opening statement, followed immediately by a summary table depicting the diseases or conditions discussed in the chapter that produce disproportionate burdens for females. The chapter then offers a discussion of a given health problem or cluster of problems, and presents a summary table showing the process of the problem or cluster across the female life span. The chapter concludes with a statement of the research needs brought into focus by the discussion and a comprehensive set of references.

Despite a common format, each chapter reflects the distinctive character of its subject and the data bases used. Thus, the internal structure of the chapters is somewhat heterogeneous. A chapter on eight different tropical infectious diseases, for example, must differ from a chapter on models of occupational and environmental health in Africa, as a chapter on a fundamental factor such as nutrition must differ from a piece on nervous system disorders.

CONCLUSIONS AND RESEARCH NEEDS

Conclusions

The committee debated whether its purview included generating a set of overarching policy recommendations related to the contextual dimensions of female health in Sub-Saharan Africa. It concluded that, first, a plethora of other organizations was already immersed in meetings and discussions of the positions they wished to take at the 1994 Cairo Conference on Population and Development and the 1995 Conference on Women in Beijing. For example, a number of women's organizations indigenous to Africa were deeply involved in many of those processes.

Second, the committee itself had been explicitly configured to include African and non-African women and men whose preeminent expertise was scientific, and that expertise would provide the strength of the final report. The committee would add no real value to the report by commenting on broad international policy issues, but a thoughtful presentation of the biomedical dimensions of female health would be a distinctive contribution.

In effect, the committee had already anticipated its principal—and only—policy recommendation. It had set out, in effect, to test the life span model and to see if it provided enough understanding of female morbidity and mortality in Sub-Saharan Africa to be worth pursuing, not only in the study region, but elsewhere as well. The committee has since concluded that the life span model is extremely useful, indeed necessary, to adequately organize data collection and analysis in more informative ways; design applied research; identify areas where significant biological factors are involved, but so poorly understood as to require fundamental research; approach decisions about development of diagnostics and therapies in the context of real needs and constraints; and to conceptualize all levels of health services as care that extends beyond the episodic and reactive.

This chapter, organized around three summary tables, is intended to cut across the entire document in three ways. First, it considers the major health problems of Sub-Saharan African females identified in the report in "Gender-Related Burden." Table 1-1 summarizes the tables that appear at the beginning of Chapters 3 through 11, and is organized by type of health problem. The remaining two tables follow the life span in organization.

The second cut analyzes those burdens and their implications in each phase of the female life span. Table 1-2 summarizes the tables in the "Conclusions" section of Chapters 3 through 11.

The third cut, shown in Table 1-3, assembles the "Research Needs" identified in each chapter of the report and arranges them according to the life span.

Gender-Related Burden

This section provides an overview of the health problems in Sub-Saharan Africa that are exclusive to females; have greater impact on females than males; and generate comparable burdens for both sexes, but have some special significance for females. "Significance" here means having an impact on health that—for biological, reproductive, sociocultural, or economic reasons—differs in its implications for females and males. The organizing table (Table 1-1) follows the order of the book chapters; order under each heading (for example, "nutrition") is alphabetical, with no other priority implied. The listing under "obstetric morbidity and mortality" merits special comment. Males obviously have no obstetric or gynecologic problems. With the exception of "genital mutilation," however, all the health problems listed under this heading do afflict males. The overriding point here is that although the sexes share an array of health problems, pregnancy and parturition exacerbate or are exacerbated by them, with the result that females suffer a greater net effect than males.

Nutrition   A comparison with other regions of the world reveals that Sub-Saharan African females appear to be better nourished than females in South Asia, but they are equally or more malnourished than females in most other parts of the world. In contrast with South Asia, there is no consistent pattern of a higher prevalence of protein-energy malnutrition (PEM) among females than among males, despite a generally higher work burden among African women. Nor is there any indication that either the prevalence or sequelae of vitamin A deficiency are worse in females than in males in the region, although the deficiency is highly prevalent in some areas.

These various deficiencies have implications for reproductive capacity and resilience in females both because of the increased nutritional demands of pregnancy and the increased and severe risks that pregnancy and childbirth pose for a woman who has been stunted by PEM. In addition, two very important deficiency disorders, iron-deficiency anemia and iodine-deficiency disorders, occur more commonly in females than in males, and put females at substantial relative disadvantage; iron-deficiency anemia is a major risk factor for maternal mortality. As life expectancy lengthens in Sub-Saharan Africa, the impact of nutritional factors beginning at birth will become manifest in degenerative diseases and other functional impairments in adult life.

Obstetric morbidity and mortality   Of all geographic regions, Africa has the highest maternal mortality ratios, and this in itself is the most significant factor in comparing health outcomes in that region by gender. The events and conditions that are associated with pregnancy, childbirth, and the puerperium for women everywhere are exacerbated in Sub-Saharan Africa by severe lack of access to appropriate care for obstetric emergencies of any kind.

There are additional conditions and events shared by females and males, in many cases at roughly equal prevalence rates, that have particularly serious consequences for females precisely because they are female and because they reproduce. These conditions and events are rarely considered in any unitary way. For that reason, they are listed in Table 1-1 as preexisting or concurrent conditions that also affect males, but are exclusively female in the way they either exacerbate risk during pregnancy and childbirth, or are themselves exacerbated by those events.

The length of this list is impressive. It includes six highly prevalent and burdensome tropical infectious diseases (dracunculiasis, or Guinea worm disease; leprosy; malaria; onchocerciasis; schistosomiasis; and trypanosomiasis); five chronic diseases (cardiomyopathies, diabetes, hypertension, rheumatic heart disease, and sickle-cell disease), including one that is clearly genetic (sickle-cell disease); three nutrition-related conditions (anemia, iodine deficiency, and protein-energy malnutrition); and three conditions related to female sexual and gender identity (HIV/AIDS, the sequelae of female genital mutilation, and the entire group of sexually transmitted diseases).

These health problems not only interact deleteriously with the gravid state and the act of parturition, but frequently with one another as well. A particularly pernicious cluster involves HIV/AIDS, the other sexually

TABLE 1-1   Health Problems in Sub-Saharan Africa: Gender-Related Burden[a]

Problem	Exclusive to Females[b]	Greater for Females	Burden for Females and Males Comparable, but of Particular Significance for Females[c]
Nutritional status (Chapter 3)			
Iodine deficiency		X	
Iron deficiency		X	
Protein-energy malnutrition			X
Nervous system disorders (Chapter 5)			
Demyelinating diseases		X	
Epilepsies		X	
Headache syndromes		X	
Impaired cognition and dementias			X
Neurologic complications of collagen diseases		X	
Toxic and nutritional disorders		X	
Mental health problems (Chapter 6)			
Psychological disorders associated with pregnancy and puerperium	X		
Cardiovascular and cerebrovascular diseases, cancers, and chronic obstructive pulmonary disorders (Chapter 7)			
Cancers			
Bladder		X?	
Breast		X	
Cervix	X		
Skin		X	
Uterine, ovarian, choriocarcinoma	X		
Cardiomyopathies associated with pregnancy	X		
Gestational diabetes mellitus	X		
Rheumatic heart disease		X	
Injury (Chapter 8)			
Domestic abuse		X	
Household burns		X	
Rape and sexual assault		X	
Adverse occupational and environmental factors (Chapter 9)[d]			
Ergonomic stressors		X	
Exposure to indoor air pollution		X	
Exposure to organic dusts from food processing		X	
Exposure to toxic wastes		X	
Job overload		X	
Lack of job control		X	
Other[e]	X	X	X
Tropical infectious diseases (Chapter 10)			
Burkitt's lymphoma		X	
Dracunculiasis		X (pelvic infection)	X
Leishmaniasis			X (stigmatization)
Leprosy		X (in pregnancy)	X (stigmatization)

TABLE 1-1 Continued

Problem	Exclusive to Females[b]	Greater for Females	Burden for Females and Males Comparable, but of Particular Significance for Females[c]
Malaria		X (in pregnancy)	X
Onchocerciasis			X (stigmatization)
Schistosomiasis		X (ages 15–44)	X
Trypanosomiasis		X (ages 0–4)	X
Trachoma		X (neonatal vaginitis)	X
Sexually transmitted diseases/HIV/AIDS (Chapter 11)			
HIV/AIDS			X
Other sexually transmitted diseases		X	
Other diseases with special implications for females			
Measles[f]		X (ages 0–4)	
Sickle-cell disease[g]	X		
Obstetric morbidity/mortality[b] (Chapter 4)			
Anemia		X	
Cardiomyopathies			X
Diabetes			X
Dracunculiasis			X
Genital mutilation, sequelae	X		
HIV/AIDS			X
Hypertension			X
Iodine deficiency/goiter		X	
Leprosy			X
Malaria			X
Onchocerciasis			X
Protein-energy malnutrition			X
Schistosomiasis			X
Sexually transmitted diseases			X
Trypanosomiasis			X

[a]The order of this table follows the order of the book chapters. Order under each rubric is alphabetical, and no priority of any kind is implied.

[b] Males obviously do not have obstetric and gynecologic problems. All the health problems listed, however, occur in both males and females. The difference is that they may be exacerbated by the processes of pregnancy and parturition. This gender differential needs to be taken into account, both in research and in application.

[c]"Significance" is defined here as having an impact on health that is different in its implications for women than for men for any reason—biological, reproductive, sociocultural, or economic.

[d]Because of limitations in what we know about adverse occupational and environmental factors in many areas of where females live and work, these designations should be considered pieces of a research agenda, a list of unanswered questions about the nature, extent, and sequelae of different exposures for female health.

[e]"Other" includes ill-fitting personal protective equipment designed for men; working under recommended exposure limits for occupational hazards designed for healthy, well-nourished men in the developed countries working an eight-hour day; exposure to malaria prophylaxis and infection not only from malaria but also from other tropical infectious diseases that pose serious risks for pregnant women or are exacerbated by pregnancy; exposure to uncontrolled chemical and ergonomic hazards that pose risks for the fetus; effects of chemicals, indoor smoke, and injury hazards that extend to infants; work-time requirements that further compromise breastfeeding and infant nutrition; and lack of sufficient "off time" to allow for appropriate rehabilitation from injury or work-related disease, thus elevating the risks from hazardous exposures or increasing female workloads.

[f]Measles is, of course, not a tropical infectious disease. It is included in this study because of measles-related research that suggests the possibility of some fundamental difference at the level of the immune system between males and females that could be relevant to the tropical infectious diseases.

[g]Sickle-cell is a genetic disease with special implications for childbearing.

transmitted diseases, and the sequelae of female genital mutilation. Anemia, malaria, and schistosomiasis form another cluster, as do diabetes and hypertension.

Nervous system disorders   This chapter assembles, for what seems to be the first time, an enormous body of information about nervous system disorders, a disease area virtually ignored in national or international health thinking. It is also the first effort to transect this set of disorders by gender.

The compilation produces two major surprises. First, the burden generated by nervous system disorders appears heavier in African communities than in comparable communities elsewhere. Second, the female portion of that burden appears to be greater in quantitative terms than the male share. The burden of the demyelinating diseases, epilepsies, headache syndromes, the neurologic complications of collagen diseases, and toxic and nutritional disorders are all larger for females than for males, and all categories produce considerable disability, as well as a nontrivial and increasing amount of mortality. Overall, these diseases reflect the contribution of complex genetic potentiation, in some cases interacting with a variety of environmental factors that, at a minimum, contribute to confounding the understanding of the etiology and processes of the disease in question.

Mental health problems   There are two striking aspects of this part of Table 1-1: one is that it contains a single listing. The other striking aspect is invisible in the table, because it has to do with what is *not* included. Well-executed, community-based studies reveal that childbearing produces significant psychological morbidity among females in Sub-Saharan Africa, the region with the highest fertility rates in the world. This is a terribly important point. It is also significant that African women, despite substantial problems, adversities, and burdens, do not exceed males in rates of defined psychological disorders, as do the women of the developed countries. Even in the case of depression, which shows the greatest evidence of an excess among females in most studies throughout the rest of the world, the African picture is quite different: males demonstrate rates of the disorder that are comparable to or higher than the rates of females. The first questions that spring to mind are linked: Why do African women find childbearing so anxiety-provoking, and what factors make them otherwise so much more psychologically resilient than women elsewhere in the world? This pair of simple queries could be vastly illuminating.

Selected chronic diseases   Of the chronic diseases considered, most are unique to females by virtue of their physiology: cervical, uterine, and ovarian cancers, and choriocarcinoma; the cardiomyopathies associated with pregnancy; and gestational diabetes. Rheumatic heart disease, which is second only to hypertension and its complications among cardiovascular disorders resulting in hospital admissions in Sub-Saharan Africa, appears to be more common and to be associated with higher rates of morbidity and mortality in Sub-Saharan African females than in males. Cancers of the skin, and possibly those of the bladder, show a disproportionate burden in females compared with males, although the finding for bladder cancer is speculative and based on the assumption that females may be at a higher occupational risk of exposure to schistosomiasis, a risk factor for bladder cancer. The evidence presented in Chapter 10, which indicates higher DALYs for schistosomiasis in males than in females, suggests otherwise. Other gender-related environmental or occupational exposures, however, such as cooking fires in enclosed spaces, may place females in the region at elevated risk for other chronic diseases, particularly chronic obstructive pulmonary diseases.

Injury   There are three categories of injury that affect females disproportionately in Sub-Saharan Africa: household burns, domestic abuse, and rape and sexual assault. Household burns might be considered a hazard of inadequate domestic technology in any country where open cooking fires are the norm. The distribution of the other injuries, however, appears similar to that in females everywhere. These injuries also appear to be underreported for domestic and cultural reasons similar to those found in the rest of the world, but the numbers are increasing nonetheless. For females in Sub-Saharan Africa, violence—in the context of civil strife, at school, at work, and at home—leads the list of the causes of morbidity and, in some cases, mortality resulting from injury. And, as indisputably "biomedical" as its sequelae may be, this violence has its roots in the very foundations of gender relationships, and its remedy will require the involvement of many other sectors and disciplines beyond the health sector, as it does worldwide. The health sector can heal, but it cannot cure what resides in the larger society.

Occupational and environmental health Until very recently, consideration of this topic has been heavily skewed toward the developed countries and male subjects. There is very little work, published or unpublished, looking specifically at women, and most treatments of the subject of work and environmental variables are not differentiated by gender. This deficit is particularly unfortunate, given that females in Sub-Saharan Africa make more substantial contributions to the world of work than their counterparts in many other regions of the world, and thus can be considered to be at elevated risk of exposure to the kinds of adverse occupational and environmental health factors associated with work in the region. Although the conclusions of this chapter had to be based on analysis and inference from trends and emergent issues found in gender-blind material combined with analysis of women's work in Africa, these data provide strong indications of a substantial number of adverse occupational and environmental factors that burden female health status disproportionately in the region. These factors include increased exposure to indoor air pollution, toxic wastes, and organic dusts from food processing; job overload; lack of job control; and ergonomic stressors, among others.

Tropical infectious diseases The first conclusion in this area is inferential and concerns what might be called "diseases of disfigurement"—dracunculiasis, leishmaniasis, leprosy, onchocerciasis, and trypanosomiasis. We presume these to be more burdensome for females than for males because of their effects on prospects for marriage and motherhood, and that these effects may be particularly cruel for adolescent girls. Adolescents tend not to present for clinical attention because they are generally asymptomatic; fear of stigma may also inhibit the seeking of care. They thus do not avail themselves of therapies that could resolve some of these diseases and prevent their lifelong sequelae. This is a special challenge to the provision of care.

Five of the tropical infectious diseases generate a burden greater for females than for males: the pelvic infection and consequent reproductive damage from dracunculiasis and the greater absolute burdens of malaria, schistosomiasis, and African trypanosomiasis for females of certain ages. The size of the absolute and relative burden of trachoma for females is frankly startling, a finding that has been treated largely by silence in the literature. That a powerful preventive tool—handwashing—is available that could diminish this burden makes the situation especially sad. In environments where water is dear, this intervention is not simple, but it is possible.

Although they are often viewed as episodic, the tropical infections produce large burdens of disability. They also act synergistically with one another and with some nonparasitic diseases to produce more severe disability and, sometimes, mortality where it might not otherwise occur. The burden of these diseases, which once weighed more heavily on males, now seems to be more evenly distributed between the sexes. Migration and changes in the division of labor appear to lead the list of factors contributing to this shift, but without solid epidemiologic longitudinal data, this conclusion remains a supposition.

The final conclusion has to do with the traditional biomedical position that the only interesting distinctions between male and female susceptibility to tropical infectious diseases lie in the relationship to female reproductive function. This preconception has biased biomedical research toward pregnancy and pregnancy outcomes, placental transmission, and maternally induced protection in the neonate; excluded understanding of nonreproductive effects; and limited gender-relevant research to diseases that produce these effects. Science must often proceed narrowly to achieve depth of understanding, and traditional research (on malaria, for example) has provided valuable insights into the workings of all parasitic diseases. Nevertheless, it is time to broaden the focus.

In addition, although differential exposure is a dominant factor in infection, there are tantalizing clues around the sequelae of parasitic infections (for example, schistosomiasis) and research on nonparasitic infections (such as cross-sex transmission of measles) that raise profound questions about the existence of genetic, physiologic, or morphologic traits associated with sex that either exacerbate or attenuate diseases in males and females. There may be basic mechanisms at the cellular level related to the relative biological strength of the sexes that will have consequences for research on sex and on infection, and may ultimately lead to improved control of severe and potentially fatal infections in general.

Sexually transmitted diseases, including HIV infection The burden of all sexually transmitted diseases (STDs) in Sub-Saharan Africa is absolutely greater for females than it is for males, and it is growing. The causes and results of that burden remain dauntingly circular. The most important gender differentials are behavioral and biological. Females are far less likely than males to be able to control the circumstances of their sexual activity. Transmission of some STDs (including gonorrhea, chlamydia, trichomoniasis, and HIV) is more efficient to females than to males for physiological and sociocultural reasons. STDs may also predispose to other STDs, and they foster HIV transmission. Women with STDs are more frequently asymptomatic than men. When symptoms do manifest in females, they are often nonspecific, and this may delay the search for medical attention. When women do seek clinical care, they are less likely to be treated effectively since the very subtlety of symptoms can confound diagnosis, making treatment less effective. Infected women are also more likely to be stigmatized as prostitutes or, at best, as promiscuous, and treated poorly. All these factors promote the possibility of complications from STDs, including infertility or, worse, full-blown HIV infection, which carries great personal, family, and societal costs.

Health Problems Across the Female Life Span: A Synthesis

The multiplicity of intermediate variables between initial causes and final outcomes makes modeling a sequential life span approach a challenging task. Analysis is complex, and it depends on very sophisticated statistical technology as well as high-quality, plentiful data—generally unavailable even in developed countries— that often must be sought deliberately for specific purposes. In addition, the numerous feedback loops and multidirectional effects can become dizzying in graphic presentations, giving the possibly false impression that everything is related to everything else. Although this may indeed be the case, articulating a problem succinctly and conceptualizing effective research or program interventions becomes difficult when all factors appear to be of equal importance.

Furthermore, in Sub-Saharan Africa some conditions start so early and manifest themselves so relentlessly throughout the female life span that they have an aura of being part some kind of "health landscape." Malnutrition and undernutrition come first to mind. Anemia in women of reproductive age, for example, tends to be multifactorial, reflecting interaction among such causal variables as pregnancy, comorbidities, dietary inadequacies and malabsorption, and depressed immunity. Some diseases appear protean; the sexually transmitted diseases, for instance, may be transmitted *in utero* or perinatally, or later in life under a variety of circumstances. Other diseases, such as hepatitis, may be similarly transmitted but remain latent or occult for years. Damage to genitourinary structure and function may result from female genital mutilation, obstructed labor, sexually transmitted disease, induced abortion, or any combination of these insults. High parity may be related to early onset of childbearing or to repeated fetal wastage, either from prior conditions or new infections.

Health Problems *in Utero* As far as we know, effects on the fetus that are either fatal or produce later morbidity and disability befall females and males in equal measure. No present indications suggest that the effects of maternal nutritional deficits, obstructed labor, or infectious diseases discriminate by sex, and our knowledge of such discrimination in relation to the genetic diseases is in its early stages.

The principal differential between males and females is in the repercussions that poor pregnancy outcomes have in later life, among the most significant the desire for replacement that, in turn, motivates high parity and its multiple sequelae. In addition, children born with birth defects or congenital disease in Sub-Saharan Africa customarily become a female responsibility, with all the attendant implications for the economic well-being of family groups and overall female life chances.

Health Problems in Infancy and Early Childhood (birth through age 4) Males are known to be disadvantaged compared with females because they lack a second X-chromosome. At birth, females thus have better possibilities of beating the odds against survival, assuming that there is no strong sex preference for male children. Since such a preference does not appear to be the general case in Sub-Saharan Africa, an African infant girl starts life with chances that surpass her brother's. Nor does the situation change throughout the early years: if their environment is not oppressed by civil strife or famine, these are the safest years for African girls. At the same time, if these earliest years include the degree of protein-energy malnutrition that produces stunting, the foundation may be laid for the inadequate pelvic development, delayed menarche, reduced fecundity, and hypertension that will produce morbidity in later years.

Health Problems in Childhood (ages 5 through 14) Whatever advantage Sub-Saharan African females have in their first five years begins to erode in the prepubescent period. These are the years of peak onset for rheumatic fever and, if malnutrition and micronutrient deficiencies are present, of the onset of the effects noted above. During these years females also enter the world of work, which exposes them to a wider spectrum of infectious diseases, a number of which (malaria and schistosomiasis, for example) contribute to anemia. Girls may also lose asymptomatic status if they have been infected earlier with trypanosomiasis, or they may convert to a chronic carrier state if there has been perinatal transmission of hepatitis. Although none of these sequelae exclusively affect females, they cumulatively ratchet up the risk as girls move toward the childbearing years. These are also years of possible sexual abuse and consequent infection. If the society is one that practices female genital mutilation, the physiologic and psychological trauma of this procedure are added.

Health Problems in Adolescence (ages 15 through 19) Adolescence can bring quantum leaps in risk. None of the health problems of the preceding period vanish, and earlier rheumatic fever may progress to full-fledged rheumatic heart disease. Rape, coerced pregnancy, and economically coerced sex appear as issues in this period. Very early marriage may also become an issue, but this custom is so variable among countries that it is difficult to detail either its distribution or a common set of reasons for its practice. Very young women are also biologically more vulnerable to STDs than older women, and are socially far more vulnerable as well. Contraceptive use among African adolescents is almost nil. The result is many early pregnancies; high rates of unsafe abortions and STDs; and accelerated, earlier, and greater prevalence of HIV infection in females than in males.[7]

From a biological standpoint, the young female body is not ready for early pregnancy, and the biological price for this untimely occurrence is high. For reasons that are not well understood, pregnancy-associated hypertensive disorder is greatest in early and first pregnancies. The disproportion in size between the young mother's still underdeveloped pelvis and the nine-month fetus is at its most extreme, so that rates of obstructed labor are highest in this age group. Rates of rectovaginal or vesicovaginal fistula in this age group are similarly high. Pregnancy both aggravates and is aggravated by iron-deficiency anemia, which is very common in this age group; iodine deficiency, which impairs pregnancy outcomes; trauma from female genital mutilation, perhaps especially traumatic for an infibulated woman experiencing her first birth; malaria parasitemia; and pelvic infection from dracunculiasis. Schistosomiasis also has severe effects on the female reproductive system that become manifest in adolescence, first in menstrual abnormalities, later in risk of fetal wastage.

There is probably no single age group that requires more attention from systems of care and governance than adolescent females, yet this age group, and the 5- to 14-year-old age group that precedes it, are virtually unattended by the formal medical system. Other than some knowledge about traditional birth attendants, we know nothing about how well other providers in the traditional medical system serve these age groups. We know almost nothing about morbidity and mortality among adolescents in rapidly urbanizing environments, where threats from some tropical infectious diseases may be fewer but other threats abound.[8]

Adulthood (ages 20 through 44) The stage for this period of life—the longest single interval in the life cycle—has been set. Depending on birth-spacing, overall parity, and nutritional intake, there may be a cumulative process of maternal depletion, with greater susceptibility to neurotoxicity in foods, drugs, and some pesticides, and reduced capacity for work. Continued anemia decreases the ability to tolerate antepartum or postpartum hemorrhage. Iodine deficiency may result in a visible goiter, and may affect the fetus. Sterility deriving from reproductive tract infections, from longer-term sequelae of female genital mutilation, or from sepsis during unsafe abortion may bring grave emotional and social consequences. Urinary and fecal incontinence may proceed from newly traumatized fistulae from female genital mutilation or previous obstructed deliveries. Perinatal cardiopathies, gestational diabetes, hypertension, viral hepatitis, pneumococcal meningitis related to sickle-cell diseases, and most of the tropical infectious diseases wait in the wings to exacerbate or be exacerbated by pregnancy.

This is a long litany of bleak possibilities. Because there is little prenatal care available to so many African

TABLE 1-2 Burden of Morbidity and Mortality Across the Female Life Span in Sub-Saharan Africa

	In Utero	Infancy/Early Childhood (birth through age 4)	Childhood (age 5 through 14)	Adolescence (age 15 through 19)	Adulthood (age 20 through 44)	Postmenopause (age 45+)
Nutrition						
Protein-energy malnutrition	Stillbirths	Low birthweights Greater susceptibility to infection/growth faltering	Stunting/pelvic subdevelopment	Obstructed labor ⟶ Structural damage Sepsis Hemorrhage	Miscarriage(s) Infertility Chronic energy deficiency	
Micronutrient deficiencies						
Iron		Low birthweights/ growth faltering	Anemia ⟶	Lowered ability to tolerate hemorrhage	Acute anemia Hypovolemic shock	
Iodine	Fetal wastage/ stillbirths	Infant mortality Congenital abnormalities (cretinism, deafness)	Impaired school performance	Impaired pregnancy outcomes	Goiter ⟶	⟶
Zinc			Impaired immune function ⟶			⟶
Obstetric morbidity and mortality						
Obstructed labor		Birth trauma (epilepsy, neuropraxia)	Rape/economically coerced sex/coerced pregnancy, very early marriage	Very early first pregnancy Obstructed labor ⟶ Fistula, urinary/fecal incontinence Structural damage Induced abortion Sepsis ⟶ Infertility Ostracism/divorce	Fistula, urinary/fecal incontinence Infertility	Childlessness/ reduced status/ loss of social support

Nervous system disorders

Toxic and nutritional disorders

Genital mutilation/ structural trauma/ Sepsis

Obstructed labor
Urinary/lower and upper genital tract infections
Stenosis

Fistula, urinary/fecal incontinence
Chronic/recurrent UTI
Infertility
Dyspareunia

Epilepsies

Headache syndromes

Demyelinating diseases
Neurologic complications of collagen diseases
Dementias

Mental health problems

Depression?
Schizophrenia?

Psychological morbidity associated with pregnancy and puerperium

Depression
Schizophrenia

Selected chronic diseases

Rheumatic heart disease

Cardiovascular diseases

Continued

TABLE 1-2 Continued

	In Utero	Infancy/Early Childhood (birth through age 4)	Childhood (age 5 through 14)	Adolescence (age 15 through 19)	Adulthood (age 20 through 44)	Postmenopause (age 45+)
Selected chronic diseases (continued)				Hypertension Cardiomyopathies associated with pregnancy → Gestational diabetes mellitis →		
					Breast cancer → Cancer of the cervix → Leukemias and lymphomas → Skin cancer → Bladder cancer →	Chronic obstructive pulmonary disease
Injury		Falls, burns, drownings, unintentional poisonings	Sexual abuse Rape	Rape Motor vehicle deaths Suicide	Motor vehicle deaths Suicide (early adulthood)	Falls
Occupational and Environmental Health		Indoor air pollution (domestic)	Child labor	Economically coerced sex ——————→		

Tropical infectious diseases

Disease				
Malaria	Low birthweight Birth defects	Anemia Cerebral malaria	Severe anemia/pulmonary edema/splenomegaly →	
			Fetal wastage →	
Schistosomiasis	Fetal wastage	Anemia/weight loss Lower genital tract disease	Delayed growth and menarche Spontaneous abortions	Infertility Cerebral edema (in pregnancy) — Chronic backache
			Liver cirrhosis → Cancer of the liver	
			Disfigurement → Cancer of the genital tract/bladder	
Dracunculiasis			Disfigurement/disability →	
			Chronic arthritis →	
Onchocerciasis		Severe pruritis/sleep loss	Deterioration of lesions in pregnancy →	
			Disfigurement → Blindness →	
Trypano-somiasis	Low birthweight Fetal wastage	Loss of asymptomatic status — Mental retardation	Organic dementia → Anemia → Myocardial involvement →	

Continued

TABLE 1-2 Continued

	In Utero	Infancy/Early Childhood (birth through age 4)	Childhood (age 5 through 14)	Adolescence (age 15 through 19)	Adulthood (age 20 through 44)	Postmenopause (age 45+)
Trachoma				Disfigurement/ disability ⟶		
Leishmaniasis			Anemia/weight loss Lower genital tract disease	Disfigurement ⟶		
Leprosy			Anemia/weight loss Lower genital tract disease	Disfigurement ⟶		
Sexually transmitted diseases						
HIV	Congenital transmission	Perinatal/ neonatal	Transmission *per* sexual abuse	Transmission via unprotected sexual activity		
Other STDs	Intrauterine transmission, adverse pregnancy outcome	Perinatal transmission Ophthalmia, inclusion conjunctivitis, trachoma	Transmission *per* sexual abuse	Infertility Enhanced HIV/other STD transmission Urethritis Fatal ectopic pregnancy	Cervical cancer	Cardiovascular (syphilis) and CNS effects

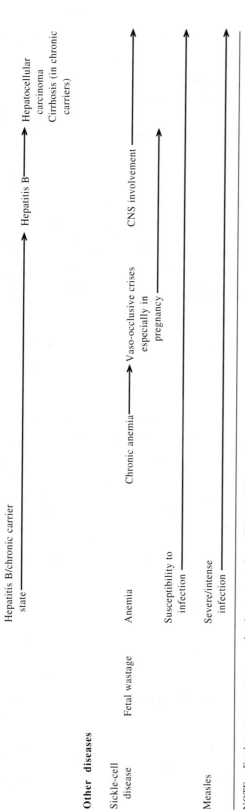

NOTE: Fetal wastage: spontaneous abortion, prematurity, stillbirth; CNS, central nervous system; UTI, urinary tract infection; PEM, protein-energy malnutrition.

women and because at least 60 percent of them bear their children outside any formal health facility, the extent to which this litany of morbidity actually plays out during these years is known only in the most fragmentary way. Indeed, the question may not even have been posed in any organized fashion, an oversight that requires prompt remedy. Another complex puzzle involving this age group is the apparent disjuncture implied by the combination of fertility that is still the highest of all regions, despite a falling trend; a large number of induced abortions; low utilization of modern contraceptives; and significant psychological morbidity around childbearing.

Menopause and Post-Menopause (age 45 onward) We know little about menopause in Sub-Saharan Africa. We can hypothesize from the view of Western medicine that menopause is a biological pathology, or from the ethnographic view that menopause is a natural, temporary, and, on balance, desirable event from the standpoint of increased status for women and decreased menstrual requirements.[9] At present, it appears likely that the latter perspective prevails in Sub-Saharan Africa, but the evidence is scanty. From a biological perspective, the cumulative effects of different nutritional deficits may contribute to earlier menopause, but again we do not know.

The number of women in Sub-Saharan Africa who reach the ages that permit full development of the degenerative diseases is increasing. Hypertension and stroke; diabetes; rheumatic heart disease; cardiomyopathies; chronic obstructive pulmonary disease; and cancers of the genital tract, breast, bladder, liver, and skin have all appeared in the region. Stroke is now recognized as an increasingly important cause of morbidity and mortality in Sub-Saharan African women, as is coronary artery disease, which seems to have a poorer prognosis for women than for men in the region. Women also display higher glucose tolerance, a precursor of full-fledged diabetes mellitus. Rates of cervical and skin cancers—already high, and rising as women live longer—are also worthy of note.

RESEARCH NEEDS

The committee was pleased to learn that its concern about inadequate information was unfounded. A great deal has been written about Sub-Saharan Africa in many areas germane to this report. At the same time, gaps and limitations will continue to constrain knowledge in areas where there really are no data; where data are currently organized in ways that limit their usefulness, but could be improved by reconsideration and reconfiguration; where additional information will be needed to properly design and assess interventions; and where current clues suggest potential breakthroughs.

The committee's conclusions take into account the current reality that funds for research, always scarce, show no signs of becoming more ample. Thus, while the need for good, insightful, systematic research remains constant, research in a resource-poor situation may prove most useful if focused on design and evaluation of interventions that aim to reduce morbidity and mortality. Intellectually, the committee does not consider research as something distinct from action; research *is* action where it makes action plausible or possible.

The committee also determined that, despite the undeniable differences between Sub-Saharan Africa and other regions, and despite the region's great heterogeneity, much research done elsewhere can serve here, at least for preliminary purposes. Work in other parts of the world on etiology, disease process, and case management of chronic diseases, for example, is sufficient for the design and testing of interventions in the African context.

The summary of the research needs identified by the committee reflects these views. Table 1-3 summarizes these requirements in four research categories: (1) epidemiologic, (2) biomedical, (3) applied/operational, and (4) ethnographic. Category 1, epidemiologic research, includes national and regional surveys, population-based studies, and certain kinds of facility-based studies. Category 2, biomedical research, includes areas of fundamental research that might produce understandings about immune response and disease process, not only in Sub-Saharan Africa, but elsewhere as well, and clinical research for the testing of low-cost preventive, curative, palliative, and diagnostic technologies and interventions. Category 3, applied and operational research, includes all research concerned with the application and evaluation of program interventions, ranging from experiments in health delivery innovation to health education approaches. Category 4, ethnographic and behavioral research, includes any research into aspects of sociocultural and socioeconomic context that affect female health, positively or negatively, as well as studies of knowledge, attitudes, and practices that are relevant to the design and assessment of any of the interventions in categories 1, 2, and 3. We ask the reader to turn to the last section of each chapter for a more detailed discussion of research needs in each biomedical area and, of course, to the text.

This report consistently calls attention to areas where research is required or advisable. In every case, the health problem in question will necessarily intersect in some fashion with the "ways of life of people." A few of these intersections have special relevance to thinking about female morbidity and mortality across the life span.

• The first is "medical distance," or gaps in knowledge about some fundamental gender- and sex-specific differences and the ways these differences affect community and individual experience of disease, episodically and throughout life. As long as such gaps persist in any major way, they will hamper health systems' efforts to encompass them in some explicit and methodical fashion. There seem to be, for example, both genetic and nongenetic aspects of differential susceptibility that have implications across the life span.

• The second issue is the manner in which females engage in health-seeking behavior across their life span, both for themselves and their families; how this varies by health problem and age; and how greater life expectancy and the experience of "new" diseases is managed. We need to approach this understanding in a more focused way, parsing "health-seeking behavior" into preventive actions and the seeking of treatment. It is possible to see these as two different domains of behavior, with different rules. Inadequate understanding of these rules may partially explain why attempts to modify behavior toward preventive goals are sometimes less than successful.

• Ethnographic research in Sub-Saharan Africa has been abundant. Nevertheless, like most such research, it has been carried out in small samples and, correctly or incorrectly, tends to be seen as anecdotal and therefore not powerful enough for the making of national policy. Thus, while it is possible to talk about traditional practices that may have extensive effects on female health status, it is not possible to determine how extensive these effects might be. Traditional dietary practices related to childbearing have a significant effect on female nutritional status, for example, but the extent of this effect is unknown. Nor is it known to what degree the use of traditional healers, in the absence of other health services, is truly deleterious to health. Methods of synthesizing what is presently available in the literature and ferreting out new data, economically yet reliably, is near the top of the list of contextual work that needs to be done. It has been possible to focus policy attention on the dilemma of female genital mutilation, with its profound biomedical implications and its equally profound cultural roots, precisely because its prevalence has been quantified to a degree that has attracted the world's attention. African women have become vigorously involved in this issue. It may be the African women, in the final analysis, who can best design the "Essential National Health," the biomedical-cum-social research to answer the many remaining questions about sex, gender, and disease.

NOTES

1. Tinker, A., P. Daly, C. Green, et al. 1994. Women's Health and Nutrition: Making a Difference. World Bank Discussion Paper 246. Washington, D.C.: World Bank. World Bank. 1994. A New Agenda for Women's Health and Nutrition. Washington, D.C.: World Bank.

2. United Nations Fund for Population Activities. 1994. Programme of Action of the United Nations International Conference on Population and Development. Cairo and New York.

3. Cf. E. Fee and N. Krieger. 1993. Understanding AIDS: historical interpretations and the limits of biomedical individualism. American Journal of Public Health 83(10):1477–1486. G. Santow. 1995. Social roles and physical health: the case of female disadvantage in poor countries. Social Science and Medicine 40(2):147–161. C. Vlassoff. 1994. Gender inequalities in health in the Third World: uncharted ground. Soc. Sci. Med. 39(9):1249–1259.

4. M. Holloway. 1994. Trends in women's health: a global view. Scientific American, August:76–83.

5. C. J. L. Murray and A. D. Lopez, eds. 1994. Global Comparative Assessments in the Health Sector: Disease Burden, Expenditures and Intervention Packages. Geneva: World Health Organization.

6. C. Vlassoff. 1994. Gender inequalities in health in the Third World: uncharted ground. Soc. Sci. Med. 39(9):1249–1259.

7. United Nations Development Programme (UNDP). 1993. Young Women: Silence, Susceptibility, and the HIV Epidemic. New York.

8. A. Mansaray. 1992. Adolescent health in Sub-Saharan Africa in the 1990s: The role of social and behavioural research. Paper presented at the First International Conference on Social Science and Medicine, Africa Network, Nairobi, Kenya, August 10–13, 1992.

9. S. Chirawatkul and L. Manderson. 1994. Perceptions of menopause in northeast Thailand: contested meaning and practice. Social Science and Medicine 39(11):1545–1554.

TABLE 1-3 Summary of Research Needs, Female Morbidity and Mortality in Sub-Saharan Africa

Epidemiologic Research	Biomedical Research	Applied/Operational Studies	Ethnographic and Behavioral Research
Continuation/expansion of internationally sponsored information on *cause-specific mortality/ morbidity*, ensuring that all data are disaggregated by sex and age, and that methods are standardized	Studies of *micronutrient deficiencies* in girls and women	Case analyses (audits, confidential inquiries) to identify *causes of maternal deaths in health care system dysfunction*; design of case management algorithms	Qualitative research on nature and magnitude of impact and management of *menopause*, and relationship of nutritional and general health status at onset
Collection of data on causes and prevalence of *disabilities*	Clinical-level recording and extra-clinical gathering of medical data on *sequelae of female genital mutilation*	Determination of feasibility and effectiveness of different preventive interventions for *stroke*, e.g., control of high blood pressure	Systematic research (quantified ethnographic studies or meta-analysis) of *local dietary practices* that impinge on diet quality during pregnancy or postpartum
Carefully designed *cohort-tracking series studies* to follow life span course in selected "population laboratories"	Study of reasons for and implications of poorer prognosis for women than men of African descent with *coronary artery disease*	Nutrition interventions designed to account for *nutrition-related toxic syndromes of the nervous system*	Synthesis of work on similarities and differences between biomedical and traditional indigenous concepts of *etiology and morbidity from different tropical infectious diseases*
Use of *sentinel disease surveillance* systems to identify and monitor changing patterns in mortality and morbidity	Study of greater frequency of *skin and other systemic disorders* related to use of skin-lightening creams and ointments containing steroids and other toxic chemicals	Research to determine how best to incorporate *management of common neurologic diseases* into primary care, and design of corresponding training	Compilation of information on *management of tropical infectious diseases*, particularly those producing disfigurement
Continued refinement of *DALYs*, and underlying assumptions and data base, and simplification of methodology for regional and local use	Confirmation of higher rates of *glucose intolerance* in SSA women than in men	Developing means to improve *nutrition for lactating mothers* and protocols for guiding them toward best lactation practice	Studies related to *STD/HIV control:* —factors determining sexual, health-seeking, and reproductive behaviors —factors determining women's social status —effects of female social status on sexual, health-seeking, and reproductive behavior
Modifications of existing longitudinal surveys of *nutrition* status, particularly child malnutrition in Sub-Saharan Africa, so that data are collected/ analyzed/ reported by age and gender	*Chronic effects of pesticides and other home chemicals* on peasant farmers and others in plantation and monocropping production	Documentation and practical cataloging of creative approaches to *better obstetric health care*, treatment guidelines and algorithms	
Collection of *nutrition* data on neglected populations: adolescent girls; nonpregnant, nonlactating women; women past reproductive age	Impact of bearing heavy weight at different ages and effects across the life span and life cycle with regard to *degenerative osteoarthritic problems*	Prevalence and trends in smoking in SSA females, and risk factors for *smoking* initiation among adolescent females, for purposes of developing appropriate intervention programs	In-depth examination of social, economic, and mental health determinants of *violence*
Population-based studies of *mortality, morbidity, and disability associated with induced abortion*	*Respiratory damage*, notably from chronic bronchitis, and reduced lung function across the life span		Mental health impact of *psychosocial stressors related to work and environment*, particularly effects of chronic fatigue
	Development of *surrogate endpoints for maternal mortality*		

TABLE 1-3 Continued

Epidemiologic Research	Biomedical Research	Applied/Operational Studies	Ethnographic and Behavioral Research
Integration of facility-based and population-based mortality and morbidity data, age- and sex-disaggregated for estimation of total impact of *injuries* in communities	Evaluation of *negative effects of lactation* on mothers	Prevention strategies for *preventing and controlling disability from injuries* of importance to SSA females, including systems of trauma care and rehabilitation techniques	Studies of decision making in *treatment-seeking behavior,* including role of stigma in disease management
Key *chronic disorders* —Rheumatic heart disease —Hypertension and stroke —Cardiomyopathies —Coronary artery disease —Leukemias, lymphomas —Cancers of cervix, breast, uterus, ovary, skin, bladder —Choriocarcinoma —Diabetes —Chronic obstructive pulmonary disorder	Study of dynamics of *differential prevalence of psychiatric disorders in SSA females* (collaborative, coordinated) Study of effects of *perinatal depression* on course of pregnancy, effects of postpartum depression on mother and neonate	Studies of magnitude, determinants, and variables affecting onset, course, and outcome of *post-traumatic stress disorders,* in order to define effective treatment approaches	
Population-based studies of *trachoma,* prevalence and risk factors	Studies of interaction of life events and expressed emotion and genesis and maintenance of *depression*	Collaborative, multidisciplinary study of causes, risk factors, and reporting of *violence,* toward design of preventive strategies and case management	
Risk factor studies Comparative surveys on risk factors for *chronic disease* —Hypertension: serum cholesterol and lipid fractions —Obesity —Nutritional risk factors Major risk factors for *stroke* in women	Research into effects of *co-infection and comorbidity with tropical infectious diseases,* e.g., impact of HIV infection on female capacity to control falciparum parasitemia	Assessment of *occupational exposure limits,* given gender and multiplicity of other environmental stressors	
Risk factors for *domestic and work-site injuries*	Development of simple, low-cost instruments for diagnosis of tropical *diseases* with similar symptomatology	*Operational research related to STD/HIV* including but not limited to: —integration of STD control with other programs —characteristics of health	
Environmental and occupational risk factors for *cancers and chronic obstructive pulmonary disease*	Cell-level research on *sex differences in severity, duration, and intensity of disease* (e.g., measles)	care systems that would better serve women's needs —counseling, testing, partner notification in	
Risk factors for *epilepsy*	Better description of natural history of *subclinical pelvic inflammatory disease*	resource-scarce, high-risk environments —program design for high-risk groups —involvement of	
Characterization of extent and severity of *nutrition-related toxic syndromes* of the nervous system	Better understanding of *impact of STDs/HIV on pregnancy outcomes,* and *influence of pregnancy on course of STDs*	traditional practitioners —development of better management algorithms for asymptomatic as well as symptomatic STD infections	

TABLE 1-3   Continued

Epidemiologic Research	Biomedical Research	Applied/Operational Studies	Ethnographic and Behavioral Research
Hospital case series investigations of higher prevalence and mortality rates for *rheumatic heart disease* in SSA females	Development of simple, cheap treatment regimens for HIV-infected pregnant women to reduce perinatal transmission Development of noninvasive, simple, rapid, affordable *diagnostic tests for identification of women with asymptomatic STD infection* Development *of female-controlled prevention methods,* e.g., safe intravaginal microbicidal agents, with or without contraceptive effect Studies of *long-term effects of childhood malnutrition on female work capacity* Studies *of functional consequences of adult malnutrition,* including, but not limited to, physical consequences	—development of simple management algorithms for opportunistic infections and neoplasms Intervention trials to help women, especially adolescents, in skills and self-esteem building to reject unsafe sexual behavior	

NOTE: DALY = disability-adjusted life year; SSA = Sub-Saharan African; and STD = sexually transmitted disease.

2

The Context of Mortality and Morbidity

THE IMPORTANCE OF CONTEXT

In 1965, microbiologist Rene Dubos commented that "the prevalence and severity of microbial diseases are conditioned more by the ways of life of people than they are by the virulence of specific etiologic agents." The same can be said of the "nonmicrobial" diseases and the growing variety of environmental hazards. It is their "ways of life," then, that explain at least part of the morbidity and mortality of populations in given geographic and social settings. For women, health as a state of total well-being is "not determined solely by biological factors and reproduction, but also by effects of workload, nutrition, stress, war and migration, among others" (van der Kwaak, 1991).

In this context, mortality and morbidity are indicators of what nations are prepared to do to affect the various dimensions of the human environment, their willingness to extend and improve the quality of life of their people by applying the resources required for longer and healthier survival—education, food, health care, jobs, and security—and to ensure equitable participation in the economic, political, cultural, and social processes that affect their lives (Sen, 1993; UNDP, 1993; World Bank, 1993). From this perspective, even though physical health is just one component of human development, it is an essential function of the development process (UNDP, 1991).

As is the case everywhere, female health, ill-health, and mortality in Sub-Saharan Africa unfold within, and are shaped by, their sociocultural, economic, and political contexts. These are horizontal and vertical: families, communities, and networks of extended kinship are embedded in regional, national, and international hierarchies and relationships. All of these affect and are affected by one another, and all have implications for human well-being.

A pivotal aspect of these horizontal and vertical dynamics is power, defined here as control or influence over, first of all, one's own life. Primary in achieving such control is access to resources—the goods, services, and information that are the intellectual, physiologic, and economic basis for healthy and productive lives. In all societies, the degree of openness or constraint of this access is affected by gender. Female morbidity and mortality are not just functions of the physical differences between males and females; whatever their evolutionary origins, they are also rooted in differences in roles and status between the sexes (Caldwell et al., 1990; Gaisie, 1990; Koblinsky et al., 1993; Mukhopadhyay and Higgins, 1988; Ubot, 1992; Vlassoff and Bonilla, 1994).

THE ISSUE OF HETEROGENEITY

Throughout this volume, statements are made about female morbidity and mortality in Sub-Saharan Africa for the purpose of comparing those indexes with the rest of the world. It cannot be emphasized enough, however, that the continent is neither homogeneous nor uniform. There are many economic, political, and sociocultural differences among East, West, central, and southern Africa; among large nations and small; highly stratified states and the more egalitarian; countries suffering wars, ethnic tensions, or other civil disturbances, and countries more serene; the economically richer and the poorer; those suffering drought and famine, and those who are not; and nations with refugees, and those without. There are also variations in religion, tribal affiliation, kinship structure, residence and household formation, language, and educational heritage.

Current statistics on economic performance, population, fertility, and education also reflect the continent's heterogeneous experience and circumstance. Gross National Product (GNP) per capita in 1987 dollars ranged from $130 in Ethiopia to Gabon's $2,700; annual average change in GNP per capita since 1965 ranged from –2.7 percent in Uganda to +8.9 percent in Botswana. Land mass varies from Sudan's 967,494 square miles to Swaziland's 6,705, and national population size from 0.7 million in Swaziland to over 100 million in Nigeria. Annual population growth rates over the past 23 years range from 1.5 percent in Mauritius to 4.2 percent in Côte d'Ivoire. Although total fertility rates are uniformly high throughout Sub-Saharan Africa, there are still major differences in absolute numbers and trends among regions and individual countries, as well as within them (Blanc, 1991; Cohen, 1993). Adult literacy in Burkina Faso is 18 percent; in Botswana it is 74 percent. Secondary school enrollment ranges from 3 percent in Rwanda and Tanzania to 51 percent in Mauritius (Feachem and Jamison, 1991; UNDP, 1993; World Bank, 1993).

Dealing with diversity is a fundamental difficulty for any study that pretends to deal with the continent as a whole. This report recognizes diversity as a fundamental fact and deals with it through the use of case material that illustrates commonalities or significant divergence in a given subject area.

THE SOCIOECONOMICS OF LIFE AND DEATH

The Variables

In its 1990 *Human Development Report (HDR)*, the United Nations Development Programme (UNDP) defined human development as the process of enlarging people's options. Of those, the most critical were the options to: (1) lead a long and healthy life; (2) acquire knowledge; and (3) have access to the resources needed for a decent standard of living. This holistic view of "human health in context" is the point of departure for this study.

It was also in the 1990 *Human Development Report* that the UNDP introduced the "Human Development Index" (HDI) as a more realistic and informative statistical measure of human development than per capita gross national product (GNP) alone. The HDI merges national income with two social indicators—adult literacy/mean years of schooling and life expectancy at birth—to yield a composite measure that makes it possible to rank the progress of nations in relation to one another. The HDI also permits measurement of how females are doing compared with males (Anand and Sen, 1992).

A great deal of analytic energy has been invested in seeking consistent patterns of causality between human mortality, and the worldwide trend of decline in that mortality, and one of the major socioeconomic factors, including income growth, education, provision of health services, ecology, and geography (cf. Feachem and Jamison, 1991). In spite of these efforts, there is still no clear picture of which of these matters most, in part because of inadequacies in the basic data and the manner of their application, and in part because of the sheer complexity in the way human health is embedded in those factors. Taking combined mortality as its lead indicator, the World Bank's *World Development Report 1993 (WDR)* finds four factors to be unremittingly important in mortality reduction: income growth, improvements in appropriate medical technology, basic education, and access to public health services and knowledge. These are not simple indicators, and there are important synergies among them. In all regions of the world, however, the main effect of income growth on health status lies in equity of income distribution and corresponding poverty reduction, as well as the extent of public investment directed toward development of human capital, both in health services and education, particularly for females.

Sub-Saharan Africa is no exception to this lack of a clear, direct association between income growth and HDI rankings. If, in frankly arbitrary fashion, we take the simple numerical midpoint (87.5) of the HDI ranking of the 173 countries, only three Sub-Saharan African countries fall into the group with the highest HDIs: Mauritius, Seychelles, and South Africa, all of which have high GNP rankings as well. A more generous cutoff adds Botswana, Congo, Gabon, Kenya, Lesotho, Madagascar, Swaziland, Zambia, and Zimbabwe, and makes the picture more complex, because all members of this group except Botswana, Gabon, and Swaziland have relatively low GNP rankings. That said, there are no dramatic exceptions at the lower HDI and GNP rankings: the very poorest countries of the Sub-Sahara have difficulty generating good HDIs. It is also the case that almost all of these lowest-ranking countries, which also have the lowest life expectancies and low health services access rates, are also the countries with low total overall adult literacy, and female literacy rates that are below 50 percent of those for males.

Nevertheless, most attempts to explain significant differentials among and within African countries in even a single phenomenon, such as infant and child mortality, founder. Part of this difficulty is generic: quantifying the contribution of admittedly crude indexes of socioeconomic development has generally found them to explain no more than half of the total variance (Blacker, 1991). Even when specific variables—for instance, maternal education—clearly and significantly correlate with mortality, the precise causal path is still unclear (Cleland and van Ginneken, 1988). The search for reasonably consistent explanations is frustrating: why, for example, if East Africa suffers the highest regional food insecurity, are the numbers of low birthweight babies and maternal mortality rates highest in West Africa?

Gender Disparities

The *Human Development Report* applies the HDI to data from 33 countries on separate female and male estimates of life expectancy, adult literacy and mean years of schooling, and wage rates, and calculates a Gender-Specific HDI for those countries. Computation of this HDI subset is not yet adjusted to account for the standard worldwide pattern of greater female longevity, and the report points to this area for further analytic attention. The data base also needs to be expanded to include a fuller range of countries; so far, data availability has permitted calculations in Sub-Saharan Africa only for Kenya and Swaziland.

The primary finding of this analysis is that when the HDI is adjusted for gender disparity, no country improves its HDI value. In other words, no country treats its women as well as it treats its men, although some countries do better than others.

The sources of gender bias in industrial and developing countries differ in important ways. In industrial countries, that bias is mainly in employment and wages, with women often getting less than two-thirds of the employment opportunities and about half the earnings of men. In developing countries, in addition to biases in the job market, there are great disparities in health care, nutritional support, and education. Those skews are exacerbated by poverty: the 1991 *HDR* notes that "Although gender discrimination is a worldwide problem, its effects are particularly harsh in the poorer countries."

Morbidity and Mortality

The overall patterns of mortality and morbidity in the Sub-Saharan region resemble those of other regions: the life expectancy of African females, like that of females virtually everywhere, is greater than that of males (Sai and Nassim, 1991; UNICEF, 1992), although life expectancy varies at different ages (that is, e_0 is not necessarily equivalent to e_{15}; see Brass and Jolly, 1993). And, as in nearly all developing countries, child mortality rates and the mortality risk for adult males are higher than they are for females (Murray et al., 1994), although differentials are usually small (Timaeus, 1991). In only two countries—Mali and Malawi—is there any evidence of excess female adult mortality. In the case of Mali, however, female mortality may have been overestimated because of adjustments made for underreporting, and Malawi may be genuinely anomalous for reasons that are unclear (Timaeus, 1991).

Still, these global similarities do not tell the whole story: the life chances of adults in Sub-Saharan Africa are extremely heterogeneous (Timaeus, 1991), and some countries of the region have mortality levels that compare favorably with individual countries of other developing regions. At the same time, although most African countries have experienced steady declines in child mortality, aggregate mortality rates for the Sub-Sahara are still the highest in the world (Sai and Nassim, 1991). The differences in this regard between Sub-Saharan African women and the majority of their global sisters are large and absolute.

In addition, avoidable mortality is considerably higher for Sub-Saharan females overall than it is for males. Avoidable deaths are those that would not occur if the rates of a given reference population were applied in the case population (Murray et al., 1994). In the Sub-Saharan case, while the mortality risk for adult males is higher than it is for females, and much higher than it is for males in the developed world, the adult female mortality risk is so elevated, and the mortality risk among adult females in the developed world so low compared with males, that a more extreme ratio is generated. Said more simply, a Sub-Saharan female has a dramatically poorer chance of survival relative to her developed-world sister than does a Sub-Saharan male compared with his developed-world brother. The odds are even poorer for Sub-Saharan African mothers: their lifetime risk of maternal death is 1 in 15, compared with the 1-in-9,850 lifetime risk of maternal death in Northern Europe—that is, 657 times as great (Graham, 1991). The statement has been made that in a context of such extreme deviation, Sub-Saharan African women are "the underside of the underside" (Ramphele, 1991).

Finally, there appear to be notable gender differences within cohorts: although the infant mortality rate for boys is somewhat higher than it is for girls in every African country with available data, the picture of mortality rates among children 1 to 5 years old is much less consistent. Mortality rates among females in this age group appear to be higher in most African countries than they are for males, for reasons that are not at all clear.

Health Services Access and Utilization and Health-Seeking Behavior

In Sub-Saharan Africa, as everywhere else, access to health services is a function of costs, measured in money, time, and distance. All of these, in turn, affect utilization and interact with perceptions of care and its quality.

Access issues are particularly acute for women, whose workload, child care responsibilities, and financial situation may all constrain their ability to utilize services for themselves and for their children to a degree not experienced by men. In addition, although women may be the chief caretakers in a residential unit, they may not be the chief decision makers. Depending on family structure and residential organization, others, particularly senior males or mothers-in-law, may be the arbiters of choices about health care (Castle, 1995; Janzen, 1978). Still, Sub-Saharan African women are numerically more likely to be the principal users of health care services. This is not the case for Muslim women, whose seclusion and inability to be attended by a male health care provider put them at comparative jeopardy, to an extent that has not been systematically studied as an issue in itself.

Quality of health services affects both utilization and compliance with preventive and curative regimens (Leslie and Gupta, 1989), although the degree of importance of inadequate quality in women's underutilization of health services remains to be systematically assessed in Sub-Saharan Africa (Mensch, 1993). Nonetheless, it is only common sense to assume that suitable clinic hours and reasonable waiting times, multiple and adequate services, courtesy, efforts to diminish social and cultural distance between providers and patients, and clarity of communication would persuade more Sub-Saharan African women to utilize health services appropriately. When these features are not the rule, which is believed to be the more typical case in the region, service utilization and regimen compliance are affected negatively (Gilson, 1995; Heggenhougen, 1991; Thaddeus and Maine, 1990).

Another, more subtle factor is what might be called "medical distance"—that is, the degree to which the health care system is equipped with the appropriate knowledge and resources to deal with the specific health needs of women. There is good reason to believe that modern medical systems worldwide may not be adequately supplied with information about gender differences, at least in part because women have been largely excluded from clinical studies of the treatments prescribed for them (A. Lucas, personal communication, 1993), and in part because of the general belief that, in most situations, women and men will not differ significantly in their responses to treatment.

At the heart of the matter is the absolute availability of all health-related services. People—male or female—cannot use, or decide to use, facilities that do not exist. The economic argument that demand will "make a market" and that consumers will, sooner or later, shape that market is questionable even in the developed world, where that assumption is at the heart of current debates about the relative roles of the public and private sectors in assuring the public health. If this is an arguable assumption in the developed world, then it would seem to be highly questionable in countries with large numbers of poor people, whose power to shape a market is infinitesimal.

The overall health service access figure for Sub-Saharan Africa is 60 percent; that is, just 60 percent of the region's population has access to any facility that might be described as modern. Only 41 percent of the total population of the region has access to safe water, and only 26 percent has access to sanitation; these are the lowest percentages of all the developing country regions (UNDP, 1993). In addition, although most of the developing world showed dramatic improvement between 1970 and 1990 in ratios of health care providers to population, Sub-Saharan Africa still has the fewest physicians and nursing persons of any region relative to population.

Table 2-1 displays variation in access indicators among and within individual countries. That variation is clearly wide. As of 1990, 11 countries in Sub-Saharan Africa had less than one hospital bed per 1,000 population. The physician/population ratio for the region as a whole was 1:23,540, with a range from 1:750 in South Africa to 1:72,990 in Rwanda. The regional nursing person/population ratio was 1:3,460, ranging from 1:600 in Zambia to 1:5,470 in Tanzania. At the same time, there is a relatively high ratio of nursing persons to physicians—5:1 for the region as a whole—with very few countries recording low ratios. Such ratios are viewed by Western health system analysts (cf. IOM, 1988; Reinhardt, 1991) as more favorable in achieving coverage, especially with public health measures, than are the lower nursing person-physician ratios that are so often a function of physician oversupply and can produce high costs to the society.

Finally, while 66 percent of Sub-Saharan African women are recorded as having some kind of prenatal care, only 38 percent of all births are attended by health facility personnel, the lowest such figure in all the developing regions. This cannot help but contribute substantially to Sub-Saharan Africa's maternal mortality ratio of 640 maternal deaths per 100,000 live births, the highest of all the world's regions (WHO, 1985). Community studies show that most maternal deaths occur outside the medical system, either at home or on the way to the hospital (Thaddeus and Maine, 1990). In response, the provision of access to high-quality emergency obstetric care is gaining recognition as the most important strategy for preventing maternal deaths in the region, in Africa, and in other developing countries where maternal mortality rates are high (Prevention of Maternal Mortality Network, 1995).

Access Bias

A severe limitation on access is urban-rural bias, which is extreme in Sub-Saharan Africa. Seventy-nine percent of the region's urban population has access to safe water; for rural areas, that figure is 28 percent. While 87 percent of the region's urban population has access to health services, over half the population in most of its countries lives more than 10 kilometers from the nearest primary care center. According to selected household surveys, of the individuals who report themselves as sick, those in urban areas obtain medical care more often than those in rural areas, and the wealthy contact a care provider more often than the poor. In Côte d'Ivoire in the mid-1980s, an urban household was nearly twice as likely to seek care as a rural household, and a family in the top income quintile within the rural population was almost twice as likely to seek care as a family in the bottom quintile (World Bank, 1993).

As for bias from other factors, there is no persuasive evidence that Sub-Saharan African females are at any significant disadvantage in being taken for clinical care in their early years. Surveys of the management of diarrheal disease, fever, and respiratory illness in infants and very young children, for example, reveal no significant differences in treatment by sex in the six African countries surveyed (Boerma et al., 1991). Nevertheless, gender bias in health services access and utilization accrues with age, as time, money, distance, and fear of stigma become matters of concern for girls and women.

TABLE 2-1 Health Infrastructure and Services, Sub-Saharan Africa and Selected Trends, 1970–1990

Country	Population per 1,000 Doctors[a] 1970	1990	Population per 1,000 Nursing Persons[a] 1970	1990	Nursing Person to Doctor Ratio[b] 1988–1992	Hospital Beds per 1,000 Population[b] 1985–1990	Percent of Births Attended by Health Staff, 1988[c]	Percent Received Antenatal Care[d]	Percent Received Delivery Assistance[d]
Sub-Saharan Africa	31,830	23,540	3,460	—	5.1	1.4	—	—	—
Angola	—	—	—	—	16.4	1.2	—	—	—
Benin	28,570	—	2,600	—	5.8	—	34	—	—
Botswana	15,220	5,150	1,900	—	—	—	52	92	77
Burkina Faso	97,120	57,320	—	1,680	8.2	0.3	—	—	—
Burundi	58,570	—	6,870	—	4.3	1.3	12	80	19
Cameroon	28,920	12,190	2,560	1,690	6.4	2.7	—	—	—
Central African Republic	44,740	25,930	2,460	—	4.5	0.9	—	—	—
Chad	61,900	30,030	8,010	—	0.9	—	—	—	—
Congo	9,510	—	780	—	—	—	—	—	—
Côte d'Ivoire	15,520	—	1,930	—	4.8	0.8	20	—	—
Ethiopia	86,120	32,650	—	—	2.4	0.3	58	—	—
Gabon	5,250	—	570	—	—	—	92	—	—
Ghana	12,910	22,970	690	1,670	9.1	1.5	73	82	40
Guinea-Bissau	17,500	—	2,820	—	—	—	16	—	—
Guinea	50,010	—	3,720	—	4.3	0.6	—	—	—
Kenya	8,000	10,130	2,520	—	3.2	1.7	—	77	50
Lesotho	30,400	—	3,860	—	—	—	28	—	—
Madagascar	10,120	8,130	240	—	3.5	0.9	62	—	—
Malawi	76,580	45,740	5,330	1,800	2.8	1.6	59	—	—
Mali	44,090	19,450	2,590	1,890	2.5	—	27	31	32
Mauritania	17,960	—	3,740	—	—	—	23	—	—
Mauritius	4,190	1,180	610	—	16.4	1.2	—	—	—
Mozambique	18,860	—	4,280	—	13.1	0.9	28	—	—

Namibia	—	4,620	—	—	—	—	—	—	—
Niger	60,090	34,850	5,610	650	11.3	—	47	57	—
Nigeria	19,830	—	4,240	—	6.0	1.4	—	—	31
Rwanda	59,600	72,990	5,610	4,190	1.7	1.7	—	64	—
Senegal	15,810	17,650	1,670	—	2.6	0.8	—	—	49
Sierra Leone	17,830	—	2,700	—	5.0	1.0	25	—	—
Somalia	—	—	—	—	7.1	0.8	—	—	—
South Africa	—	1,750	300	—	4.5	4.1	—	—	—
Sudan	14,520	—	990	—	2.7	0.9	20	71	69
Tanzania	22,600	24,880	3,310	5,470	7.3	1.1	74	—	—
Togo	28,860	—	1,590	—	6.2	1.6	—	81	54
Uganda	9,210	—	—	—	8.4	0.8	—	87	38
Zaire	—	—	—	—	2.1	1.6	—	—	—
Zambia	13,640	11,290	1,730	600	6.0	—	—	—	—
Zimbabwe	6,300	7,180	640	1,000	6.1	2.1	69	91	70

[a]Derived from World Health Organization data, supplemented by data obtained directly by the World Bank from national sources. Data refer to a variety of years, generally no more than two years before the year specified. Nursing persons include auxiliary nurses, as well as paraprofessional personnel such as traditional birth attendants.

[b]Each value refers to one particular but unspecified year within the time period denoted.

[c]Refers to births recorded where a recognized health service worker was in attendance. Data are from WHO, supplemented by UNICEF data, based on national sources, primarily from official community reports and records of hospitals of a wide range of size and sophistication. These figures should be used very cautiously.

[d]Data are from Demographic and Health Surveys, 1986–1990.

SOURCES: Blanc, 1991; World Bank, 1993.

Health-Seeking Behavior

Throughout the world, individuals and families are adaptive, pragmatic, and pluralistic in patterning their health-seeking behavior, depending on time and circumstance (see Bastien, 1992; Cosminsky, 1983; Finkler, 1994; Heggenhougen and Sesia-Lewis, 1988; Janzen, 1978; among many examples). Sub-Saharan women resort to various home remedies, over-the-counter and prescription pharmaceuticals, and medicines purchased from traditional healers. Similarly, they seek recourse through the categories of healers, including modern allopathic medical practitioners, traditional or folk healers, and trained and untrained traditional birth attendants (TBA). These resources are used serially or concurrently in different combinations and sequences; selecting among them is a complex process based on habit, cost, perception of risk or urgency, familiarity, and ease of access. The general perspective is that traditional and modern health systems are not seen as in conflict, but rather as two different, but valid, roads to recovery. At the same time, traditional healers in Africa have only rarely "straddled" the two systems in the same way Ayurvedic practitioners do in parts of Asia, and their patients rarely receive whatever benefits modern medicine may confer (Caldwell and Caldwell, 1993).

Although understanding this process and the behaviors associated with it would seem to be valuable to the design of preventive and curative interventions, there has been little systematic field research in the Sub-Saharan region into the ways females of different ages and educational histories manage their armamentarium of preventive and curative strategies across the spectrum of health problems and across the life span. Fortunately there is an increasing number of exceptions: the work done on mothers' management of illness in their youngest children, which offers some insight about their own health-seeking behavior; the body of behavioral and epidemiologic research that is accumulating in connection with the HIV infections and sexually transmitted diseases; data beginning to emerge from the Safe Motherhood Initiative; and the series of annual papers on gender and the tropical diseases sponsored by Canada's International Development Research Centre (IDRC). One hypothesis suggested by this still uneven body of research is that women may be most likely to attempt to access the modern medical system in connection with illness in a very young child, and least likely to do so when there is a potential for some kind of stigma—for example, for family planning services, diagnosis and treatment of either sexually transmitted diseases or tropical infectious diseases that seem to be sexually transmitted (for example, urinary schistosomiasis), or conditions that might have social repercussions if disclosed (such as leprosy).

The Dynamics of Female Education

The *World Development Report* is unequivocal on the centrality of education in human health, stating flatly that "Households with more education enjoy better health, both for adults and for children, [a result that] is strikingly consistent in a great number of studies, despite differences in research methods, time periods, and population samples" (World Bank, 1993).

The key link in that causal chain is women's central role in the health of their households, a centrality that prevails in virtually every society, even though patterns of decisionmaking and external power may differ greatly. Women's own health and their efficiency in using available resources are absolutely crucial to the health of others in the family, particularly children. The weight of the literature is toward a clear association between low levels of maternal education and increased child mortality (Cleland, 1990; Elo, 1992; Harrison, 1986). This seems to be particularly true for female children, especially when they are disvalued by the larger society.

In addition, it appears that a child's health is affected much more by the mother's schooling than by the father's; furthermore, the child benefits from maternal schooling even before its birth. Data for 13 African countries between 1975 and 1985 show that an increase of just 10 percent in female literacy rates reduced child mortality by an equivalent 10 percent, whereas changes in male literacy had little influence (Hobcraft, 1993). To take a specific country case, a calculation has been made for Kenya that 2 maternal deaths and about 45 infant deaths would be averted for every 1,000 girls provided with one extra year of primary schooling (World Bank, 1993).

There is broad general agreement on the major dimensions of the advantages of female education for household health. Female education increases knowledge about the importance of health and health care. It enhances the propensity and ability to get health information and act on it, as well as to seek, demand, and use health services wisely. It enhances access to income and the capacity and willingness to pay for health care, and is frequently correlated with access to such health-enhancing services as improved household water supplies. Better-educated women marry and start their families later, diminishing the risks associated with early pregnancies, and they tend to make greater use of prenatal care and delivery assistance and to produce fewer low-birthweight babies (Harrison, 1986; Hobcraft, 1993; Kennedy, 1992). Children of educated mothers enjoy such health-enhancing advantages as better food and domestic hygiene and more immunization, which in different ways reduce risk of infection. Mothers with more schooling also tend to be more effective in regimen compliance, use of health technologies, and overall case management (Vlassoff and Bonilla, 1994). Female education is also clearly linked to a woman's social standing, decisionmaking power, autonomy, and her own health status. In contrast, illiterate women do not do very well. Data from Ethiopia, for example, indicate that, regardless of whether or not abortion deaths were included in the calculation, illiterate women still suffered the most mortality (Kwast et al., 1986). While this is all very compelling, it is important to keep in mind that maternal education and most co-variates, such as child and maternal mortality, utilization of health services, and the like, are greatly confounded with income levels (Zimicki, 1989).

Table 2-2 presents data on adult literacy, mean years of schooling, and male-female primary and secondary school enrollment ratios. It also includes data on average age at first marriage and percentages of women in the labor force. The message is that Sub-Saharan Africa as a whole does not do well compared with other regions of the world; Sub-Saharan females do even less well. Although female enrollment in precollege formal education did increase substantially over the past 15 years, the percentage of female children enrolled is far less than the proportion of females in the school-age population of every country for which data are available, and the rates of growth in female enrollment are less than the rates of growth in the female primary-school-age population, suggesting that over time a growing number of girls lack access to schooling. Representation of females at higher educational levels is small to begin with, and rates of attrition are high. Part of the problem is that enrollments have been stagnating in Africa and the quality of education at all levels has been declining in the wake of the economic decline that started in the mid-1970s, and continues with the economic hardships associated with structural adjustment and other austerity programs of the 1980s (World Bank, 1989). There are other reasons as well: academic factors that do not favor girls in such subject matter areas as mathematics and sciences; cultural and societal expectations around gender roles; early marriage and pregnancy; and, for both males and females, lack of relevant or sufficiently rewarding employment in their fields of expertise (Beoku-Bettes and Ikubolajeh Logan, 1993).

Access Bias

It is crucial to note that, as in the case of health services, all difficulties and biases are multiplied for three major population categories: those who reside in isolated rural areas, where distance is the primary impediment; lower socioeconomic groups, where cost and foregone earnings are of concern; and girls. When there is substantial male emigration, leaving female heads of household with correspondingly larger responsibilities for agricultural subsistence labor, it is customary for such women to delegate at least some of their traditional responsibilities for household chores and care of younger siblings to school-age daughters. These tasks are not perceived as suitable for boys, a perception that is hardly exclusive to Sub-Saharan Africa. It is a view that is prevalent in most societies and is closely tied to cultural views about appropriate gender roles and female identity.

Still, while evidence is anecdotal, there appear to be signs of change, at least in some parts of the region. In northern Nigeria, where seclusion has been thoroughly embedded in all parts of community and household structure for centuries, one observer noted over a decade ago that:

> [Although] patterns of sexual inequality are extremely entrenched. . . . It is already apparent from observations over only five years that girls are being sent to school and kept there [by their parents] beyond the traditional age of marriage. . . . [This] could place women in line for jobs in the formal sector and lead to a whole sequence of demands and changes which are still quite remote from the perspectives of most Third World women. (Schildkrout, 1984)

TABLE 2-2 Educational Profile of Females in Sub-Saharan Africa

Country	Adult Literacy Rate (as of age 15+)			Mean Years of Schooling (25+)			Average Age at First Marriage (females, years), 1980–1989	Enrollment Ratios[a]		Women in Labor Force (percentage, total labor force), 1990–1992
	Total 1992	F 1992	M 1992	Total 1992	F 1992	M 1992		Primary (gross), 1950	Secondary (gross), 1990	
Mauritius	80	75	85	4.1	3.3	4.9	23.8	108	54	30
Seychelles	—	—	—	4.6	4.4	4.8	23.0	—	—	43
Botswana	75	66	85	2.5	2.5	2.6	26.4	119	45	39
S. Africa	—	—	—	3.9	3.7	4.1	26.1	—	—	39
Gabon	62	50	76	2.6	1.3	3.9	17.7	—	—	38
Swaziland	—	—	—	3.8	3.4	4.1	—	108	46	34
Maldives	—	—	—	4.5	3.9	5.1	17.9	—	—	20
Lesotho	—	—	—	3.5	4.1	2.8	20.5	116	31	44
Zimbabwe	69	61	76	3.1	1.8	4.5	20.4	116	46	48
Congo	59	45	72	2.1	1.1	3.1	21.9	—	—	39
Cameroon	57	45	70	1.6	0.8	2.6	18.8	95	23	30
Kenya	71	60	82	2.3	1.3	3.1	20.3	93	25	40
Namibia	—	—	—	1.7	—	—	—	126	47	24
Madagascar	81	74	90	2.2	1.7	2.6	20.3	91	18	40
Ghana	63	54	74	3.5	2.2	4.9	19.4	70	20	40
Côte d'Ivoire	56	41	69	1.9	0.9	2.9	18.9	58	14	32
Zambia	75	67	83	2.7	1.7	3.7	19.4	92	15	29
Nigeria	52	41	63	1.2	0.5	1.7	18.7	63	17	33
Zaire	74	63	86	1.6	0.8	2.4	20.1	64	15	36
Senegal	40	26	55	0.9	0.5	1.5	18.3	—	11	26
Liberia	42	31	53	2.1	0.8	3.3	19.4	—	—	31
Togo	45	33	59	1.6	0.8	2.4	18.5	87	12	37
Tanzania	—	—	—	2.0	1.3	2.8	18.5	68	4	48
Equatorial Guinea	52	38	66	0.8	0.3	1.3	19.1	—	—	36
Sudan	28	13	45	0.8	0.5	1.0	20.9	43	20	29
Burundi	52	42	63	0.4	0.3	0.7	21.7	66	4	53
Rwanda	52	39	67	1.1	0.5	1.5	21.2	70	7	54
Uganda	51	37	65	1.1	0.6	1.6	17.7	—	—	41
Angola	43	29	57	1.5	1.0	2.0	17.9	70	—	39
Benin	25	17	35	0.7	0.3	1.1	18.3	45	7	24
Malawi	—	—	—	1.7	1.1	2.4	17.8	60	3	51
Mauritania	35	22	48	0.4	0.1	0.7	19.5	43	10	22
Mozambique	34	21	46	1.6	1.2	2.2	17.6	52	6	48
C. African Republic	40	26	55	1.1	0.5	1.6	18.4	52	7	47

Ethiopia	—	—	—	1.1	0.7	1.5	18.1	30	11	41
Djibouti	—	—	—	0.4	0.3	0.7	—	31	36	—
Guinea-Bissau	39	25	53	0.4	0.1	0.7	18.3	42	4	42
Somalia	27	16	41	0.3	0.2	0.5	20.1	—	—	39
The Gambia	30	18	43	0.6	0.2	0.9	—	53	13	41
Mali	36	27	43	0.4	0.1	0.7	16.4	17	4	16
Chad	33	20	46	0.3	0.2	0.5	16.5	35	3	17
Niger	31	18	44	0.2	0.2	0.4	15.8	21	4	47
Sierra Leone	24	12	35	0.9	0.4	1.4	—	39	12	33
Burkina Faso	20	10	31	0.2	0.2	0.3	18.4	28	5	49
Guinea	27	15	39	0.9	0.3	1.5	16.0	24	5	30
All developing countries	69	58	79	3.9	3.0	4.9	20.8	90	34	35
Least-developed countries	46	34	58	1.6	0.9	2.2	18.7	55	12	38
Sub-Saharan Africa	—	—	—	1.6	1.0	2.2	19.0	60	15	37
Industrial countries	—	—	—	10.0	—	—	24.5	—	—	43
World	—	—	—	5.2	—	—	21.0	—	—	37

a The gross enrollment ratio is the number of students enrolled in a level of education, whether or not they belong in the relevant age group for that level, as a percentage of the population in the relevant age group for that level. All figures in this column are expressed in relation to the male average, which is indexed to equal 100. The smaller the figure, the bigger the gap; the closer the figure to 100, the smaller the gap.

SOURCE: UNDP, 1994.

Access to Assets, Employment, and Income

A cursory inspection of world health suggests that the single most important factor determining survival is income (World Bank, 1994). Lower income characteristically predicts poor health status, both among and within countries. At the same time, wealth does not necessarily bring health: issues of equity and political commitment are transcendent (World Bank, 1994).

In the 1991 edition of the *Human Development Report*, the UNDP predicted that Africa's share of the world's poor would overtake Asia's, to rise from 30 percent to 40 percent by the year 2025. The *HDR* added that, while Africa had made important human development gains since independence, the world economic crisis in the early 1980s, slow economic growth on the continent during the rest of the decade, and population increases of 3.2 percent annually had combined to produce declines in per capita GNP at an average annual rate of 2.2 percent over the decade; real wages declined by 30 percent over the same period. As a result, the social gains on the continent since independence were "reordered" (Bassett and Mhloyi, 1991). An analysis of the economic experience in seven diverse African countries (Botswana, Ghana, Kenya, Nigeria, Senegal, and Uganda) concluded that their economic reversals have indeed had demographic effects and that the lives of many Africans were affected as they suffered the deaths of their children and made decisions to delay or forgo marriage and parenthood (NRC, 1993a).

To respond to the economic crises of the 1970s and 1980s, a number of the Sub-Saharan countries were required to change their economic policies and adopt macroeconomic and microeconomic reforms designed to produce price stability, sustainable monetary balance, efficient resource use, and faster economic growth. These changes generally involved cuts in public spending and liberalization of prices, areas of special relevance to the health sector. To support the reforms, the World Bank and the International Monetary Fund extended "adjustment lending" to cushion developing economies during transition to new growth paths; the effects of these "structural adjustments" have spun off a swirl of controversy and analysis (World Bank, 1993).

The UNDP view is that these economic reforms have yet to bear fruit in human development (UNDP, 1993), and the *World Development Report* agrees that the health costs of slow economic growth (as expressed in declining per capita incomes and increasing percentages of the population defined as living in poverty) have been high. Although, for example, child health has been improving everywhere in the developing world, gains have been much less rapid in countries with slow income growth. More severely stated, evidence suggests that the adjustment process in itself is associated with less favorable child mortality outcomes than would have been predicted by long-term trends (Cornia et al., 1987). Had economic growth in Africa been as fast in the 1980s as it was in the preceding two decades, 7 percent of total infant deaths in the region would have been averted (World Bank, 1993).

Assessing the specific effects of structural adjustment on health sector funding is more complicated. The nature and degree of impact seem to vary with the timing of the process and the ways in which spending cuts were designed. Although, in countries both with and without adjustment loans, health sector spending as a percentage of total country income declined in the early 1980s in relation to the average for the decade, it recovered in the rest of the decade much faster in countries that undertook and sustained major policy reforms (World Bank, 1993, 1994).

Whatever the long-term costs and benefits of adjustment policies, there appears to be some consensus in parts of the African policy community (SOMANET, 1992) that these policies have been more acutely problematic for the poor and for women. Cliff (1991), in her study of destabilization in Mozambique, suggests that:

> Structural adjustment has an in-built gender bias against women. As Elson (1987:3) shows, "the success of the macroeconomic policy in reaching its goals may be won at the cost of a longer and harder working day for women. This cost will be invisible to the macroeconomic policy makers because it is unpaid time. But the cost will be revealed in statistics on the health and nutritional status of such women."

She adds that poor urban women—and particularly female-headed households—are particularly vulnerable to the effects of adjustment. Poor urban women tend to be in low-wage, low-status jobs, with few skills that make them eligible for wage employment in the formal sector. When the formal labor market shrinks in response to adjustment, females tend to be the first to be laid off and to leave school, and must then take lower-paying jobs or enter the informal labor market to patch together family subsistence.

Other costs associated with adjustment policies include increases in drug prices and the establishment of user fees for both education and health services. Analysis of clinic utilization at a referral center for sexually transmitted diseases in Kenya indicated that user fees had a dampening effect on clinic utilization, particularly for women (Moses et al., 1992). Case studies in Swaziland and Zimbabwe found that these fees led to substantial drops in clinic utilization for immunizations, preventive care, and maternal and antenatal series (Loewenson et al., 1991; Yoder, 1989). A series of 11 multidisciplinary situation analyses of facilities providing emergency obstetric care in Ghana, Nigeria, and Sierra Leone found marked declines in utilization of nonemergency services and in numbers of normal deliveries at a sample of clinics that had established or increased user fees for drugs and specific services. User fees and, somewhat ironically, lack of drugs and supplies at these facilities also contributed to unacceptably long waiting times between admission and treatment of complicated cases. At some sites, these delays were associated with increases in the numbers of maternal deaths (Ekwempu et al., 1990; Prevention of Maternal Mortality Network, 1995). At the same time, a recent and very thorough study of the Tanzanian health system suggests that user fees would not be a disincentive were the facility to provide services of reasonable quality (Gilson, 1995).

Widowhood and Its Sequelae

Another byproduct of adjustment appears to have been decreased care of the elderly, particularly widows, whose status is already fragile enough. A number of factors affect the status of women who have been widowed; these, in turn, affect their physical, economic, and mental well-being. Among these influences are household arrangements, whether or not she has children (particularly sons), age, advent of menopause, property rights, land rights, and the culturally prescribed length of mourning periods.

Legal status is crucial, particularly in connection with laws of inheritance. The tradition in patrilineal societies is for a widow to become the property of her late husband's brother or cousin (the levirate), and it is under that circumstance that she will be able to keep her children with her. Otherwise, she can only hope that the children will transfer to her some portion of their own patrilineal inheritance (Henn, 1984). Should she not acquiesce to the dictates of tradition, she may also face the possibility of ostracism by her deceased husband's family. If, as is the case in some subcultures, a widow is blamed for her husband's death, her ostracism is complete (U. Amazigo, personal communication, 1992). The levirate seems to be declining rapidly where AIDS is the probable cause of death, but the dynamics and implications of that change are unknown (Fortney, personal communication, 1994). Inheritance, however, remains a major issue in patrilineal societies, and women's rights groups are forming around attempts to understand attitudes toward traditional law, with an eye toward reform.

Economic hardship, whether or not it is related to structural adjustment programs, in combination with increased urbanization has also resulted in decreased care of the elderly. Again, widows are at particularly high risk, because customary practices of support, either by a woman's children or by the brothers of a widow's husband, tend to attenuate in rapidly urbanizing settings; in some places, they have disappeared altogether (Adamchak et al., 1991). Widows may be utterly abandoned by their relatives and acquire a new, and detrimental, urban identity. In an urban area of Kenya, widows living alone are widely recognized as being available for any man, and the incidence of rape against widows is said to be very high (Raikes, 1989). In polygamous societies, younger widows may find refuge in remarriage, but there are accounts of older single women or elderly widows without the protection of nearby children being accused of witchcraft, murdered, and their possessions taken (P. Masanja, personal communication, 1991).

Widows may also find themselves compelled to resort to commercial sex work for economic survival. While the sample is not representative, the following figures are interesting: a study at a family planning clinic in Nairobi found a prevalence of HIV infection of 4.3 percent among married women, 8.5 percent in single women, and 11.8 percent in widowed and divorced women (D. Hunter, Department of Epidemiology, Harvard School of Public Health, personal communication, 1993). The intervening variable appears to be economic status: in general, women of lower socioeconomic status, including lower-status commercial sex workers, are at higher risk of contracting sexually transmitted diseases (Brunham and Embree, 1992).

Finally, war leaves widows, and may often leave them without their children as well. In a survey of elderly women in centers for displaced persons, 64 percent in Mozambique and 74 percent in Zimbabwe were widows (Ramji, 1987). The same study found that the proportion of severe malnutrition among Mozambican women over age 45 was 21 percent, using a weight of under 40 kilograms as a cutoff point; the corresponding percentage for men in the same age group was 5 percent. This suggests that the health status of older women may be especially threatened in conditions of displacement.

POWER, CONTROL, EQUITY, AND STATUS

In an analysis of reproduction and social organization, Lesthaeghe (1989) comments on the effects of postcolonial and postindependence developmental dynamics in Sub-Saharan Africa:

> The development of the migrant labor system created new roles and responsibilities for the wives of migrants and for migrant women. To a considerable extent, these have become accepted and institutionalized both culturally and legally. This and related developments, such as the spread of female education, have greatly enhanced women's status. Nevertheless, their responsibility for child-rearing, restricted access to land, exclusion from inheritance, and lack of opportunities for paid employment mean that most women, whether married or not, remain dependent on relationships with men to obtain the means of survival.

In Sub-Saharan African societies, as elsewhere in the world, women are likely to have a status subservient to that of men, with less control over family resources; minimal access to cash; and, in general, inferior social power. Some analysts claim that in several African countries, women have the status of minors and tend to be reduced to wards of their fathers or husbands (Sacks, 1982). At the same time, there is heterogeneity across Africa in the structure of family power. Circumstances range from the powerlessness described by Sacks to the greater independence found in western and middle Africa, for example. This greater autonomy can be partially credited to high levels of polygyny, which render each wife and her children a separate economic unit. This independence is compromised, however, when a wife must seek money from her husband or a child's father for such expenses as medical treatment, which then involves him in the health decision-making process (Caldwell and Caldwell, 1993).

One very important source of variation is the organization of family labor. In 1982, Ifeka concluded from her ethnographic work that when gender relationships are reciprocal rather than oppositional, as she suggests they often are, the balance of power—and control—tends to be more equitable. Considered as a hypothesis, this is neither simple nor trivial and merits further inquiry in other national and subnational contexts.

Other sources of female-male power and status differential are employment, class, educational level, and the relative social position of ethnic groups. For instance, compared with the majority of their female counterparts elsewhere in Africa, market women in West Africa have considerably more access to cash income; greater control over that cash, as well as over their own freedom of movement; and, perhaps correspondingly, enhanced social status. Among the Hausa, recognition is given to women who neither remarry after divorce nor engage in prostitution, but support themselves through other income-earning activities and live with their families (Coles and Mack, 1991; Pittin, 1983). In 1980, such single urban and rural Ugandan women were described as being in the forefront of social change and, even when they were not university women, they commanded prestige and respect (Obbo, 1980).

In many African countries the processes of marrying and negotiating for the most suitable partner are real factors in social change. Education, often with considerable maneuvering to obtain it, is a factor in forming unions in which women will have greater autonomy and more equity with their spouses, particularly among the elite (Bledsoe, 1990; Obbo, 1987). Additional education, such as adult evening classes, is also seen as a means to empowerment for older women, even as they remain within their traditional roles (Osuala, 1990).

Fostering

Older women may also achieve enhanced status through the widespread practice of child fostering, which is largely in the hands of women.   Studies in Ghana found that the percentages of households with fostered-in children ranged from 17 percent for households headed by a male of working age to as high as 74 percent if the head were a woman age 60 or older (Lloyd and Brandon, 1991). The practice has a variety of social and economic functions for both the fostering-out and the fostering-in families. The foster parent benefits from the child's company and labor in furtherance of her own economic and social advancement and, more broadly, the reinforcement of the larger female social hierarchy (Castle, 1995; NRC, 1993b). "Purposive fostering" (as opposed to "crisis fostering") is intended to advance a child's short- and long-term life-chances, with schooling one of the major objectives (Goody, 1982).   The picture of how well that objective is achieved is mixed. Fostered-in children, especially girls, have much lower enrollment rates than do "own children," or even their nonfostered sisters in their households of origin. In theory, girls should have more options as a consequence of fostering; in practice, this might not be the case, but there is no quantification that permits a claim in either direction. It is perhaps indicative of the benefits that can accrue to female participants in kinship fostering arrangements that they are being replicated.   Informal fostering arrangements based on friendship and mutual assistance are critical for women attempting to cope with the harshness of life in urban squatter settlements.

Kinship and Residence

Power may also vary according to rules of kinship and residence. Female status is enhanced in matrilineal as opposed to patrilineal societies, and several features of matrilineality contribute to women's economic and social security (Henn, 1984; MacCormack, 1989). A woman in such a society is less likely to move away from her maternal village upon first marriage and, under certain circumstances, her husband may begin to farm there. If the marriage dissolves, a divorced woman who has moved away can reactivate land rights in her maternal village much more easily than a divorced woman in a patrilineal society. In addition, her children remain with her because they belong by right to their maternal rather than their paternal kin, and she has greater assurance of continued support from her children, irrespective of the course of her marriage (NRC, 1993b). Greater power and social status also accrue to women when they move beyond the age of childbearing; this seems to be especially true, although not exclusively so, in matrilineal groups (Ngubane, 1987).

Ironically, modernization may reverse this situation. Lesthaeghe (1989) suggests that the integration of rural and urban economies and the emergence of human capital as a movable economic asset have combined to weaken the control of lineages over economic resources and decision making. The significance of the lineage has been threatened from several directions from colonial times, and women are distinctively threatened by deterioration in the power of the matriliny:

> The new family code undermines the juridical basis of the matrilineal extended family which Lemba women view as the basis of their continuing social support networks. . . . The government's cultural engineering project, polygyny, strong patriarchal authority, and female subordination are lauded as "authentic," "traditional" social forms, while independent women are sometimes made scapegoats for economic ills. . . . The cultural autonomy of the Lemba may be undermined at the same time that their economic base can no longer support them. (Schoepf, 1987)

It is also important to inspect some of the correlates of low social status. Low female status often means that not only are families less willing to expend scarce resources on the health of their girls and women, but also that those same women may accept this perspective as appropriate. As noted in the preceding section, inequality may well be exacerbated by widowhood. Status issues also affect health care practice. In some cultural settings, women are less likely than men to become physicians, and they may be unable to work in rural areas if they are unmarried. In turn, the lack of female physicians deters many women from seeking medical care, particularly in Muslim societies.

HIV and AIDS

The impact of the sexually transmitted diseases, including HIV/AIDS, on female morbidity and mortality is becoming increasingly well known and is discussed at length in Chapter 11 and in the Appendix to this volume. Its interactions with female roles and status have become a growing issue as the heterosexual dimensions of the epidemic have become more apparent.

Among those dimensions, perhaps the most critical touches differential power between males and females, a differential that has several interrelated origins. One is age. Women tend to become infected with HIV-1 at earlier ages than men because of the greater biological efficiency of male-to-female transmission than the reverse, an efficiency that is enhanced if either partner has another sexually transmitted infection. Infectivity in younger women is also enhanced because their partners are generally older; they thus have a higher cumulative risk of infection than the female partners of their male contemporaries. This feature of the epidemic is being translated into more severe increases in mortality among women at younger adult ages (Gregson et al., 1994).

In an analysis of the contributions of the balance of power between women and men to HIV transmission, Mason (1994) examines each possible variable. A fundamental contributor is the imbalance in standards of sexual obligations, the "double standard." As Western as the term is thought to be, it is amazingly ubiquitous. It simply means that males are generally understood to have more sexual freedom than females, and thus more sexual partners (Mason, 1994). University women in Nairobi, interviewed in a brief informal study in 1992, reported that "women get AIDS in their own bedrooms"; in other words, they are infected by husbands who have extramarital sexual partners (Amazigo, personal communication, 1992). Several studies suggest that increasing numbers of women may be choosing not to marry, anticipating that they will have more control over their ability to demand protection from potential infection in an extramarital relationship than might be the case in a marriage (Akeroyd, 1990; Bassett and Mhloyi, 1991; Carovano, 1991; Krieger and Margo, 1991). The net result is that women are faced with almost diametrically opposed options (Bassett and Mhloyi, 1991). Whatever new status single women may have acquired in some Sub-Saharan African contexts, the dominant model for an African woman, her social insurance, is maternity. To renounce that role is a kind of social death; to contract AIDS is, of course, a biological death.

Another effect of gender inequality is to increase STD prevalence: first, because women are constrained from either asking about or controlling their husband's sexual activities; second, because women are inequitably served by appropriate health facilities, or constrained by fear of stigma or inability to pay for services; third, because they may view reproductive ill-health fatalistically as part of their natural female lot; and fourth, women's limited economic opportunities may have made some sort of exchange of sex for money a necessary option. One surprising conclusion from the analysis is that the relationship of gender inequality to the use of condoms is ambiguous to a degree that commands solid, thoughtful research involving African researchers, community women, and commercial sex workers.

Despite frequent calls for a body of national and regional information concerning patterns of sexual behavior and their determinants, there remains the dilemma of heterogeneity and the risks of undue reliance on aggregate data. There are highly significant variations in sexual behavior among different population subgroups, including differentiation by residence in urban or rural areas; educational level; use and nonuse of family planning methods; and marital status, although the last is an inadequate proxy for exposure (Rutenberg et al., 1994). One of the great challenges to research will be to locate some middle-level, cost-effective, and technically modest approaches to understanding sexual behavior patterns in some practical way in this swirl of differentiation.

SOCIAL DISRUPTION AND HEALTH STATUS

War and Civil Strife

In Angola, Burundi, Chad, Liberia, Mozambique, Somalia, South Africa, Sudan, Togo, and Zaire, civil strife and general violence have been the *status quo* for decades. Up to 90 percent of war-related fatalities in such conflict situations have occurred among civilians (Werner, 1989), and females are at particular risk. Cliff (1991) paints a harrowing picture of the situation of women and girls in Mozambique. Because of their responsibilities for gathering firewood, hauling water, and farm work, they are in constant danger of kidnapping, repeated rape, use as forced laborers, and eventual death. UNICEF (1989) estimated that 494,000 "excess" deaths in children occurred between 1980 and 1988 in Mozambique as a result of guerrilla activities; over 1.5 million people were internally displaced, and the majority of those were female (Bread for the World, 1992; Cole et al., 1992; Forbes-Martin, 1991; Shipton, 1990).

A less obvious consequence of civil instability is the need to siphon off money for defense from other sectors, usually the social sectors, which have the potential to be especially supportive of women and children (Dodge, 1990; Gellhorn, 1984; Ityavyar and Ogba, 1989; Ogba, 1989). Mozambique's annual per capita expenditure on health in 1981 was US$4.00; by 1988, it was US$0.05. In addition, the involvement of large numbers of males in military activities drastically reduced agricultural production and, consequently, GDP. The military movements of those same males were also the major factor in increasing rates of sexually transmitted diseases, including HIV/ AIDS (Bastos dos Santos et al., 1992).

Refugee Status

Both war and famine produce refugees. In 1990, one-third of the world's 16.5 million refugees were in Africa, a figure that only grows. The UNDP estimated that there were 19 million refugees worldwide by 1994 (UNDP, 1994). To this must be added the 11 million internally displaced people in Mozambique, South Africa, and Sudan, and the uncounted millions in other African countries with internal displacements of one sort or another (Bread for the World, 1992; Forbes-Martin, 1991).

Once again, females suffer greatly, and they do so in large numbers. The current estimate is that 75 percent of the world's refugees are women and girls (Overhagen, 1990, cited in Heise, 1993); in Sub-Saharan Africa, that figure surpasses 80 percent (Cole et al., 1992; Shipton, 1990). As individuals with no country, they essentially have no rights to special protection; unlike their husbands, brothers, or fathers who may be fighting in the same conflict that produced their refugee situation, women and children are not protected by the Geneva Convention.

The situation of refugee girls and women is one of extreme vulnerability. They are subject to sexual violence and the possibility of abduction at every step of their exodus, from flight, to border crossings, to life in the camps (Heise, 1993). In 1984, Aitchison reported that virtually all women from Ethiopia and Somalia entering Djibouti were raped, almost as a matter of course. Given the lack of ability to earn income in any other manner, it is not surprising that refugee women come to view prostitution as self-protection, even survival; women note bitterly that the end result is the same, and they might as well earn the money. Violence follows refugee women even after resettlement in a new country: women who are raped during their journey to freedom are, for reasons that are probably of exquisite complexity, more likely to be victims of domestic violence in their new homes (Kuoch et al., 1992).

Gender Violence

Article 2 of the 1993 United Nations declaration on violence against women defines the term "gender violence" as including, though not limited to, physical, sexual, and psychological violence occurring in the family and in the community, including battering, sexual abuse of female children, dowry-related violence, marital rape, female genital mutilation and other traditional practices harmful to women, nonspousal violence, violence related to exploitation, sexual harassment, intimidation at work, trafficking in women, forced prostitution, and violence perpetrated or condoned by the state. The central notion is that of physical and psychological harm rather than the express intent of the perpetrator (Heise et al., 1994).

Table 2-3, which displays the manifestations of gender violence across the life cycle on a global basis, makes it sadly clear that there is no stage of that cycle in which the females of the world, as a group, are categorically exempt. There are three very considerable manifestations that do not seem to be part of life in Sub-Saharan Africa: there is no reliable evidence for sex-selective abortion, female infanticide, or differential access to food or medical

TABLE 2-3 Gender Violence Throughout the Life Cycle, All Countries

In Utero	Infancy/ Early Childhood (birth through age 4)	Childhood (ages 5–14)	Adolescence (ages 15–19)	Adulthood (ages 20–44)	Postmenopause (age 45+)
Sex-selective abortion	Female infanticide	Child marriage	Dating and courtship violence	Abuse by intimate male partners	Abuse of widows
Battering during pregnancy	Emotional/physical abuse	Genital mutilation	Economically coerced sex	Marital rape	Elder abuse
Coerced pregnancy	Differential access to food and medical care for girl infants	Sexual abuse by family members and strangers	Partner homicide	Dowry abuse and murder	
	Differential access to food and medical care	Sexual abuse in the workplace	Psychologic abuse		
	Child prostitution	Rape	Sexual abuse in the workplace		
		Sexual harassment	Sexual harassment		
		Forced prostitution	Rape		
		Trafficking in women	Abuse of women with disabilities		

care for female infants in the region. At the same time, other areas indicated in the table are of great concern. Table 2-4 reports on one of those areas, spousal abuse. The percentages of women who report it are terribly high, and a number of other sources indicate that it is prevalent across the entire region (Levinson, 1989). Whether alcoholism as a subset of substance abuse is a major problem in Sub-Saharan Africa is an open question (Heath, 1993). If it proves to be a significant issue, it may be expected that, as elsewhere, women will suffer disproportionately, primarily because of the drain on family income that could otherwise be used for food, health services, and school fees. Substance abuse is known to be significantly correlated with accidents (Feachem et al., 1991), homicide rates, and domestic violence and spouse abuse (Malik and Sawi, 1976).

Estimates of rape incidence are highly speculative in the developing world overall, but there are some data, and they are chilling. Rates of rape in South Africa are extremely high. In 1988, although 19,308 rapes were documented in police reports, the National Institute of Crime Prevention and the Rehabilitation of Offenders estimated that only 1 in 20 rapes is reported. If that is indeed the case, the true total would be close to 386,160 (Russel, 1991; Vogelman, 1990). That is an average of one rape every minute and a half, or 34 rapes per 1,000 adult women, compared with the U.S. rate of 18 per 1,000 women (Heise, 1993).

The question of the extent of the association between rape and sexism and how that might be defined in the African context is unknown. African female voices increasingly attest to the presence of sexism (Mazrui, 1991; Ngaiza and Koda, 1991; Osaki, 1990; *Weekly Review*, 1991). Public reaction to the 1991 rape of 71 girls in Meru District, Kenya, was muted in ways that have been interpreted by some analysts as sexist, and the Kenyan Public Law Institute and the Women's Bureau have issued *A Guide to Women of Kenya on Rape and the Legal Process* (*Weekly Review*, 1991). The entire issue of rape in Africa, its prevalence, a more precise definition of its causes and correlates, and the nature of its impact on cohorts of females is beginning to be examined. Whatever the responses to these questions, there is little doubt that rape is profoundly bad for female emotional and physical health; what is in doubt is the ability of health and social services in Sub-Saharan Africa to deal with it in an adequate fashion.

Early Marriage

The Africa-wide perception of women as primarily wives and mothers reinforces patterns of premature childbearing and high parity. Early adolescent marriage and subsequent early motherhood are all too often negative events in the health trajectory of young Sub-Saharan African women, reflected most vividly in mounting rates of abortion among adolescents. Of those women, nearly 50 percent are married by age 18, some by age 15 (UNDP, 1991). Ages at entry into a regular sexual union vary widely across the region: proportions of women who are still single between the ages 15 to 19 range from 10 to more than 90 percent, and corresponding mean ages at first union range from about 16 to more than 21 years. Links between formation of a union and motherhood in most Sub-Saharan countries are close: women are almost as likely to have their first birth before age 20 as they are to marry before age 20. That some young women are single does not mean that they are not having sexual intercourse and, in some cases, that they are not having babies. In most of the 16 countries included in the Demographic and Health Surveys (DHS), a large proportion (37–78 percent) of single women ages 15–24 have already had a sexual relationship; 26–53 percent are currently involved in a sexual relationship; and 2–42 percent have already had a child (Alan Guttmacher Institute, 1995). In general, the median age of women at first birth in Sub-Saharan Africa is approximately two years younger than it is in North Africa, Asia, or Latin America (Arnold and Blanc, 1990).

The two primary determinants of these early liaisons are the influence of Islam and the practice of polygyny, so often a feature of patrilineal societies (Lesthaeghe, 1989). In contrast, matrilineal social structure, higher levels of female education, and urbanization are three cultural factors associated with later marriage (NRC, 1993b). Polygyny "presupposes a large age difference between spouses and . . . a combination of late marriage for men and early marriage for women" (NRC, 1993b). The Islamic influence is identified with a more stringent social control of women, a control more likely to be assured through early first marriages for girls (Goody, 1973, 1976; Lesthaeghe et al., 1992). Among the many consequences of early marriage is the simple actuarial probability that

TABLE 2-4 Prevalence of Spouse Abuse, Selected Countries, Sub-Saharan Africa

Country and Author	Sample	Sample Type	Findings	Comment
Kenya (Raikes, 1990)	733 women from Kissi District	District-wide cluster	42% beaten regularly	Taken from contraceptive prevalence survey
Tanzania (Sheikh-Hashim and Gabba, 1990)	300 women from Dar es Salaam	Convenience, from 3 districts (interviews)	60% had been physically abused by a partner	
Uganda (Wakabi and Mwesigye, 1991)	80 women (16 from each of Kampala's 5 divisions)	House-to-house written survey; 7 women refused to answer	46% of 73 women responding reported being physically abused by a partner	An additional 7 women reported beatings by family members and another 5 reported assaults or rapes by outsiders
Zambia (Phiri, 1992)	171 women ages 20–40	Convenience, women from shanty compounds, medium- and high-density suburbs of Lusaka and Kafue Rural	40% beaten by a partner; another 40% mentally abused	17% said they thought that physical abuse was a normal part of marriage

SOURCE: Heise et al., 1994.

women often will be widowed quite early in their lives. Because widowhood in itself is a threat to female health, as noted earlier in this chapter, the net result is usually negative.

Another negative effect of early marriage derives from the insufficient development of most adolescent bodies for the physical burdens of pregnancy. Women in early adolescence are at the highest risk of all age groups for the cephalopelvic disproportion that causes obstructed labor, the single greatest reported cause of maternal mortality (see Chapter 4).

In addition to the increase it generates in mortality risk, early childbearing also produces physiologic sequelae that contribute to higher accrued morbidity across the female life span. One very durable effect is the development of vesico-vaginal and recto-vaginal fistulae, which are ruptures in the tissue between the bladder or rectum and the vagina (Harrison, 1983). Women with unrepaired fistulae are far more likely to experience urinary or fecal incontinence, which can sometimes be ostracizing to the point of divorce. Yet repair of such tissue traumas requires a level of surgical sophistication not widely available in the region, and perhaps out of the financial reach of women in the lower socioeconomic strata.

Finally, the early onset of childbearing extends the time span of possible pregnancy and birth. A childbearing span that begins at age 15 lasts for approximately 22 years, compared with the average 7-year span in developed countries, where the range is from ages 23 through 30. In Sub-Saharan Africa, the region with the highest parity in the world, early initiation of childbearing does more than just increase the number of children a woman will conceive and bear. Grandmultiparity also increases her chances for developing the condition that has come to be called "maternal depletion syndrome." Although definition of "maternal depletion" and the mechanisms and timing of its contribution to disability are subjects of controversy (Winkvist et al., 1992), one thing that is clear is the hazardous relationship between very early childbearing and mortality: the risk of maternal mortality for women under age 20 is twice the rate for women between ages 20 and 34 (UNDP, 1991; WHO, 1992).

Traditional Medicine

There are cultural dimensions to every part of human life. While culture always matters, there are circumstances in which it quite overwhelms other fundamental dimensions of human existence such as economic dynamics, physical environment, and other seemingly more objective facts of life.

There are large areas of female life in Sub-Saharan Africa in which cultural expectations and responses dominate health status, either enhancing that status or limiting it. Much of the data that correspond to these areas are found in ethnographic accounts of relatively small human groups and are dismissed as anecdote, usually for reasons of sample size and sampling procedure. Yet it is these essentially cultural accounts that provide the clues to the thought, values, and behavior that can submerge the noblest and most "rational" attempts to enhance health status—in our case, female health status.

As everywhere, illness and disease in Sub-Saharan Africa are both cultural and biomedical constructs, so that there is a wide range in the ways illness and disease are generated, defined, explained, and managed (Dagnew, 1984; Fosu, 1981; Gaisie, 1990; Janzen, 1978; Kloos et al., 1987).

The National Traditional Healers Association of Zimbabwe has defined 'traditional medicine' as follows:

> The sum total of all the knowledge and practices, whether explicable or not, used in diagnosis, treatment, prevention and elimination of physical, mental or social imbalance and relying exclusively on practical experience and observation handed down from generation to generation, whether verbally or in writing. Traditional medicine might also be considered as a solid amalgamation of dynamic medical know-how and ancestral experience. (Chavundaka, 1984)

What this definition does not address explicitly is the very fundamental matter of etiology—that is, the cultural explanations of why disease befalls humankind. Traditional medicine is built on a deeply rooted structure of belief and theory about the origins of illness and the maintenance of health, a structure that takes into account both spiritual and physical causation. One of these beliefs is the almost fatalistic view that physical suffering is intrinsic to the female condition. Another widely distributed explanatory structure is the set of beliefs around humoral balance in the human body and the importance of equilibrium between conditions typically described as "hot" and "cold" (Logan, 1977). Even when the definitions of these states of being and the strategies for dealing with them vary—as they often do, from society to society—the concept of mental and physical balance is found in virtually every region of the world. Although the idea of balance is a reasonable medical and societal premise for healthy lives and is the basis for a large number of beneficial traditional health interventions, it is often ignored by Western medical practice.

Throughout Sub-Saharan Africa, traditional medicine is a lively and pervasive component of everyday life, and an estimated 90 percent of the population rely on traditional healers as primary health care providers (WHO, 1982). This may be because of the heritage of respect this category of health practitioner has acquired across the generations, the very positive nature of many of the health interventions such healers provide or reinforce, because such practitioners constitute the only accessible resource, or some combination of all of these factors.

Traditional Practices

Within the system that is traditional medicine are sets of what we chose to call "traditional practices," which are employed in the maintenance or restoration of what is culturally defined as "health." Some of these are tightly integrated into aspects of Sub-Saharan culture and society and may reinforce them across the life span. In childhood and adolescence, the most notable practices are early marriage and female genital mutilation; in adulthood, they include traditional practices linked to pregnancy, birth, and the postpartum period; and, in later years, they involve practices associated with widowhood.

The degree to which these practices affect female health, either positively or negatively, is almost completely unquantified. Analysis has been based largely on the amassing of anecdote, a very few in-depth studies, and extrapolations from experience elsewhere. This base of information, although incomplete, suggests that certain traditional practices in the Sub-Saharan region are strongly supportive of female health. The positive view of breastfeeding is a good example; the prescription for an ample postpartum rest period for new mothers is another. Still others remain to be identified and more systematically characterized so that they can be maintained as valued components of national and local systems of medical care or, in the cases of traditional practices that are injurious to female well-being, discouraged.

Food Prescriptions and Proscriptions

Cultural prescriptions and proscriptions of certain foods have the potential to influence female nutritional status, particularly in areas where high levels of malnutrition, iron-deficiency anemia, chronic malaria, goiter, and helminthic infestations have been documented. The ethnographic record in Sub-Saharan Africa reflects patterns of food prescriptions and proscriptions, particularly for pregnant women, that are not unlike such prescriptions and proscriptions elsewhere in the world, where they fall into three categories of concern: (1) possible harm to the fetus; (2) a precipitated miscarriage; or (3) a difficult delivery, including concerns about an overly large fetus.

At the same time, researchers do not yet have a good grasp of the volume, duration, and quality of either the positive or the deleterious effects of these traditional practices. This is partly because it is difficult to separate the effects of traditional dietary practices from the effects of overall food shortages, and partly because the monitoring and logging of actual food intake in largely illiterate human groups is difficult and costly. While these restrictions cause no harm in areas of considerable dietary diversity and affordable dietary substitutes, food proscriptions in food-deficient circumstances may affect dietary quality for pregnant women and their imminent offspring. For women of already poor nutritional or health status, any resulting undernutrition could not be helpful.

One aspect of prenatal nutritional intake that appears to reach beyond anecdotal levels toward real potential significance is the concern for keeping fetal size down. In Ethiopia, traditional birth attendants (TBA) advise pregnant women to restrict their intake of foods, including milk and vegetables, that are believed to increase the weight of both mother and baby (UNDP, 1991). Whether the intake of nonprescribed foods is adequate is unknown. It may be that nothing detrimental is happening, but since rates of low birthweight are so high in the region, some inquiry would be useful.

Pregnancy, Labor, and Delivery

Maternal mortality rates are high in Sub-Saharan Africa, and at least some of that mortality and related morbidity can be attributed to traditional practices that need to be categorized as harmful. A recent study in Nigeria concluded that 4 percent of reported maternal deaths were attributable to such practices (WHO, 1991) and noted that, because such a large proportion of births and deaths in Sub-Saharan Africa occur outside hospital, the 4 percent figure may be a significant undercount. At the same time, the accuracy of cause-of-death attributions are so highly questionable in general that it might be more useful—and culturally neutral—to look initially in some systematic way at the practices themselves and ask whether they are, in themselves, appropriate even for populations of women in optimum health.

A crucial function in the childbearing sequence and in the perpetuation of traditional practices is the role of the TBA, trained or untrained. Because that is so directly an obstetric topic, it is addressed as such in Chapter 4.

Female Genital Mutilation

The term "female circumcision," until recently in general use, has been largely replaced by the more collective term "female genital mutilation" (FGM). FGM comprises a variety of operations that, in their most prevalent forms, go beyond circumcision of the clitoris to excision of most of the external female genitalia (Gordon, 1991).

Whatever terminology is employed, the topic is highly charged and highly complex. Not only are these traditional procedures of considerable biomedical importance (see Chapter 4), but they also exemplify the profound integration between what is medical and what is cultural, and between what is modern and what is traditional.

As preface to any scrutiny of the biomedical aspects and effects of these practices, it is important to look at what is known about their prevalence and to place them in the context to which they are so intimately and, in some cases, precisely tied. FGM is practiced extensively throughout Sub-Saharan Africa, in Oman, South Yemen, the United Arab Emirates, Malaysia, India, and Pakistan, as well as in large immigrant communities in Europe, the United Kingdom, and the United States. Somewhere in the range of 84 to 94 million girls and women in the world today have undergone some form of genital excision (Cutner, 1985; Lightfoot-Klein, 1989; Rushwan, 1990). Kouba and Muasher (1985) estimated that 5.5 million children or adolescents are operated on annually, primarily in Africa. One source (Hosken, 1992) calculates that the practice is found in at least 20 Sub-Saharan countries, and that the percentage of women who have undergone the procedure ranges from nearly 100 percent of women in Somalia and Djibouti to under 5 percent in Uganda and Zaire.

It is vital to recognize that there are differences in the extent of the practice among and within the Sub-Saharan countries. For example, approximately 70 percent of women in Burkina Faso have been genitally excised; the percentage in neighboring Ghana is around 30 percent (Hosken, 1992). There is also variation within countries: in northern Sudan, for example, 89 percent of ever-married women ages 15-49 are infibulated, while the procedure is rare in southern Sudan (Kheir et al., 1991). (The types of FGM are described from a biomedical perspective in Chapter 4.)

CONCLUSIONS

The purpose of this report, as stated in its opening chapter, is to assemble as much as possible of what is known about the biomedical dimensions of female morbidity and mortality in Sub-Saharan Africa. This has not been done before in a systematic way, and the committee believes that just as it is perilous to limit thinking about human health to biology alone, it is similarly perilous to focus on larger environments without understanding the biologic organisms with which they interact. It is surely true that there is no pharmaceutical remedy for inequitable economic and educational opportunity or for the easy victimization of females. It is equally true, however, that biomedical understanding can produce at least some of the solutions to human health problems that will persist in even the most equitable societal settings for a very long time.

REFERENCES

Aaby, P. 1992. Influence of cross-sex transmission on measles mortality in rural Senegal. Lancet 340:388–391.

Adamchak D. J., A. O. Wilson, A. Nyanguru, and J. Hampson. 1991. Elderly support and intergenerational transfer in Zimbabwe: an analysis by gender, marital status, and place of residence. Gerontologist 31(4):505–513.

Agarwal, B., T. D. Bare, et al. 1990. Engendering Adjustment for the 1990s: Report of a Commonwealth Expert Group on Women and Structural Adjustment. London: Commonwealth Secretariat.

Aitchison, R. 1984. Reluctant witnesses: the sexual abuse of refugee women in Djibouti. Cult. Surv. Q. 8(2):26–27.

Akeroyd, A. V. 1990. Sociocultural aspects of AIDS in Africa: topics, methods and some lacunae. Paper presented at the Conference on AIDS in Africa and the Caribbean: The Documentation of an Epidemic, Columbia University, New York, 5 November 1990.

Alan Guttmacher Institute. 1995. Women, Families and the Future: Sexual Relationships and Marriage Worldwide. New York and Washington, D.C.: Fact Sheets.

Anand, S., and A. Sen. 1992. Human Development Index: methodology and measurement. Background paper for Human Development Report 1993. New York: United Nations Development Programme.

Anderson, R. 1991. The efficacy of ethnomedicine: research methods in trouble. Med. Anthropol. 13:1–17.

Arnold, F., and A. K. Blanc. 1990. Fertility trends and levels. Demographic and Health Surveys Comparative Studies 2: Fertility. Columbia, Md.: Institute for Resource Development.

Bantje, H. F. W. 1988. Female stress and birth seasonality in Tanzania. J. Biosoc. Sci. 20(2):195–202.

Barnes-Dean, V. L. 1985. Clitoridectomy and infibulation. Cult. Surv. Q. 9(2):26–30.

Bassett, M. T., and M. Mhloyi. 1991. Women and AIDS in Zimbabwe: the making of an epidemic. Intl. J. Hlth. Svcs. 21(1):143–156.

Bastien, J. W. 1992. Drum and Stethoscope. Salt Lake City: University of Utah Press.

Bastos dos Santos, R., E. M. Pereira Folgosa, and L. Fransen. 1992. Reproductive tract infections in Mozambique: a case study of integrated services. In Reproductive Tract Infections: Global Impact and Priorities for Women's Reproductive Health, A. Germain, K. K. Holmes, P. Piot, and J. N. Wasserheit, eds. New York: Plenum.

Beoku-Betts, J., and B. Ikubolajeh Logan. 1993. Developing science and technology in Sub-Saharan Africa: gender disparities in the education and employment processes. In Science in Africa: Women Leading from Strength. Washington, D.C.: American Association for the Advancement of Science.

Bhargava, A., and J. Yu. 1992. A longitudinal analysis of infant and child mortality rates in Africa and non-African developing countries. Background paper prepared for the Africa Health Study, Africa Technical Department, World Bank, Washington, D.C.

Blacker, J. G. C. 1991. Infant and child mortality: development, environment, and custom. In Disease and Mortality in Sub-Saharan Africa, R. G. Feachem and D. T. Jamison, eds. New York: Oxford University Press for the World Bank.

Blanc, A. K. 1991. Demographic and Health Surveys World Conference, August 5–7, 1991: Executive Summary. Columbia, Md.: Institute for Resource Development/Macro International.

Bledsoe, C. 1990. The politics of children: fosterage and the social management of fertility among the Mende of Sierra Leone. In Births and Power: Social Change and the Politics of Reproduction, W. P. Handwerker, ed. Boulder, Colo.: Westview.

Bledsoe, C., and B. Cohen, eds. 1993. The Social Dynamics of Adolescent Fertility in Sub-Saharan Africa. Washington, D.C.: National Academy Press.

Boddy, J. P. 1989. Wombs and Alien Spirits: Women, Men, and the Zar Cult in Northern Sudan. Madison.: University of Wisconsin Press.

Boerma, J. T., A. E. Sommerfelt, and S. O. Rutstein. 1991. Childhood morbidity and treatment patterns. Demographic and Health Surveys, Comparative Studies No. 4. Columbia, Md.: Institute for Resource Development/Macro International.

Bohannan, P. 1960. African Homicide and Suicide. Princeton, N.J.: Princeton University Press.

Bonair, A., P. Rosenfield, and K. Tengvald. 1989. Medical technologies in developing countries: issues of technology development, transfer, diffusion, and use. Soc. Sci. Med. 28:769–781.

Brass, W., and C. L. Jolly, eds. 1993. Population Dynamics of Kenya. Washington, D.C.: National Academy Press.

Bread for the World, Institute on Hunger and Development. 1992. Hunger 1993—Uprooted People, Third Annual Report on the State of World Hunger, Washington, D.C.

Brown, R. C., J. E. Brown, and O. B. Ayowa. 1992. Vaginal inflammation in Africa. N. Engl. J. Med. Aug. 20, 1992:572.

Brunham, R. C., and J. E. Embree. 1992. Sexually transmitted diseases: current and future dimensions of the problem in the Third World. In Reproductive Tract Infections: Global Impact and Priorities for Women's Reproductive Health, A. Germain, K. K. Holmes, P. Piot, and J. N. Wasserheit, eds. New York: Plenum.

Caldwell, J. C., and P. Caldwell. 1990. High fertility in Sub-Saharan Africa. Sci. Am. May 1990: 118–125.

Caldwell, J. C., and P. Caldwell. 1993. Roles of women, families, and communities in preventing illness and providing health services in developing countries. In The Epidemiological Transition: Policy and Planning Implications for Developing Countries. Washington, D.C.: National Research Council.

Caldwell, J., S. Findley, P. Caldwell, G. Santow, et al., eds. 1990. What We Know about Health Transition: The Cultural, Social, and Behavioural Determinants of Health. Health Transition Series, Vol. I. Canberra: Australian National University.

Caplan, P. 1989. Perceptions of gender stratification. Africa 59(2):196–208.

Carovano, K. 1991. More than mothers and whores: redefining the AIDS prevention needs of women. Intl. J. Hlth. Svcs. 21(1):131–142.

Castle, S. E. 1995. Child fostering and children's nutritional outcomes in rural Mali: the role of female status in directing child transfers. Soc. Sci. Med. 40(5):679–693.

Chavundaka, G.L. 1984. The Zimbabwe National Traditional Healers Association (ZINANTHA). Harare.

Christian Medical Commission. 1984. Women and health: women's health is more than a medical issue. Contact, Issue 80. Geneva: World Council of Churches.

Clark, G. 1992. Flexibility equals survival. Cult. Surv. Q. 16(4):21–24.

Cleland, J. 1990. Maternal education and child survival: further evidence and explanations. In What We Know about Health Transition: The Cultural, Social, and Behavioural Determinants of Health, J. Caldwell, S. Findley, P. Caldwell, et al., eds. Health Transition Series, Vol. I. Canberra: Australian National University.

Cleland, J., and J. K. van Ginneken. 1988. Maternal education and child survival in developing countries: the search for pathways of influence. Soc. Sci. Med. 27(12):1357–1368.

Cliff, J. 1991. The war on women in Mozambique—health consequences of South African destabilization, economic crisis, and structural adjustment. In Women and Health in Africa, M. Turshen, ed. Trenton, N.J.: Africa World Press.

Cohen, B. 1993. Fertility levels, differentials, and trends. In Demographic Change in Sub-Saharan Africa, K. A. Foote, K. H. Hill, and L. G. Martin, eds. Washington, D.C.: National Academy Press.

Cole, E., O. M. Espin, and E. D. Rothblum, eds. 1992. Refugee Women and Their Mental Health: Shattered Societies, Shattered Lives. New York: Harrington Park.

Coles, C., and B. Mack. 1991. Hausa Women in the Twentieth Century. Madison: University of Wisconsin Press.

Constantinides, P. 1979. Women's spirit possession and urban adaptation in the Muslim northern Sudan. In Women United, Women Divided, A. P. Caplan and J. Bujra, eds. Bloomington: Indiana University Press.

Cornia, A., R. Jolly, and F. Stewart. 1987. Adjustment with a Human Face. Oxford, U.K.: Clarendon.

Cosminsky, S. 1983. Medical pluralism in Mesoamerica. In Heritage of Conquest, Thirty Years Later, C. Kendall, J. Hawkins, and L. Bossen, eds. Albuquerque: University of New Mexico Press.

Counts, D. A. 1987. Female suicide and wife abuse: a cross-cultural perspective. Suicide and Life-Threatening Behavior 17(3):194–204.

Cutner, L. P. 1985. Female genital mutilation. Obstet. Gynecol. Sur. 40:7.

Dagnew, M. B. 1984. Patterns of health care utilisation in a small rural Ethiopian town. Ethiopian Med. J. 22:173–177.

Danquah, S. A. 1978. Some aspects of mental health of Ghanaian women: female psychoneuroses and social problems. Paper presented at Women in Development Seminar, Trinity College, Legon, Ghana.

Davies, W. 1985. Slow progress on women's health. New Afr. 215:42

Dodge, C. P. 1990. Health implications of war in Uganda and Sudan. Soc. Sci. Med. 31(6):691–698.

Dubos, R. 1965. Man Adapting. New Haven, Conn.: Yale University Press.

Ekwempu, C. C., D. Maine, M. B. Olorukoba, E. S. Essien, and M. N. Kisseka. 1990. Structural adjustment and health in Africa (letter). Lancet 336(8706): 56–57.

El Dareer, A. 1982. Women, Why Do You Weep? London: Zed.

Elo, T. I. 1992. Utilization of maternal health-care services in Peru: the role of women's education. Hlth. Trans. Rev. 2(1): 49–69.

Elson, D. 1987. The Impact of Structural Adjustment on Women: Concepts and Issues. IFAA 1987 Conference on the Impact of IMF and World Bank Policies on the People of Africa, London.

Falola, T., and D. Ityavyar, eds. 1992. The Political Economy of Health in Africa. Ohio University Center for International Studies, Monographs in International Studies, Africa Series #60. Athens.

Feachem, R. G., and D. T. Jamison, eds. 1991. Disease and Mortality in Sub-Saharan Africa. New York: Oxford University Press for the World Bank.

Feierman, S., and J. M. Janzen, eds. 1992. The Social Basis of Health and Healing in Africa. Berkeley: University of California Press.

Ferguson, A. 1986. Women's health in a marginal area of Kenya. Soc. Sci. Med. 23(1):17–29.

Ferguson, A. 1988. Schoolgirl Pregnancy in Kenya. Nairobi: Ministry of Health, Division of Family Planning.

Finkler, K. 1994. Sacred health and biomedicine compared. Med. Anthr. Q. 8(2):178–197.

Forbes-Martin, S. F. 1991. Refugee Women. London: Zed.

Fosu, G. B. 1981. Disease classification in rural Ghana: framework and implications for health behavior. Soc. Sci. Med. 15B:471–482.

Gaisie, S. 1990. Culture and health in Sub-Saharan Africa. Pp. 609–627 in What We Know about Health Transition: The Cultural, Social, and Behavioural Determinants of Health, J. Caldwell, S. Findley, et al., eds. Proceedings of an International Workshop, Canberra, May 1989, Vol. II. Canberra: Australian National University.

Gellhorn, A. 1984. National security and the health of people: human needs and the allocation of scarce resources. Soc. Sci. Med. 19:307–332.

Gilson, L. 1995. Management and health care reform in Sub-Saharan Africa. Soc. Sci. Med. 40(5):695–710.

Good, B. 1993. Medicine, Rationality and Experience: An Anthropological Perspective. New York: Cambridge University Press.

Goody, E. N. 1982. Parenthood and Social Reproduction: Fostering and Occupational Roles in West Africa. New York: Cambridge University Press.

Goody, J. 1973. Polygyny, economy, and the role of women. In The Character of Kinship, J. Goody, ed. New York: Cambridge University Press.

Goody, J. 1976. Production and Reproduction—A Comparative Study of the Domestic Domain. New York: Cambridge University Press.

Gordon, D. 1991. Female circumcision and genital operations in Egypt and the Sudan: A dilemma for medical anthropology. Med. Anthr. Q. 5(1):3–28.

Graham, W. J. 1991. Maternal mortality: levels, trends, and data deficiencies. In Disease and Mortality in Sub-Saharan Africa, R. G. Feachem and D. T. Jamison, eds. Washington, D.C.: Oxford University Press for the World Bank.

Gregson, S., G. Garnett, R. Shakespeare, G. Foster, and R. Anderson. 1994. Determinants of the demographic impact of HIV-1 in Sub-Saharan Africa: the effect of a shorter mean adult incubation period on trends in orphanhood. In Health Transition Review: AIDS Impact and Prevention in the Developing World: Demographic and Social Science Perspectives, Supplement to Vol. 4. Canberra: Australian National University.

Harrison, K. A. 1983. Obstetric fistula: one social calamity too many (commentary). Brit. J. Ob. Gyn. 90: 385–386.

Harrison, K. A. 1986. Literacy, parity, family planning and maternal mortality in the Third World. Lancet 2(8511):865–866.

Heath, D. 1993. Beverage alcohol in developing regions. Paper prepared for the International Mental Health Policy Project, Department of Social Medicine, Harvard Medical School.

Heggenhougen, H. K. 1991. Perceptions of health-care options and therapy-seeking behaviour. In The Health Transition, Methods and Measures, J. Cleland and A. Hill, eds. Proceedings of an International Workshop, London, June 1989. Canberra: Health Transition Centre, The Australian National University.

Heggenhougen, H. K. 1992. The interlocking web of development, environment and health. In Health and Environment in Developing Countries, A. Manu, ed. Oslo: Centre for Development and Environment, University of Oslo Press.

Heggenhougen, H. K., and L. Gilson. In press. Perceptions of efficacy and the use of traditional medicine, with examples from Tanzania. In Medicine and Social Criticism: A Festschrift for Charles Leslie, F. Zimmerman and B. Pfleiderer, eds. Berkeley: University of California Press.

Heggenhougen, H. K., and P. Sesia-Lewis. 1988. Traditional Medicine and Primary Health Care: An Introduction and Selected Annotated Bibliography. London: London School of Hygiene and Tropical Medicine.

Heise, L. 1993. Violence against women: The missing agenda. In The Health of Women: A Global Perspective, M. A. Koblinsky et al., eds. Boulder, Colo.: Westview.

Heise, L., J. Pitanguy, and A. Germain. 1994. Violence against Women: The Hidden Health Burden. World Bank Discussion Paper 255. Washington, D.C.: World Bank.

Henn, J. 1984. Women in the rural economy: past, present, and future. In African Women South of the Sahara, M. Hay and S. Stichter, eds. London: Longman.

Hobcraft, J. N. 1993. Women's education, child welfare, and child survival: a review of the evidence. Health Trans. Rev. 3(2).

Hosken, F. P. 1992. The Hosken Report: Genital and Sexual Mutilation of Females. WIN News 18(4).

Ifeka, C. 1982. The self viewed from "within" or "without": twists and turns in gender identity in a patrilineal society. Mankind 13(5):401–415.

Inter-African Committee (IAC) on Traditional Practices Affecting the Health of Women and Children (Addis Ababa). 1992. Editorial. IAC Newsletter 13:1.

IOM (Institute of Medicine). 1988. The Future of Public Health. Washington, D.C.: National Academy Press.

Isiugo-Abanihe, U. 1985. Child fosterage in West Africa. Population and Development Review 11:53–73.

Ityavyar, D. A. and L. O. Ogba. 1989. Violence, conflict and health in Africa. Soc. Sci. Med. 28(7):649–657.

Janzen, J. 1978. The Quest for Therapy in Lower Zaire. Berkeley: University of California Press.

Jeffreys, M. D. W. 1952. Samsonic suicide or suicide of revenge among Africans. Afr. Stud. 11:118–122.

Kabeer, N., and A. Raikes. 1992. Gender and health: an introduction. In Gender and Primary Health Care: Some Forward-Looking Strategies, A. Raikes and N. Kabeer, eds. IDS Bull. 23(1).

Kandrack, M. A., K. R. Grant, and A. Segal. 1991. Gender differences in health-related behaviour: some unanswered questions, Soc. Sci. Med. 32(5):579–590.

Kanji, N. 1989. Charging for drugs in Africa: UNICEF's Bamako Initiative. Hlth. Pol. Plan. 4(2):110–120.

Kennedy, E. 1992. Effects of gender of head of household on women's and children's nutritional status. Paper presented at workshop on Effects of Policy and Programs on Women, January 16, International Food Policy Research Institute, Washington, D.C.

Kennedy, E. T., and B. Cogill, 1987. Income and nutritional effects of the commercialization of agriculture in Southwestern Kenya: Research Report 63. Washington, D.C.: International Food Policy Research Institute.

Kennedy, J. G. 1967. Nubian zar ceremonies as psychotherapy. Human Organization 26:185–194.

Kheir, E. H. 1991. Female Circumcision: Attitudes and Practices in Sudan. Paper presented at the Demographic and Health Surveys World Conference, Washington, D.C.

Kisekka, M. N. 1990. Gender and mental health in Africa. Women and Therapy 10(3):1-13.

Kloos, H., E. Etea, A. Degefa, H. Aga, et al. 1987. Illness and health behavior in Addis Ababa and rural central Ethiopia. Soc. Sci. Med. 25(9):1003–1019.

Koblinsky, M. A., O. M. R. Campbell, and S. D. Harlow. 1993. Mother and more: a broader perspective on women's health. Women's Health: A Global Perspective, M. J. Koblinsky, J. Timyan, and J. Gay, eds. Boulder, Colo.: Westview.

Koblinsky, M. J., J. Timyan, and Y. J. Gay, eds. 1993. Women's Health: A Global Perspective. Boulder, Colo.: Westview.

Kouba, L., and Muasher, J. 1985. Female circumcision in Africa: An overview. African Studies Rev. 28(1):95–110.

Krieger, N., and G. Margo. 1991. Women and AIDS: introduction: Intl. J. Hlth. Serv. 21(1):127–130.

Kruks, S., and B. Wisner. 1984. The state, the party and the female peasantry in Mozambique. J. S. Afr. Stud. 1 (11):106–127.

Kuoch, T., S. Wali, and M. F. Scully. 1992. Foreword. In Refugee Women and Their Mental Health—Shattered Societies, Shattered Lives, E. Cole, O. M. Espin, and E. D. Rothblum, eds. New York: Harrington Park.

Kwast, B., R. W. Rochat, and W. Kidane-Mariam. 1986. Maternal mortality in Addis Ababa, Ethiopia. Stud. Fam. Plan. 17(6):288–301.

Lado, C., 1992. Female labour participation in agricultural production and the implications for nutrition and health in rural Africa. Soc. Sci. Med., 34(7):789–807.

Last, M. 1979. Strategies against time. Sociology of Health and Sickness: A Journal of Medical Sociology 1:306–317.

Leslie, J. 1992. Women's lives and women's health: using social science research to promote better health for women. J. Women's Hlth. 1(4):307–318.

Leslie, J., and G. R. Gupta. 1989. Utilization of Formal Services for Maternal Nutrition and Health Care in the Third World. Washington, D.C.: International Center for Research on Women.

Lesthaeghe, R. J., ed. 1989. Reproduction and Social Organization in Sub-Saharan Africa. Berkeley: University of California Press.

Lesthaeghe, R. J., C. Verleye, and C. Jolly. 1992. Female education and factors affecting fertility in Sub-Saharan Africa. IPD-Working Paper 1992-2. Belgium: Interuniversity Programme in Demography.

Levinson, D. 1989. Violence in Cross-Cultural Perspective. Newbury Park, Calif.: Sage.

Lewis, I. M. 1971. Ecstatic Religion: An Anthropological Study of Spirit Possession and Shamanism. Middlesex: Penguin.

Lightfoot-Klein, H. 1989. Prisoners of Ritual: An Odyssey into Female Genital Circumcision in Africa. New York: Harrington Park Press.

Lloyd, C., and A. Brandon. 1991. Children's living arrangements in developing countries. Working Paper No. 31. New York: Population Council.

Loewenson, R., D. Sanders, and R. Davies. 1991. Challenges to equity in health and health care: a Zimbabwean case study. Soc. Sci. Med. 32(1079).

Logan, M. H. 1977. Anthropological research on the hot-cold theory of disease: some methodological suggestions. Med. Anthr. 1(4):87–112.

MacCormack, C. P. 1989. Health and the social power of women. Soc. Sci. Med. 26(7):677–683.

Mair, L., 1980. Women, health and development. World Health, June:3–5.

Malik, M. O., and O. A. Sawi. 1976. A profile of homicide in the Sudan. Forensic Sci.

Malterud, K. 1987. Illness and disease in female patients. Scand. J. PHC 5:204–216.

Manderson, L., and P. Aaby. 1992. Can rapid anthropological procedures be applied to tropical diseases? Hlth. Pol. Plan. 7:46–55.

Mason, K. O. 1994. HIV transmission and the balance of power between women and men: a global view. In Health Transition Review: AIDS Impact and Prevention in the Developing World: Demographic and Social Science Perspectives, Supplement to Vol. 4. Canberra: Australian National University.

Mastroianni, A., R. Faden, and D. Federman, eds. 1994. Women and Health Research: Ethical and Legal Issues of Including Women in Clinical Studies, Vol. 1. Washington, D.C.: National Academy Press.

Mazrui, A. 1991. The black woman and the problem of gender. Weekly Review, 9 Aug.:16–18.

Mbacke, C. 1991. Sex differentials in health status and health care utilization in Mali. Paper presented at Demographic and Health Surveys World Conference, August 5–6, 1991, Washington, D.C. Columbia, Md.: IRD/Macro International.

Mburu, F. M. 1986. The African social periphery. Soc. Sci. Med. 22:785–790.

Mechanic, D. 1976. Sex, illness, illness behavior, and the use of health services. Soc. Sci. Med. 12B:207–214.

Mensch, B. 1993. Quality of care: a neglected dimension. In The Health of Women: A Global Perspective, M. Koblinsky, J. Timyan, and J. Gay, eds. Boulder, Colo.: Westview.

Mhango, C., et al. 1986. Reproductive mortality in Lusaka, Zambia, 1982–83. Stud. Fam. Plan. 17(5):243–251.

Michaelson, E. H. 1991. Adam's rib awry: women and schistosomiasis. In Women and Tropical Diseases, P. Wijeyaratne, E. M. Rathgeber, and E. St. Onge, eds. Ottawa: IDRC.

Moses, S., F. Manji, J. E. Bradley, N. J. Nagelkerke, M. A. Malisa, and F. A. Plummer. 1992. Impact of user fees on attendance at a referral centre for sexually transmitted diseases in Kenya. Lancet 340:463–466.

Mukhopadhyay, C. C., and P. J. Higgins. 1988. Anthropological studies of women's status revisited: 1977-1987. Ann. Rev. Anthr. 17:461–495.

Murray. C. J., A. D. Lopez, and D. T. Jamison. 1994. The global burden of disease in 1990: Summary results, sensitivity analysis, and future directions. Bull. WHO 72(3):495–509.

NRC (National Research Council). 1993a. Economic Reversals in Sub-Saharan Africa. Washington, D.C.: National Academy Press.

NRC (National Research Council). 1993b. Factors Affecting Contraceptive Use in Sub-Saharan Africa. Washington, D.C.: National Academy Press.

Ngaiza, M. K., and B. Koda, eds. 1991. The Unsung Heroines—Women's Life Histories from Tanzania. Dar es Salaam: WRDP.

Ngubane, H. 1987. The consequences for women of marriage payments in a society with patrilineal descent. In Transformation of African Marriage, D. Parkin and D. Nyamwaya, eds. Manchester: Manchester University Press for the International African Institute.

Nigerian Federal Office of Statistics and Institute for Resource Development. 1992. Nigeria Demographic and Health Survey 1990. Lagos, Nigeria: Federal Office of Statistics; Columbia, Md.: Institute for Resource Development/Macro International.

Obbo, C. 1980. African Women: Their Struggle for Economic Independence. London: Zed.

Obbo, C. 1987. The old and the new in East African elite marriages. In Transformation of African Marriage, D. Parkin and D. Nyamwaya, eds. Manchester: Manchester University Press for the International African Institute.

Ogba, L. O. 1989. Violence and health in Nigeria. Hlth Pol. Plan. 4:82–84.

Oppong, C., ed. 1983. Female and Male in West Africa. London: Allen and Unwin.

Osaki, L. T. 1990. Siti binti Saad: herald of women's liberation. SAGE 7(1):49–54.

Osuala, J. D. C. 1990. Nigerian women's quest for role fulfillment. Women and Therapy 10(3):89–98.

Panos Institute. 1990. Triple Jeopardy: Women and AIDS. London: Panos.

Peacock, N. 1984. The Mbuti of Northeast Zaire: women and subsistence exchange. Cult. Surv. Q. 8(2):15–18.

Pittin, R. I. 1983. Houses of women: a focus on alternative life-styles in Katsina City. In Female and Male in West Africa, C. Oppong, ed. London: Allen and Unwin.

Plitcha, S. 1992. The effects of woman abuse on health care utilization and health status: a literature review. Women's Health (Jacobs Institute of Women's Health) 2(3): 154–161.

Potash, B., ed. 1986. Widows in African Societies. Stanford, Calif: Stanford University Press.

Prevention of Maternal Mortality Network. 1995. Situation analyses of emergency obstetric care: examples from eleven operations research projects in West Africa. Soc. Sci. Med. 40(5):657–667.

Raikes, A. 1989. Women's health in East Africa. Soc. Sci. Med. 28(5):447–459.

Ramalingaswami, V. 1986. The art of the possible. Soc. Sci. Med. 22:1097–1103.

Ramji, S. 1987. Growing Old in Mozambique Under Fire: A Study of Displaced Mozambican Elderly Living in Mozambique and Zimbabwe. Maputo:Help the Aged.

Ramphele, M. 1990. Women and rural development: the debate about appropriate strategies. SAGE 7(1):9–12.

Ramphele, M. 1991. Empowerment and the politics of space. In Women Transforming Societies: Sub-Saharan Africa and Caribbean Perspectives, M. Ramphele, E. Okeke, and V. Anderson-Manley, eds. Cambridge, Mass.: Radcliffe College.

Rashed, A. H. 1992. The fast of Ramadan. Brit. Med. J. 304(6830):521–522.

Reinhardt, U. E. 1991. Health manpower forecasting: the case of physician supply. In Health Services Research: Key to Health Policy, E. Ginzberg, ed. Cambridge, Mass.: Harvard University Press.

Rodin, J., and J. R. Ickovics. 1990. Women's health: review and research agenda as we approach the 21st century. Am. Psychol. 45:1018.

Rodney, W. 1972. How Europe Underdeveloped Africa. London: Bogle-L'Ouverture.

Rodriguez-Trias, H. 1992. Editorial: women's health, women's lives, women's rights. Am. J. Pub. Hlth. 82(5):663–664.

Rosenfield, A., and D. Maine. 1985. Maternal mortality—a neglected tragedy: Where is the M in MCH? Lancet 2(8446):83–85.

Royston, E., and S. Armstrong, eds. 1989. Preventing Maternal Deaths. Geneva: WHO.

Rushwan, H. 1990. Female circumcision. World Health (April/May).

Russel, D. 1991. Rape and child sexual abuse in Soweto: An interview with community leader Mary Mabaso. Seminar presented at the Centre for African Studies, University of Cape Town, South Africa, March 26.

Rutabanzibwa-Ngaiza, K. Heggenhougen, and J. G. Walt. 1985. Women and Health in Africa. Evaluation and Planning Centre Publication 6. London: EPC/London School of Hygiene and Tropical Medicine.

Rutenberg, N., A. K. Blanc, and S. Kapiga. 1994. Sexual behaviour, social change, and family planning among men and women in Tanzania. In Health Transition Review: AIDS Impact and Prevention in the Developing World: Demographic and Social Science Perspectives, Supplement to Vol. 4. Canberra: Australian National University.

Sacks, K. 1982. Overview of women and power in Africa. In Perspectives on Power: Women in Africa, Asia, and Latin America, J. F. O'Barr, ed. Duke University Center for International Studies Occasional Paper 13. Durham, N.C.

Sai, F. T. 1986. Family planning and maternal health care: A common goal. World Health Forum 7(4).

Sai, F. T., and J. Nassim. 1991. Mortality in Sub-Saharan Africa: an overview. In Disease and Mortality in Sub-Saharan Africa, R. G. Feachem and D. T. Jamison, eds. New York: Oxford University Press for the World Bank.

Schildkrout, E. 1984. Schooling or seclusion: choices for northern Nigerian women. Cult. Surv. Q. 8(2):46–48.

Schoepf, B. G. 1987. Social structure, women's status and sex differentials in nutrition in the Zairian copper belt. Urban Anthr. 16(1):73–102.

Sen, A. 1993. The economics of life and death. Sci. Am. 268(5):40–47.

Shipton, P. 1990. African famines and food security: anthropological perspectives. Ann. Rev. Anthr. 19:353–394.

Sicoli, F. 1980. Women in rural development: recommendations and realities. CERES 75:15–22.

Soejarto, D. D., A. S. Bingel, M. Slaytor, and N. R. Farnsworth. 1978. Fertility regulating agents from plants. Bull. WHO 56(3):343–352.

SOMANET. 1992. Proceedings of the African Regional Social Sciences and Medical Meeting, Nairobi, Kenya, August 10–14, 1992.

Staudt, K. A. 1981. Women's politics in Africa. In Women and Politics in Twentieth-Century Africa and Asia. Studies in Third World Societies 16:1–28.

Strauss, J., P. Gertler, O. Rahman, and K. Fox. 1992. Gender and life-cycle differentials in the patterns and determinants of adult health. Prepared for the Government of Jamaica. Santa Monica, Calif.: RAND.

Tambiah, S. J. 1989. Bridewealth and dowry revisited: The position of women in Sub-Saharan Africa and North India. Curr. Anthr. 30(4):413–435.

Tahzib, F. 1983. Epidemiological determinants of vesicovaginal fistulas. Br. J. Obstet. Gynaecol. 90:387–391.

Thaddeus, S., and D. Maine. 1990. Too Far to Walk: Maternal Mortality in Context. New York: Columbia University Center for Population and Family Health.

Timaeus, I. M. 1991. Adult mortality. In Demographic Change in Sub-Saharan Africa, K. A. Foote, K. H. Hill, and L. G. Martin, eds. Washington, D.C.: Oxford University Press.

Toubhia, N. 1993. Female Circumcision. A Call for Global Action. New York: Women, Ink.

Turshen, M. 1983. The study of women, food and health in Africa. In Third World Medicine and Social Change, J. H. Morgan, ed. Lanham, Md.: University Press of America.

Turshen, M., ed. 1991. Women and Health in Africa. Trenton, N.J.: Africa World Press.

Turton, D. 1988. Anthropology and development. In Perspectives on Development: Cross-disciplinary Themes in Development Studies, P. L. Lesson and M. M. Minogue, eds. Manchester, U.K.: Manchester University Press.

Ubot, S. S. 1992. Social science and medicine in Africa. The Political Economy of Health in Africa, T. Falola and D. Ityavyar, eds. Athens: Ohio University Press.

UNICEF (United Nations Children's Fund). 1989. Children on the Frontline. The Impact of Apartheid, Destablization and Warfare on Children in Southern and South Africa. New York.

UNICEF (United Nations Children's Fund). 1992. The State of the World's Children. New York: Oxford University Press.

UNICEF, WHO, and the World Bank. 1987. La Contribution de la Planification Familiale à l'Amélioration de la Santé des Femmes et des Enfants. Report of a conference held in Nairobi, Kenya.

UNDP (United Nations Development Programme). 1990. Human Development Report 1990. New York: Oxford University Press.

UNDP (United Nations Development Programme). 1991. Human Development Report 1991. New York: Oxford University Press.

UNDP (United Nations Development Programme). 1992. Human Development Report 1992. New York: Oxford University Press.

UNDP (United Nations Development Programme). 1993. Human Development Report 1993. New York: Oxford University Press.

UNDP (United Nations Development Programme). 1994. Human Development Report 1994. New York: Oxford University Press.

van der Kwaak, A., et al. 1991. Women and health. Vena J. 3(1):2-33.

van Ginneken, J. K., and A. S. Muller, eds. 1984. Maternal and Child Health in Rural Kenya: An Epidemiological Study. London: Croom Helm.

Vaughan, M. 1991. Curing Their Ills—Colonial Power and African Illness. Stanford, Calif.: Stanford University Press.

Vlassoff, C., and E. Bonilla. 1994. Gender-related differences in the impact of tropical diseases on women: what do we know? J. Biosoc. Sci. 26:37–53.

Vogelman, L. 1990. Violent crime: rape. In People and Violence in South Africa, B. McKendrick and W. Hoffman, eds. Cape Town: Oxford University Press.

Walker, A., and P. Parmar. 1993. Warrior Marks: Female Genital Mutilation and the Sexual Blinding of Women. New York: Harcourt Brace.

Ware, N. C., N. A. Christakis, and A. Kleinman. 1992. An anthropological approach to social science research and the health transition. In Advancing Health in Developing Countries: The Role of Social Research, L. C. Chen, A. Kleinman, and N. C. Ware, eds. New York: Auburn House.

Weekly Review. 1991. Sexism in Kenya. August 9:4–7.

Werner, D. 1989. Health for no one by the year 2000: the high cost of placing "national security" before global justice. Paper for the International Health Conference, National Council on International Health, Arlington, Virginia, June 1989.

Williams, B. 1993. Female Circumcision in Sub-Saharan Africa. Photocopy.

Winkvist, A., K. M. Rasmussen, and J. P. Habicht. 1992. A new definition of maternal depletion syndrome. Am. J. Pub. Hlth. 82(5):691–694.

World Bank. 1989. Sub-Saharan Africa: From Crisis to Sustainable Growth. Washington, D.C.

World Bank. 1993. World Development Report 1993: Investing in Health. New York: Oxford University Press.

World Bank. 1994a. Better Health in Africa: Experience and Lessons Learned. Washington, D.C.

World Bank. 1994b. Adjustment in Africa: Reforms, Results, and the Road Ahead. New York: Oxford University Press.

WHO (World Health Organization). 1982. The extension of health services coverage with traditional birth attendants: a decade of progress. WHO Chronicle 36(3):92–96.

WHO (World Health Organization). 1983. Apartheid and Health. Geneva.

WHO (World Health Organization). 1984. Apartheid and Mental Health. Geneva.

WHO (World Health Organization). 1985. Maternal Mortality Rates: A Tabulation of Available Information. Geneva.

WHO (World Health Organization). 1991. Maternal Mortality: A Global Factbook. Geneva.

WHO (World Health Organization). 1992. Women's Health: Across Age and Frontier. Geneva.

WHO/UNICEF. 1978. Alma Ata 1978: Primary Health Care, Health for All, Series 1. Geneva.

Whyte, S. R., and P. W Kariuki. 1991. Malnutrition and gender relations in Western Kenya. Hlth. Trans. Rev. 1(2):171–187.

Yoder, R. A. 1989. Are people willing and able to pay for health services? Soc. Sci. Med. 29(1):35–42.

Zimicki, S. 1989. The relationship between fertility and maternal mortality. In Contraceptive Use and Controlled Fertility: Health Issues for Women and Children (Background Papers). Washington, D.C.: National Research Council.

3

Nutritional Status

As in most developing countries, the nutritional status of girls and women in Sub-Saharan Africa is compromised by the cumulative and synergistic effects of many risk factors, including limited availability of, or access to, food resources because of natural and human-made disasters; lack of control over inputs and resource allocations at the household level; traditional feeding practices and other customs that limit women's consumption of certain energy- and nutrient-rich foods; the energy demands of heavy physical labor; the nutritional demands of frequent cycles of pregnancy and lactation; a high burden of infections; and limited access to preventive or curative care.

Available data on nutrition in Sub-Saharan Africa emphasize preschool children and women of reproductive age. Thus, our analysis, despite its emphasis on a life span perspective, is limited by the scarcity of reliable data on the female population outside these age groups. In addition, only rarely are the available data nationally representative or comparable over time. The hope in this chapter, as in other chapters of this volume, is that a first attempt to assemble much of what is known about the nutritional situation of women and girls in Sub-Saharan Africa will lead to interim recommendations that may be useful to policymakers and program planners. Even more important, it is hoped that this review will suggest hypotheses and stimulate interest in conducting multidisciplinary, applied research concerning the extent, causes, and consequences of nutrition-related problems among Sub-Saharan African females throughout their life span. The committee also hopes that such research will provide a stronger foundation for the design of appropriate, cost-effective interventions to improve the nutrition and health situation of women and girls in the region.

This chapter begins with an analysis of some of the major determinants of the nutritional status of females in Sub-Saharan Africa, focusing particularly on household and individual factors that determine energy intake and expenditure. The reader is also referred to Chapter 2 for a discussion of macro-level factors that affect nutrition. The chapter then summarizes available data on the extent and types of malnutrition that affect females in Sub-Saharan Africa, including a section assessing the extent of gender differences. The chapter pays particular attention to conditions that burden females disproportionately; these are listed in Table 3-1. Protein-energy malnutrition (PEM) is discussed in light of the increased nutritional demands of pregnancy and the increased risks that pregnancy and childbirth impose on a woman who is stunted as a result of PEM. The chapter also gives careful consideration to two deficiency disorders—iron-deficiency anemia and iodine-deficiency disorders—that occur more commonly in females than in males. The third section of the chapter uses a life span perspective to examine the functional consequences of malnutrition among Sub-Saharan African females. The chapter concludes with some preliminary research recommendations.

TABLE 3-1 Nutritional Disorders Adversely Influencing Health in Sub-Saharan Africa: Gender-Related Burden

Disorder	Exclusive to Females	Greater for Females than for Males	Burden for Females and Males Comparable, but of Particular Significance for Females
Iodine deficiency (goiter)		X	
Iron-deficiency anemia		X	
Protein-energy malnutrition		X	

NOTE: Significance defined here as having impact on health that, for any reason—biological, reproductive, sociocultural, or economic—is different in its implications for females than for males.

WOMEN'S ROLES AND FEMALE NUTRITIONAL STATUS IN SUB-SAHARAN AFRICA

Crucial conflicts face poor women in low-income countries as they try to fulfill their economic, biological and social roles at each stage in the life cycle, particularly during the childbearing years. Changes in behavior that enhance their contribution to one area can have crucial negative effects on their other roles and activities. This role conflict relates to the tremendous time, energy, and money-resource constraints facing these women. . . . Conflicts between the economic, reproductive, and cultural roles of women can have detrimental effects on their nutrition and/or that of their families. (McGuire and Popkin, 1989, p. 53)

Standard models of determinants of the nutritional status of both children and women include quality and quantity of dietary intake, presence of infection, and energy expenditure as proximate determinants, which are themselves seen to be determined by a range of household, community, national, and global variables related to wealth, food production, education, and availability of health services, among other matters (see Kennedy et al., 1992; Leslie, 1991; Merchant and Kurz, 1993). In this first section, we focus on the implications of three interrelated variables that are particularly significant determinants of the nutritional status of Sub-Saharan African women and, indirectly, of the nutritional status of their children. These include women's central role as food producers, their high fertility, and their high level of energy expenditure, which is, in part, a consequence of the first two variables.

Effects of Household Food Production and Acquisition Strategies on the Nutritional Status of Women and Children

Women's agricultural labor in Sub-Saharan Africa is extremely important, both as a percentage of total agricultural labor and as a percentage of women's total labor force participation. Almost 80 percent of economically active women in Sub-Saharan Africa are working in agriculture (UN, 1991). Throughout most of the region, not only do women put in longer workdays overall than men (Juster and Stafford, 1991; Leslie, 1989), but women also spend more hours a week in agricultural work (McGuire and Popkin, 1989; UN, 1991). Women's responsibility is at least equal to that of men in determining the quantity of food available at the household level, and it is significantly greater in determining the variety and palatability of the household diet (Holmboe-Ottesen et al., 1989).

Findings from a study in Malawi of the gender division in agricultural decision making are reasonably representative for the region as a whole (Lamba and Tucker, 1990). The study found that husbands make most of the decisions regarding major farm inputs and have almost complete control over decisions concerning cash-crop production. Women have significant input into decisions regarding the production of food crops and full responsibility for decisions about the cultivation of selected vegetables—such as pumpkins and beans—that are used in food preparation. With respect to the use of income, men appeared to have control over formal, more regular sources of income (for example, income from the sale of cash crops or from employment), while women tended to manage the income from the sale of beer, fruits, or cooked food items. In Sub-Saharan Africa, women's dominant role in both subsistence food production and food preparation may give them more control over their own and their children's dietary consumption than women in some other regions of the world, but this control comes at the cost of extremely long and energy-demanding workdays (Bleiberg et al., 1980; Holmboe-Ottesen et al., 1989).

Subsistence agriculture remains the basis of food consumption patterns throughout most of rural Africa, which leaves the populations vulnerable to famine when crop failures caused by natural disasters are compounded by inadequate government response (see Chapter 2). At the same time, however, traditional food production and security strategies are rapidly evolving in the region because of population increases, deteriorating environmental conditions, and changing market circumstances, alterations that have led to significant urban migration and increased linkages between rural communities and major urban centers. This adaptation process has brought significant changes in food production patterns, the distribution and acquisition of food, and household food consumption. There is some evidence that gender asymmetries in access to productive resources have meant that women are less able to take advantage of agricultural intensification strategies (Dey, 1992).

Effects of Commercial Agriculture

Concerns have also been raised about the effects of agricultural intensification strategies on the health and nutritional well-being of women and children (Ferguson, 1986; Lado, 1992; Raikes, 1989). Some studies have suggested that expansion and intensification of commercial agriculture in Sub-Saharan Africa have contributed to gradual declines in food production levels and reductions in the amount of food available for household consumption. It has also been argued that women and children may be adversely affected by a shift to cash-cropping because of increased demands on women's labor for agricultural activities and reductions in women's individually earned income, and that children, in particular, may be adversely affected by earlier weaning and a reduced frequency of meals during the peak of the agricultural season. Conversely, it has been theorized that a shift to cash-cropping will ultimately produce higher household incomes that will lead to better household diets, and thus to improved nutritional status for all members of the household.

The most rigorous examination of the effects of cash-crop production on child health and nutrition comes from a comparative analysis of six methodologically similar studies carried out by researchers associated with the International Food Policy Research Institute, four of which were in countries of Sub-Saharan Africa (Kennedy et al., 1992)—The Gambia, Kenya, Malawi, and Rwanda—while the other two study sites were in Guatemala and the Philippines. Findings from the four African countries comparing child outcomes in households that participated in a cash-cropping scheme with otherwise similar, nonparticipating households found no evidence of a negative effect on child nutritional status from household participation in cash-cropping, but only very weak evidence of a positive effect. Comparison with the findings from the Guatemala study is illuminating: Guatemala was the only one of the six study sites where household participation in cash-cropping was significantly associated with better child health and nutrition outcomes, and this was attributed to the decision of the vegetable production and marketing cooperative to directly invest some of its profits in community health and social services.

A separate and earlier analysis of data from the same study in Kenya examined the effects of the commercialization of agriculture on allocation of time and patterns of food consumption by women, as well as on their nutritional status (Kennedy and Cogill, 1987). The central findings were that women from sugarcane-producing households did not spend more time away from home than women from non-sugarcane-producing households; there were no significant differences in the amount of time spent on the various household activities (the amount of time women spent on sugarcane production was negligible); and the mean weights of women from sugar- and non-sugar-producing households were similar. In sum, these studies suggest that agricultural intensification strategies do not necessarily affect child nutritional status adversely.

Seasonality

The seasonal patterns of the agricultural cycle in Sub-Saharan Africa impose different demands on women's energy expenditure throughout the year and have a significant influence on household food availability and women's energy intake and nutritional status. The periods of greatest nutritional stress for rural women usually occur during the preharvest period (generally known as the "soudure" or "lean" months), when household food stocks are low, the energy demands of agricultural work are highest, and energy intake is below normal levels (Bailey et al., 1992; Bleiberg et al., 1980; Holmboe-Ottesen et al., 1989; Lamba and Tucker, 1990; Loutan and Lamotte, 1984). When there are two or more poor harvests in a row, particularly in areas where there is only one rainy season annually, the lean period will not be limited to just one or two months, but may stretch throughout most of the year and can lead to true famine (see Chapter 2). In urban areas, periods of nutritional stress are more frequently linked to the market availability of basic food supplies and occur when market prices of basic food commodities are highest.

The effect of seasonality on women's nutritional status in Sub-Saharan Africa is particularly well illustrated by a study carried out in southern Benin on the effects of seasonal changes in food availability on women's nutritional status in both rural and periurban areas (Fakambi, 1990). Findings were reported for a sample of 567 nonpregnant (but lactating) women, of whom 366 lived in rural areas and 201 lived in a periurban setting. The study found significant nutritional status changes between what was defined as Phase I (November, the preharvest season) and Phase II (May–June, the postharvest season), as well as noteworthy differences in seasonal effect between rural and periurban settings. In rural areas, household food stocks were at their lowest during Phase I, because households had been forced to sell much of the produce from the big harvest (of June–July) because of inadequate household storage facilities to preserve food during the humid months. In contrast, most of the production from the second harvest (in December) could be stored during the subsequent dry season, thus ensuring adequate food supply between Phase I and Phase II. Twenty-five percent of the rural women gained more than two kilos between Phase I and Phase II, and average body mass index (BMI) also increased significantly during this period. In the periurban setting, the pattern was different. Phase I was characterized by relatively low food prices because of an excess supply of basic food commodities in the market. Between Phase I and Phase II, however, food prices began to rise, and periurban women were increasingly less able to buy adequate amounts of food. In contrast to the rural women, 25 percent of periurban women lost more than 2 kilos between Phase I and Phase II, and their BMI decreased, although the decrease was not statistically significant.

The Benin study indicates that the food security and nutritional consequences of seasonal changes in food availability can differ significantly between rural women, who depend mostly on food from their own production, and periurban women, who purchase a large proportion of their food. The findings of this study are significant in view of the growing integration of rural populations into national cash economies and the consequent increase in the number of families in both rural and urban areas who are not direct producers of food for home consumption.

Dietary Intake and Energy Expenditure of Pregnant and Lactating Women

With an average regional fertility rate of 6.5 in 1990, women in Sub-Saharan Africa experience significantly higher fertility than women in any other region of the world (World Bank, 1992b). Studies of food consumption during pregnancy and lactation in Sub-Saharan African countries indicate that macronutrient intakes are low, in the range of 1,400 to 2,000 kilocalories (Kcal) of energy and 25 to 50 grams of protein daily, while vitamin and mineral intakes are often extremely low as well (McGuire and Popkin, 1989; Prentice, 1980). Nevertheless, several detailed, country-specific studies suggest that when the energy cost of activity, reproduction, and lactation can be partially met by mobilization of maternal tissue stores, the impact of low energy intake on fetal growth and lactation performance is less than might be anticipated (Kusin et al., 1984; Lawrence et al., 1985, 1987a). Given that the energy demands of lactation are higher than those of pregnancy, however, it is essential to increase energy intake and/or reduce energy expenditure during breastfeeding in order to protect women's long-term nutritional status (Parker et al., 1990).

Kusin and colleagues (1984) analyzed cross-sectional data on food consumption in the Machakos area of Kenya among pregnant, nonpregnant, and lactating women over the period from October 1977 to December 1979, and found that the diets of pregnant women, and to a lesser extent lactating women, were inadequate when compared by the World Health Organization (WHO) with both the daily intakes it recommends, and the diets of nonpregnant, nonlactating women in the same population. Compared with the *WHO recommended daily intakes*, pregnant women received adequate amounts of protein, thiamin, and ascorbic acid, but their energy intakes were low, with median values ranging from 70 percent of recommended intake during the first trimester to 62 percent during the third trimester. An even larger deficit was recorded in the median calcium, iron, retinol equivalents, and riboflavin intakes of pregnant women. The authors could not explain clearly why food intake was reduced in the last trimester of pregnancy, but they suggested that cultural factors could be major determinants, because food availability was not a constraint in the region.

Similarly, the Machakos data indicated that the dietary intake of lactating women was found to be inadequate in energy and all nutrients except protein and ascorbic acid. The deficits noted were lower, however, than the deficits among pregnant women. The study found that mean weights remained the same during the first and second trimesters of pregnancy, and were only two kilos higher in the third trimester. The mean weight-for-height of lactating women at 15 to 24 months was slightly lower than the mean for women during the first year of lactation. Kusin and colleagues concluded from these findings that there was deterioration in the nutritional status of women as pregnancy and lactation progressed.

Studies of European and American women report significant increases in skinfold thickness at triceps and subscapular sites of the body between 10 and 20 weeks of pregnancy. Comparable analyses of changes in skinfold thickness at various stages of pregnancy in Africa are rare. A study of pregnant Nigerian women is one of the few published on the subject (Hussain and Akinyele, 1980). It provides an excellent analysis of the magnitude and patterns of subcutaneous fat deposition at triceps and subscapular sites in a group of "normal" pregnant Yoruba women living in low socioeconomic conditions in rural areas. All the women in the study had experienced multiple pregnancies, their mean age was 27 years, and, on the average, each woman had completed four pregnancies at the time of the study. Other anthropometric measurements collected on the women included arm circumference, weight, height, age, and parity number. In keeping with the findings from the Kenya study and other research from Sub-Saharan Africa, low weight gains during pregnancy were found; total mean weight gain between 20 and 30 weeks of pregnancy was 3.8 kilos, which was about half that reported for elite Nigerian women in Ibadan. The study also reported gradual declines in arm circumference, triceps, and subscapular skinfold thickness throughout pregnancy; the average total decline for the group was 4.1 millimeters. Thus, instead of showing the expected increase between 20 and 30 weeks of pregnancy, both individual and combined skinfold thickness at the triceps and subscapular sites among low-income pregnant Nigerian women declined. The authors interpret these declines as indicating a continuous depletion of energy stores during the course of pregnancy to compensate for inadequate dietary intake. In addition, the study found a negative correlation between parity and subscapular skinfold thickness, which was interpreted to mean that the ability of pregnant women to store body fat at the subscapular site decreased as parity increased.

There is mixed evidence concerning the extent to which women reduce energy expenditure to compensate for the increased energy demands of pregnancy or lactation. The majority of research has found little evidence of a change in activity patterns or energy expenditure during pregnancy or lactation by women in Sub-Saharan Africa or elsewhere in the developing world (IOM, 1992; Lamba and Tucker, 1990). Nevertheless, a recent detailed study of the functional consequences of malnutrition among the Embu in Kenya found that reduction in energy expenditure during the third trimester was a major mechanism used by pregnant women to achieve reasonable infant birthweights in the face of inadequate dietary intake (Neumann et al., 1992). Evidence of the contribution of energy-sparing mechanisms to partially meet the additional energy demands of pregnancy has also emerged from a series of studies of women in three rural Gambian villages.

Although expenditure of energy by pregnant women on activities with relatively low energy demands did not appear to change over the course of pregnancy, activities with higher energy demands were reduced during the second and third trimesters (Heini et al., 1991; Lawrence et al., 1987a; Lawrence and Whitehead, 1988). A similar finding of a reduction in energy-intensive activities in one, but not both, of the Zairian tribal groups studied is reported by Peacock (1992). Among Efe women, who are seminomadic foragers, the proportion of time spent in the most energy-intensive activities was reduced during pregnancy, and diminished further during lactation. No compensatory reduction in energy expenditure was found among the pregnant or lactating Lese women, who work as swidden cultivators.

The general problem of meeting the nutritional demands of pregnancy and lactation on top of the already substantial energy demands of a long and energy-demanding workday is particularly acute during seasonal periods of food shortage. This is well illustrated by research in The Gambia. Fifty women subsistence farmers were followed through pregnancy (during which some were provided with food supplements), and seasonal changes in basal metabolic rate (BMR), body fat, activity patterns, and total energy expenditure were assessed (Lawrence et al., 1987b). Seasonal variations in body fat content occurred in all women, whether pregnant or not, and pregnancy fat gain in individual women was found to be dependent upon the times of the year through which the pregnancy progressed. Seasonal fluctuations in body fat content of rural Gambian women were as large or larger than the changes resulting from pregnancy. Weight loss during the rainy season among unsupplemented, nonpregnant, nonlactating women averaged 5 kilos, most of which was adipose tissue. Among pregnant women, unsupplemented women who gave birth at the end of the rains (when agricultural activity was intense and food supplies were very low) lost 4.7 kilos of body fat, whereas those who were pregnant during the dry season (when little agricultural work was done and the food supplies increased) gained as much as 3 kilos of body fat. The interaction between seasonality and supplementation was highly significant. In supplemented women, neither weight nor fat gain during pregnancy varied as much with season as in the unsupplemented group. Overall, supplementation increased fat gain during pregnancy by about 2 kilos and gave some protection against seasonal weight loss. Lawrence and colleagues interpreted their combined findings concerning changes in BMR, fat deposition, and energy expenditure as demonstrating that maternal nutritional status is significantly compromised in rural Gambian women by pregnancy during the rainy season.

Given the marginal food availability in most of rural Sub-Saharan Africa and the need for women to continue with heavy physical work throughout most, if not all, of the time they are pregnant and lactating, the importance of ensuring an adequate interval to replenish maternal reserves of fat and other nutrients after the end of lactation and before the next pregnancy cannot be overemphasized. It is estimated, for example, that even when food intake is adequate, it may take two years to replenish body iron stores after a pregnancy (WHO, 1992). In addition, efforts to reduce the energy demands on women through easier access to needed resources and labor saving devices—during the preconception period as well as during pregnancy and lactation—would be extremely beneficial.

EXTENT OF MALNUTRITION AMONG FEMALES IN SUB-SAHARAN AFRICA

Our brief analysis of the nutritional implications of the multiple demands of time and energy of the roles of Sub-Saharan African women, particularly when considered within the broader context of the health and welfare risks reviewed in other chapters of this volume, would lead the reader to anticipate a high prevalence of malnutrition among Sub-Saharan African females. As this section makes clear, girls and women in this region are, indeed, severely malnourished. Given their limited economic resources and their physically arduous lives, however, it is surprising that their nutritional status is not even worse than it is.

Micronutrient Disorders

Protein-Energy Malnutrition

The United Nations Administrative Committee on Coordination/A System of National Accounts (ACC/SCN) recently published the most thorough and up-to-date global review available of the nutritional situation of women of reproductive age as part of its *Second Report on the World Nutrition Situation.* The ACC/SCN report provides the starting point for this chapter's assessment of the nutritional status of females in Sub-Saharan Africa.[1]

The four anthropometric measures of nutritional status that the ACC/SCN was able to use to make regional estimates of prevalence of PEM among women were height, weight, body mass index (BMI = weight in kilos/ height in meters squared), and arm circumference. Women in Sub-Saharan Africa were found to be surprisingly tall. Average height was 158 centimeters, only 3 centimeters less than the average height of 161 centimeters for European women, while mean female height in South America and most of Asia was only about 151 centimeters. Although these differences might be assumed to be attributable to differences in genetic potential, the finding that mean female height in China was exactly the same as for Sub-Saharan African women suggests that factors other than genetic potential must be important determinants.

Short stature or stunting among adults is usually taken as an indicator of cumulative malnutrition during childhood and adolescence, and it is associated with a range of negative functional outcomes, including reduced work capacity and poorer reproductive outcomes (Buzina et al., 1989; Royston and Armstrong, 1989). The cutoff point for the definition of stunting used by the ACC/SCN is a height of 145 centimeters, which is quite conservative. (As will be discussed in greater detail later, increased obstetrical risk has been associated with short stature, even at heights well above 145 centimeters.) Using this cutoff point, fewer than 5 percent of women in Sub-Saharan Africa were classified as stunted, compared with more than 15 percent in Middle America and Asia (excluding China), and about 12 percent in South America.

The three other anthropometric measures of nutritional status included in the ACC/SCN report are interpreted as indicative of current nutritional status. By these measures, women in Sub-Saharan Africa also do fairly well compared with other regions, but the differences are not so striking as they are for height. Absolute weight, of course, is highly correlated with height. Using 45 kilos as the cutoff point (again, quite conservatively), the ACC/SCN study finds 20 percent of African women to be underweight, about the same percentage as in Middle America and China. This is a larger segment than is found in South America, but a significantly lower percentage than in Asia (excluding China). It was found that 45 percent of women in Southeast Asia and a shocking 60 percent of women in South Asia are underweight. The percent of women with arm circumference below 22.5 centimeters could only be calculated for Sub-Saharan Africa, South Asia, and Southeast Asia, and these percentages followed very closely those for weight below 45 kilos. The relative position of women in Sub-Saharan Africa is least good when BMI, a measure of relative thinness, is considered. Using BMI below 18.5 as the cutoff point, fewer than 20 percent of women in Middle America, South America, and China; slightly more than 20 percent of women in Sub-Saharan Africa; and about 40 percent of women in South and Southeast Asia were excessively thin.

It is helpful to compare the regional information on child nutritional status from the *Second Report on the World Nutrition Situation* with the information on women's nutritional status, although unfortunately the ACC/SCN does not report child nutritional status disaggregated by gender. Anthropometric indicators of child nutrition have been more routinely collected than information on adult nutritional status, so it is possible to estimate regional trends in child nutrition over the past 20 years. It is when trends in child nutrition are examined that the basis for the current concern about the nutritional situation in Sub-Saharan Africa becomes clearer. While between 1975 and 1990 all other regions of the developing world show a marked decline in the prevalence of underweight preschool children (defined as the percent below two standard deviations from the mean weight-for-age in the age range from birth to 5 years), ranging from a 50 percent decline in South America to a 10 percent decline in South Asia, their prevalence in Sub-Saharan Africa appears to have remained essentially unchanged. Because of the continuing rapid rates of population growth in Sub-Saharan Africa, the absolute number of undernourished preschool children increased from 18.5 million in 1975 to 28.2 million in 1990. This means that there are now almost as many undernourished preschool-age *girls* in Sub-Saharan Africa as there were total undernourished preschool children in the region in 1975. It also appears that the relative nutritional status of children is somewhat less favorable than that of women in Sub-Saharan Africa when compared with other regions of the developing world. Perhaps, given their smaller size and less mature immune systems, children have been less able than adults to withstand the particularly harsh conditions that have been endured by most Sub-Saharan Africans over the last decade.

Any attempt to assess the nutritional situation of women and girls in individual countries, or to compare one part of the region with another beyond the aggregate regional estimates of PEM in Sub-Saharan Africa available from the *Second Report on the World Nutrition Situation*, becomes more problematic. Although a substantial amount of research has been carried out to investigate the nutritional situation in Sub-Saharan Africa during the postcolonial period, the number, scope, and quality of nutrition studies vary substantially from one country to another, and many otherwise excellent studies (particularly of child malnutrition) do not report gender-disaggregated results. Two approaches have been taken in this chapter to begin to disaggregate the extent and diversity of nutritional problems of females within the Sub-Saharan African region.

The first approach is to examine three indirect indicators related to women's nutritional status that are available for essentially all countries in the region: the daily per capita energy supply, the percent of infants with low birthweight, and the maternal mortality rate for all countries in Sub-Saharan Africa for which such data could be found (see Table 3-2).[2]

Daily per capita energy supply is not specific to individual households, much less to females within those households, but countries with a per capita energy availability below 2,100 kilocalories are usually designated as food insecure and believed to be at risk of having a substantial number of food-deficient households (FAO and WHO, 1992). We also know that in the Sub-Saharan African region, women who live in the most food-deficient households are usually the women who do the most physically demanding work and who are pregnant with and breastfeed the largest number of infants. Therefore, without being able to estimate a specific number, it seems safe to assume that in any country with a per capita energy supply below 2,100 kilocalories, there will be a reasonably high prevalence of female malnutrition. Of the 37 countries in Table 3-2 with available kilocalorie estimates of daily per capita energy supply in 1989, 12, or about one-third, were below 2,100 kilocalories.

Several studies in Sub-Saharan Africa (as well as many studies from other parts of the world) have demonstrated a relationship between women's nutritional status—both current and past—and the birthweight of their infants (Harrison et al., 1985; Neumann et al., 1992; Prentice et al., 1987). Although low birthweight can occur in the absence of maternal malnutrition, and moderately malnourished women can give birth to infants of adequate birthweight, the correlation between poor maternal nutritional status and low birthweights at the aggregate level is sufficiently strong that it is appropriate to use the percent of low-birthweight infants as an indirect indicator of female nutritional status. In general, we would expect to find a substantial degree of malnutrition among women of reproductive age (both stunting and thinness) in countries reporting a rate of more than 10 percent low-birthweight infants. Of the 37 countries in Table 3-2 for which low-birthweight data are given, 26, or approximately two-thirds, reported more than 10 percent low-birthweight infants in the mid-1980s.

The maternal mortality ratio is also a reasonable indicator of maternal nutritional status, particularly in the absence of adequate, accessible prenatal and childbirth services. Stunting is associated with a greater risk of obstructed labor, and both obstructed labor and anemia are among the major causes of maternal mortality in Sub-Saharan Africa (see Chapter 5, Obstetric Morbidity and Mortality). Therefore, while the maternal mortality ratio does not differentiate among the different kinds of nutritional problems that may affect girls and women, a high maternal mortality ratio is strongly suggestive of a high prevalence of female malnutrition. Virtually all of the countries in Table 3-2 had maternal mortality ratios in 1980 over 100 maternal deaths per 100,000 live births, and 11 of 36 had maternal mortality ratios above 500.

Comparisons among countries and even subregions of Sub-Saharan Africa based on the data in Table 3-2 must be made quite cautiously because of missing data and some lack of comparability among the data (for example, maternal mortality ratios for some countries are based entirely on hospital data). In addition, there is some inconsistency in data between the two sources used to compile this table. Nonetheless, with these caveats in mind, the data in Table 3-2 do present some slightly surprising findings when the four subregions are compared. In food availability, Table 3-2 suggests that eastern Africa and middle Africa are the two most food-insecure parts of the region. In both subregions, more than half the countries have a daily per capita energy supply below 2,100 kilocalories, and for most of the remainder of the countries, per capita energy availability is only slightly above the 2,100 kilocalorie level. Food availability appears to be distinctly better in southern and western Africa.

When the other two indicators related to female nutritional status are examined, however, a somewhat different picture emerges. Based on percentage of low-birthweight infants and maternal mortality ratios, female malnutrition seems to be greatest in western Africa (this is consistent with the estimated subregional prevalences of anemia, as shown in Table 3-4). In western Africa, 10 of the 13 countries for which there are data have more than 10 percent of infants born with low birthweights, and the remaining three are at the 10 percent level. Similarly, in maternal mortality ratios, 6 of 13 countries in western Africa have more than 500 maternal deaths per

TABLE 3-2 Selected Health and Agricultural Indicators Related to Female Nutritional Status in Sub-Saharan Africa

Country	Daily per Capita Energy Supply (1989)[a]	Percent Babies with Low Birthweight (1985)[b]	Maternal Mortality Rate (per 100,000 live births) (1980)[b]
Eastern Africa			
Burundi	**1,932**	14/18	800
Comoros	(89%)	7	460
Ethiopia	**1,667**	13	360
Kenya	2,163	13/18	170[c]
Madagascar	2,158	10	300
Malawi	2,139	10	250
Mauritius	2,887	9/8	99
Mozambique	**1,680**	15/11	479/300[d]
Rwanda	**1,971**	17	210
Somalia	**1,906**	—	1,100
Uganda	2,153	10	300/500
United Republic of Tanzania	2,206	14/13	185
Zambia	**2,077**	14	110
Zimbabwe	2,299	15/6	90
Middle Africa			
Angola	**1,807**	17/21	
Cameroon	2,217	13	303
Central African Republic	**2,036**	15	600
Chad	**1,743**	11	700/1,000
Congo	2,590	12	200
Gabon	2,383	16\8	130
Zaire	**1,991**	16	800
Southern Africa			
Botswana	2,375	8	300/200
Lesotho	2,299	10	370
Namibia	**1,946**	—	—
South Africa	3,122	12	550[e]
Swaziland	(110%)	7	—

Continued

100,000 live births, 6 fall into the range of 100 to 500, and the data for one, Mauritania, are difficult to interpret. The situation in middle Africa appears to be similarly poor in the percentage of low-birthweight infants—all seven countries have in excess of 10 percent low-birthweight infants—and only slightly better in maternal mortality, with three countries recording more than 500 maternal deaths per 100,000 live births, and three in the 100 to 500 range.

In contrast, the situation in eastern Africa looks noticeably better. Of the 13 countries for which there are data on low birthweight, 7 have percentages above 10; 3 are at 10 percent; 2 are below 10 percent; and 1, Zimbabwe, is difficult to classify because the rates given in the two sources, 15 percent and 6 percent, are so different. In maternal mortality ratios, only two countries in eastern Africa have a rate above 500 per 100,000 live births, 10 are in the 100 to 500 range, and 2 have rates below 100. The number of countries for which there are data in southern Africa is small, but both percentage of low-birthweight infants and maternal mortality rates seem to be similar to, or slightly better than, those in eastern Africa.

TABLE 3-2 Continued

Country	Daily per Capita Energy Supply (1989)[a]	Percent Babies with Low Birthweight (1985)[b]	Maternal Mortality Rate (per 100,000 live births) (1980)[b]
Western Africa			
Benin	2,305	10	1,680[d]
Burkina Faso	2,288	18/11	600
Cape Verde	(112%)	—	107
Côte D'Ivoire	2,577	14/15	—
The Gambia	(97%)	—	1,034
Ghana	2,248	17	1,070[d]
Guinea	2,132	18	—
Guinea Bissau	(105%)	14	400
Liberia	2,382	—	173
Mali	2,314	17/13	—
Mauritania	2,685	10	119/1,100
Niger	2,308	20	420
Nigeria	2,312	25	1,500
Senegal	2,369	10	530[f]
Sierra Leone	**1,700**	14	450
Togo	2,214	20	418

[a]Entries in kilocalories are from the 1992 World Development Report (WDR). Those printed in bold face are below 2,100 kilocalories/person/day, which a recent FAO/WHO document labels as indicative of household food insecurity based on a very low level of average food consumption (FAO and WHO, 1992). For countries with populations of less than one million, no data were available from the WDR, and the estimated daily per capita energy supply in 1985 as a percentage of the requirement from Better Health in Africa (BHA) is given. Although figures vary from country to country based on the age and sex distribution of the population, the daily per capita energy supply needs to be about 2,300 to be equivalent to 100 percent of average requirements.

[b]Where two numbers are given, the first is from the WDR and the second from BHA. Where only one number is given, the two sources agreed or only one source had an entry for that indicator and country.

[c]Before 1980.

[d]Hospital data only.

[e]Rural data only.

[f]Hospital data only, before 1980.

SOURCE: All data are from World Bank, 1992a,b.

Unlike daily per capita energy availability, both the percentage of infants born with low birthweights and maternal mortality ratios are specific to females. Therefore, Table 3-2 appears to suggest that western and middle Africa are the two subregions where female malnutrition is the most prevalent, despite better overall food security. An issue that may warrant further investigation is whether there are any dietary or behavioral factors in eastern Africa that contribute to protecting female nutritional status within the context of extremely low household food availability, or factors in western or middle Africa that are significantly detrimental. Alternatively, it may be that access to health care is better in eastern and southern Africa, thus to some extent compensating for the negative effect of food insecurity.

Data are presented in Table 3-3 that measure the nutritional status of women more directly, using BMI as a measure of chronic energy deficiency. Table 3-3 also presents the available BMI data for men, but discussion of the gender differences shown in Table 3-3 is reserved for later in this section. Although different cutoff points have been recommended, in general a BMI below 18 or 18.5 is considered excessively thin, and a person below this mark is categorized as suffering from chronic energy deficiency (CED).[3] Among the countries in eastern Africa with BMI data, it is clear that the situation is most severe in Ethiopia, where half the women suffer from CED. Twelve percent of women in the Zimbabwe study, and probably a similar percentage in the Kenya study, would be considered malnourished. For middle Africa, data are only available from two studies done in Zaire. Although the data are not presented in percentages below a cutoff, the relatively low range of the mean BMI values (19.7 to 21.7) suggests that the percentage of women suffering from CED in these Zairian populations would be lower than in Ethiopia, but higher than in Zimbabwe or Kenya. In western Africa, except for Côte d'Ivoire, where the mean BMI of women is similar to that found in the Kenya study, the BMI data support the conclusion of substantial female malnutrition suggested by the indirect indicators in Table 3-2. The data in Table 3-3 are consistent with the estimated regional average of 21 percent of women in Sub-Saharan Africa with a BMI below 18.5 (UN, 1992).

It seems reasonably clear from the information presented in Tables 3-2, 3-3, and 3-5 (see below) that the problem of protein-energy deficiency is of considerable magnitude among females in Sub-Saharan Africa, with somewhere in the range of 5–10 percent of girls suffering from acute PEM, and 20–40 percent suffering from chronic PEM. Among adult women, somewhere in the range of 1–6 percent may suffer from severe CED (chronic energy deficiency based on low BMI), and 10–40 percent may have mild to moderate CED. During acute famine, of course, the proportion of females suffering from acute PEM will be much higher.

Obesity

While inadequate energy intake is certainly the major macronutritional problem among females in Sub-Saharan Africa, it is important to consider the prevalence of excess energy intake, or obesity. Obesity is known to substantially increase the risk of many chronic diseases (see Chapter 8, Chronic Diseases) and, with the decline in rates of many infectious diseases and increasing life expectancy, a rapid increase in the prevalence of noncommunicable diseases can be expected in the near future in Sub-Saharan Africa (Feachem et al., 1991). The prevalence of obesity is an issue that has received little attention from researchers concerned with nutrition in Sub-Saharan Africa; relevant data are thus extremely limited. One of the few studies to examine simultaneously the prevalence of CED and obesity in the same population groups was a comparative study of adult nutritional status in India, Ethiopia, and Zimbabwe (Ferro-Luzzi et al., 1992). In the Ethiopian population, there was a high prevalence of CED (58 percent of women had BMI below 18.5; 6 percent were below 16) and essentially no obesity, defined as BMI greater than 25. In contrast, in the Zimbabwean population, 12 percent of women had a BMI below 18.5 (only 1 percent were below 16), and 17 percent were defined as obese, with 2.5 percent having a BMI over 30. It is clear that a high prevalence of CED is correlated with a low prevalence of obesity and vice versa, but also that a moderate prevalence of each can be found in the same population.

In Zimbabwe, the average BMI for females was reported to be 22 (SD, 2.3). This figure is not dissimilar to the average BMI reported for females in a number of other Sub-Saharan African populations (see Table 3-3). Therefore, it seems probable that in at least some countries in the region we could expect to find a prevalence of obesity among adult females in the range of 5–10 percent.

Micronutrient Deficiencies

Iron-Deficiency Anemia Iron-deficiency anemia is the most common nutritional deficiency in the world, and given that it particularly affects preschool children and reproductive-age women, it is certainly the most widespread nutritional problem affecting girls and women in Sub-Saharan Africa. It is generally accepted that about half of worldwide anemia is the result of iron deficiency, and there is emerging evidence that low iron stores, even in the absence of anemia, can have negative functional consequences (UN, 1992; WHO, 1992). Therefore, the prevalence of iron-deficiency anemia can be taken as a minimum estimate of both the problems of anemia and of iron deficiency.[4]

A 1992 publication prepared jointly by the Maternal Health and Safe Motherhood Programme and the Nutrition Programme of WHO offers the most recent estimates of the prevalence of nutritional anemias in the world's women, based on studies carried out since 1970 (WHO, 1992). Table 3-4 presents the WHO data on the number and percentage of women with hemoglobin levels below the norm for the four Sub-Saharan African subregions; most of the anemia is attributable to iron deficiency.[5] The relative nutritional situation of women

TABLE 3-3 Body Mass Index (BMI) of Women, Selected Sub-Saharan African Countries (nonpregnant, nonlactating)

Region/Country	BMI Women	Men	Comments	Source
Eastern Africa				
Ethiopia	19.15	18.42[a]	Significant seasonal variation; lowest BMI in March/April	Vesti and Witcover, 1993
Ethiopia	58% < 18.5 BMI (42% BMI 18.5 to 24.9)	50% < 18.5 BMI (51% BMI 18.5 to 24.9)	0.7% of women and no men were classified obese (BMI 25.0)	Ferro-Luzzi et al., 1992
Kenya	22.08	—		Kennedy and Garcia, 1993
Zimbabwe	12% < 18.5 BMI	15% < 18.5 BMI	17.4% of women and 5.6% of men were classified obese (BMI 25.0)	Ferro-Luzzi et al., 1992
Middle Africa				
Zaire	LESE: 21.7 EFE: 20.2	LESE: 21.6 EFE: 20.2	Significant seasonal variation in weight loss, December to June	Bailey et al., 1992
Zaire	TEMBO: 19.7 NTOMBA: 21.1 HIGHLAND: 21.35	—		Caräel, 1978
Western Africa				
Benin[b]	11.5% < 18.0 BMI	—	22.0% of women had BMI > 23.0; significant seasonal variation in rural areas; lower BMI in May/June	Fakambi, 1990
Côte d'Ivoire	22.50	22.23		Thomas et al., 1992
The Gambia	20.6	—		Kennedy and Garcia, 1993
Ghana	20.38	19.39		Kennedy and Garcia, 1993
Ghana	18.8% 18.6 BMI (60.6% BMI 18.6 to 23.8)	40.1% 19.9 BMI (54.8% BMI 19.9 to 25.0)	20.6% of females had BMI > 23.8 5% of males had BMI > 25.0	Alderman, 1990
Guinea	20.52	—	23.5% of women had BMI < 18.6%; 9.7% had BMI > 23.8	Mock and Konde, 1991
Mali	20.8	20.0	11.9% of women and 12.4% of men were malnourished, BMI < 18.	Dettwyler, 1992

[a]Indicates BMI of males was significantly lower than BMI of females.
[b]All women in sample were lactating.

TABLE 3-4   Estimated Prevalence of Anemia among Women in Sub-Saharan Africa by Region (hemoglobin below norms; circa 1988)

Region	Percent	Number (000s)	Percent	Number (000s)	Percent	Number (000s)
Eastern Africa	47	3,380	41	13,540	42	16,920
Middle Africa	54	1,290	43	5,330	45	6,620
Southern Africa	35	380	30	2,500	30	2,880
Western Africa	56	4,170	47	15,120	48	19,290

SOURCE: Figures are taken from Table 2 (page 10), WHO, 1992.

regarding nutritional anemia by subregion is quite similar to the profile of indicators related to female undernutrition more generally, presented in Table 3-2. Table 3-4 suggests that although women in western Africa experience the highest prevalence of nutritional anemia, the prevalences in western Africa, middle Africa, and eastern Africa are quite similar, while women in southern Africa are definitely less anemic. The better situation of women in southern Africa has been attributed by some to the widespread use of iron cooking pots in this region (WHO, 1992).

One disturbing finding reported in the *Second Report on the World Nutrition Situation* is the apparent increase in iron deficiency in Sub-Saharan Africa, as well as in many other regions of the developing world (with the exception of the Near East, North Africa, and South America). While the United Nations cautions that estimates of trends over time in prevalence of anemia should be considered quite tentative, their data suggest that the prevalence of anemia among nonpregnant adult women of reproductive age in Sub-Saharan Africa was around 37 percent from the mid-1970s to the mid-1980s, and had increased to about 46 percent by the late 1980s. Given the population increase over this time, an unavoidable conclusion is that the absolute number of anemic women in Sub-Saharan Africa has probably increased quite dramatically in the past decade. Part of the reason for the deteriorating profile for iron-deficiency anemia is that the iron density in the diet appears to be decreasing rather than increasing in Sub-Saharan Africa, along with most other parts of the developing world. Although dietary iron density in Sub-Saharan Africa appears relatively good compared with other parts of the developing world (between 7 and 8 mg/1,000 kilocalories), the percentage of dietary iron from animal sources is lower than for any region except South Asia, and the general bioavailability of the dietary iron must be quite low.

Anemia during pregnancy is widely recognized as one of the major health and nutritional problems among pregnant women in Sub-Saharan Africa (Royston and Armstrong, 1989). Factors that contribute to the high incidence of anemia among pregnant women in the region include poor dietary practices during pregnancy, infection, malabsorption, malaria, and increased fetal demand. A case-control study of 122 pregnant anemic women in Nigeria by Elegbe and colleagues (1984) reported two particularly interesting findings. Pregnant women's traditional views and practices of treating anemia—wearing black rings presoaked in traditional medicine on their middle fingers as a prophylactic against dizziness—significantly increased rather than decreased the incidence of anemia among those who wore the rings compared with those who did not. In addition, despite a significant increase in the mean hemoglobin levels of all the women in the study, the difference in anemia levels persisted among the two groups even after two months of drug therapy and nutritional counseling (with ferrous gluconate, 300 milligrams three times daily; folic acid; weekly antimalarial drug; and regular individual nutrition counseling). The authors concluded that the wearing of the black rings among the pregnant women, although not effective as a preventive measure, indicates that the women were aware that they were at high risk of anemia.

Iodine-deficiency disorders   Iodine deficiency exists in most regions of the world, although usually in pockets rather than throughout entire countries. Iodine-deficient environments are those where iodine, normally supplied from soil and water, has been leached from the topsoil by rain, flooding, glaciation, or snow; these environments tend to be inland mountainous regions or floodplains. Iodine deficiency is less correlated with food insecurity than are PEM and iron-deficiency anemia. It is rare to encounter iodine deficiencies in populations living near the sea or where the soil has adequate iodine, no matter how impoverished or subject to seasonal food shortages they may be. The main manifestations of iodine deficiency are goiter; impaired mental function; and increased rates of fetal wastage, stillbirths, and infant deaths. Severe mental and neurological impairment, known as cretinism, occurs among infants born to mothers who are seriously iodine-deficient.

The extent of iodine-deficiency disorders (IDD) is usually assessed by the prevalence of goiter in affected populations, although this understates the number of people affected by IDD, particularly if those suffering from the reversible lethargy or mild mental impairment associated with iodine deficiency are included. The United Nations estimates that goiter prevalence is about 8 percent in Africa. There are 39 million people with goiters in Africa, half a million suffer from overt cretinism, and another 227 million are estimated to be at risk of IDD (Hetzel, 1988; UN, 1992). The ratio of those at risk of IDD to those with goiter is extremely high in Africa. This reflects, in part, the lack of control programs, suggesting that IDD will continue to be a serious public health problem in the region for many years to come.

IDD among women is of particular concern for two reasons. First, the range of functional consequences of iodine deficiency is broader for women than for men, because it includes severe negative reproductive outcomes for both mothers and infants (Hetzel, 1988). In addition to the broader range of functional consequences, the prevalence of goiter appears to be significantly higher among females than males in virtually all studies with gender-disaggregated data (Simon et al., 1990). One Africa-specific study that reported gender-disaggregated data is a study from Zaire (Thilly et al., 1977, cited in Simon et al., 1990). Thilly and his colleagues found a significantly higher prevalence of goiter among females than among males, beginning at age 10. The prevalence of visible and voluminous goiter in the age range of peak prevalence (20 to 30 years) was almost 50 percent among females and about 20 percent among males.

Vitamin A Deficiency   Vitamin A deficiency, defined by eye damage (ranging from reversible night blindness, through ulceration of the cornea, to permanent scarring and blindness) has been identified as a widespread public health problem in at least 37 countries (UN, 1992). Each year it is estimated that between 250,000 and 500,000 preschool children go blind from vitamin A deficiency, and that within months of going blind, two-thirds of these children die (UN, 1992). In addition, there is growing evidence that even children who do not necessarily have eye signs may have a subclinical vitamin A deficiency that puts them at greater risk of morbidity and mortality from infectious diseases. While all children above the age of 6 months, as well as pregnant and lactating women, are at risk of vitamin A deficiency, the peak prevalence seems to occur between the ages of 2 and 4 years (Eastman, 1987, cited in Levin et al., 1993). There seems to be a general finding of a higher prevalence of eye damage from vitamin A deficiency among preschool-age boys compared with girls (Levin et al., 1993). It is not well established whether adult males are similarly at greater risk compared with adult females, because relatively few studies have been done of vitamin A deficiency among adults.

In Africa, about 7.2 percent, or 1.3 million, preschool children are estimated to have eye damage because of vitamin A deficiency, and another 7.2 million suffer from a mild to moderate deficiency (Levin et al., 1993; UN, 1992). The proportion of the preschool-age population affected in Africa is similar to the proportion in most other parts of the developing world. Within the Sub-Saharan African region, the areas most affected are eastern Africa, southern Africa, and the Sahelian parts of western Africa. Populations living where red palm oil is produced or distributed—that is, along the coastal parts of western Africa and in some parts of central Africa—are reasonably well protected against vitamin A deficiency. As far as gender differences in vitamin A deficiency are concerned, a small number of somewhat older country-specific studies from Sub-Saharan Africa report not only higher rates of ocular signs of vitamin A deficiency among preschool-age boys compared with preschool-age girls, but also among adult males compared with adult females (South Africa: May and McLellan, 1971; Ethiopia: May and McLellan, 1970; Rwanda: May and McLellan, 1965).

Gender Differences in Malnutrition Throughout the world, differences between males and females in the prevalence of micronutrient deficiencies appear to be substantially attributable to biological differences between the sexes. The higher prevalence of iron-deficiency anemia found among adolescent girls and adult women, for example, is primarily the product of increased iron losses associated with menstruation and the increased iron demands of pregnancy and lactation. This biological risk can be exacerbated by female diets that are lower in animal protein or, in some cases, by a higher prevalence among females of hookworm or schistosomiasis. Similarly, the higher prevalence of IDD among adult women and the higher prevalence of vitamin A deficiency among preschool-age boys (and perhaps among older males) is documented by studies carried out in many different cultural settings and appears to be primarily physiological, although the specific mechanisms are less well understood than in the case of iron-deficiency anemia, and there may be local dietary practices that enhance or reduce the biological gender differences.

In contrast, as far as micronutrient disorders are concerned, there are no underlying physiological reasons to expect a higher prevalence of thinness or obesity among males or females. Where such a pattern does emerge, explanations must be sought in behavioral and cultural factors. While there are significant differences in the roles and opportunities of males and females in Sub-Saharan Africa, no widespread pattern of gender differences in PEM has emerged from studies to date (Kennedy and Bentley, 1993; Svedberg, 1990). Based on recent, gender-disaggregated demographic and health survey data for children presented in Table 3-5, BMI data for adult males and females (see Table 3-3), a secondary analysis of somewhat older height and weight data from Eveleth and Tanner's (1976) *Worldwide Variation in Human Growth* undertaken by Svedberg (1990), and other research reviewed by the committee (see, for example, Alderman, 1990; Strauss, 1990; Thomas, 1991), it seems clear that, in contrast to the situation in South Asia, in Sub-Saharan Africa there is no significant pattern of female disadvantage in anthropometric measures of nutritional status.

In his extensive analysis of gender bias in undernutrition in Sub-Saharan Africa, Svedberg (1990) proposes that the slight anthropometric advantage shown by girls and women in many countries may suggest a historical pattern of preferential treatment of females because of the high value placed on women's agricultural labor. Given that there are also a number of studies in Sub-Saharan Africa that report dietary discrimination against females (see, for example, Caplan, 1989; Trueblood, 1970, cited in Ravindran, 1986; Zumrawi, 1988), however, any conclusion of a nutritionally advantaged position for females in the region seems premature.

One particularly interesting report of gender differences in dietary intake comes from a study of child feeding practices in Zinder, Niger. Field research conducted by CARE on traditional knowledge and practices related to child care and feeding revealed that, in some villages, male and female children are weaned at different ages, with girls weaned one month later than boys. It is traditionally believed that an excess of breastmilk will make a child stupid; boys are weaned earlier "so that they will be intelligent," and have a better chance of success in school (Swimmer, 1990). Although this particular practice may be beneficial to girls' nutrition in the short run, it is actually motivated by the lower value placed on education for females, which may be detrimental to female health and nutritional status in the longer run. It is quite likely that the aggregate finding of little gender difference in anthropometric measures of PEM in Sub-Saharan Africa reflects the cumulative effect of a number of specific behaviors and practices, some of which may favor females, while others may favor males, and that in specific settings and during certain seasons significant gender differences may emerge.

FUNCTIONAL CONSEQUENCES OF FEMALE NUTRITIONAL STATUS: TAKING A LIFE SPAN PERSPECTIVE

Malnutrition is multifactorial in its etiology and cumulative in its manifestations. Merchant and Kurz (1993, p. 73) note that "A nutritional problem is generally the consequence of earlier problems and the cause of later problems." Some of the most important functional consequences of female malnutrition (for example, the obstetrical risks associated with short stature and iron-deficiency anemia) have been studied directly in Sub-Saharan African populations. Many other functional consequences of nutritional status (both positive and negative) have not been studied directly to any great extent among Sub-Saharan African females, but reasonable extrapolations can be made based on studies of men and studies from other parts of the world.

TABLE 3-5 Child Health and Nutrition Status Indicators by Gender, Selected Sub-Saharan African Countries (late 1980s)

Region/ Country	Child Mortality[a]		Height-for-Age[b]		Weight-for-Height[b]		Weight-for-Age[b]		Children with Diarrhea (%)[c]		Children Taken to Health Facility for Diarrhea (%)	
	Male	Female	Male	Female	Male	Female	Male	Female	Male	Female	Male	Female
Eastern Africa												
Burundi	101.0	113.8	48.3	47.8	6.2	5.1	37.5	39.0	17.7	17.0	12.8	11.7
Uganda	97.3	86.0	47.3	41.6	1.8	1.9	23.1	23.4	25.4	23.2	13.8	15.8
Zimbabwe	30.2	32.5	29.9	28.0	1.4	1.3	11.3	11.9	20.5	19.0	33.5	33.2
Western Africa												
Ghana	78.3	79.4	30.2	29.8	9.0	6.9	30.3	31.1	27.0	26.1	40.8	45.6
Mali	166.0	174.0	23.8	24.9	12.0	9.8	30.0	32.2	35.7	33.0	68.4	68.3
Nigeria	93.7	89.1	43.4	42.7	9.8	8.3	35.8	35.7	19.4	16.4	23.6	26.8
Senegal	131.0	129.7	24.8	20.6	7.6	4.1	22.5	20.6	38.9	36.9	19.4	19.4
Togo	74.9	90.1	32.2	26.9	6.2	4.4	25.0	23.8	29.6	29.2	24.2	26.7

NOTE: Data were kindly provided by Kenneth Hill of the World Bank. They are assembled from Demographic and Health Survey Reports and are for all Sub-Saharan African countries for which data on these indicators were available.

[a]Child mortality is usually considered most indicative of child nutritional status.
[b]For children 3–36 months old, percent below 2 standard deviations.
[c]Percent of children under age 5 with diarrhea during the two weeks preceding the survey.

Mortality and Morbidity

Mortality

The ultimate consequence of severe malnutrition is death. Malnutrition is a particularly significant contributing cause of infant and child mortality, and of maternal mortality. Based on estimates made by UNICEF and others, it seems likely that at least one-third of infant and child deaths in Sub-Saharan Africa are partially attributable to PEM (Pinstrup-Andersen et al., in press). In times of famine, both the rates of infant and child mortality and the proportion of total deaths attributable to malnutrition increase dramatically (WHO, 1990).

Low birthweight, which can be the result of either prematurity or intrauterine growth retardation (IUGR), is the most significant nutritional risk factor for subsequent infant and child mortality. It has been estimated that maternal nutritional factors account for approximately half the influence of established determinants of intrauterine growth retardation in developing countries (Kramer, 1987, cited in Merchant and Kurz, 1993). Current or past maternal malnutrition—as evidenced by short stature, low weight-for-height, poor quality dietary intake, and excessive energy expenditure—is a significant risk factor for bearing infants of low birthweight, a relationship that shows a direct intergenerational transmission of malnutrition.

Stunting and wasting among preschool-age children, whether attributable to low birthweight, poor diet and disease postnatally, or both, significantly increases risk of death. A study in Iringa, Tanzania, for example, found a sharp increase in mortality risk at weight-for-age below 60 percent of the median, weight-for-height below 70 percent of the median, and height-for-age below 85 percent of the median (Yambi, 1988, cited in Pinstrup-Andersen et al., in press). Another analysis, based on data from six countries, concluded that infant and child mortality increase at a compounded rate of 7.6 percent for every 1 percent deterioration in weight-for-age, even when the weight deficit is not severe (Pelletier et al., in press, cited in Habicht, 1992). The finding of an increased mortality risk even among mildly to moderately malnourished children has important programmatic and policy implications, given the much larger number of such children compared with those who are severely malnourished.

After infants and preschool-age children, those most at risk of mortality associated with malnutrition are women during pregnancy and childbirth. Given the extremely high rates of maternal mortality in Sub-Saharan Africa (see Table 3-2), assessing and reducing as many of the major causes of maternal death as possible will be a particularly important component of improving women's health in this region (see Chapter 5).

Obstructed labor and its sequelae are the most important causes of maternal death in Sub-Saharan Africa (Royston and Armstrong, 1989). The risk of experiencing obstructed labor, in which the birth canal is too small or too deformed to allow passage of the baby, is directly related to maternal age, developmental stage, and stature. Growth of the birth canal is not complete until about three years after height growth ceases, and PEM both slows down the rate at which girls mature, and, in many cases, permanently stunts their growth. Thus, PEM directly increases the risk of obstructed labor, particularly among adolescent mothers. A study in Nigeria found that among a group of primigravidae who received prenatal care, the proportion who required operative delivery because of a small pelvis ranged from 40 percent among women under 1.45 meters, to 14 percent among those of at least 1.50 meters, to less than 1 percent among those who were 1.60 meters or taller (Fortney, 1986, cited in Royston and Armstrong, 1989). A population-based case-control study in Harare, Zimbabwe, reported similar findings. Controlling for other factors, women of short stature (less than 1.60 meters) were twice as likely as taller women to have an operative delivery (caesarean section, vacuum extraction, or forceps) because of cephalopelvic disproportion (Tsu, 1992). Given the relatively low rate of stunting among women in Sub-Saharan Africa compared with other regions of the developing world, the importance of obstructed labor as a cause of maternal mortality may seem somewhat surprising. The proportion of births in Sub-Saharan Africa among young mothers who are not yet fully physically mature is part of the explanation. Even more significant is the widespread lack of access to timely medical intervention in the case of obstructed labor.

The other nutritional deficiency that significantly increases the risk of maternal mortality is anemia. When anemia is acute, it can cause death directly through heart failure or shock. Fortunately, even among malnourished women, anemia this severe is quite rare. Yet, while less severe anemia may not be a direct cause of maternal death, it is a significant contributory cause. Anemic women are much less able to tolerate hemorrhage, both antepartum and postpartum, and hemorrhage is one of the four leading causes of maternal deaths in Sub-Saharan Africa (Royston and Armstrong, 1989). Anemia is estimated to account for one-fifth to one-tenth of all maternal deaths in many countries of the region; in the extreme circumstances of two refugee camps in Somalia, over 90 percent of maternal deaths were associated with anemia (WHO, 1992). Again, however, it is probably more accurate to say that it is the combination of preexisting anemia, hemorrhage, and lack of access to medical care that causes women to die.

Morbidity

Scientific studies relating malnutrition to both infectious and noncommunicable diseases have proliferated over the past decade. A large number of micronutrient deficiencies have been found to impair the function of the immune system, particularly through their effect on cellular immunity (Buzina et al., 1989; Rose and Martorell, 1992). The negative effect of zinc deficiency on the immune system seems to be particularly notable. As far as noncommunicable diseases are concerned, the effect of malnutrition is cumulative, and primarily manifests itself in disease outcomes during the postreproductive years. Obesity, and probably excess dietary fat, are risk factors for both diabetes and coronary heart disease, while low consumption of the antioxidant vitamins—A, E, and C— increases the risk of developing most, if not all, cancers (Slater and Block, 1991; UN, 1992).

Although the negative impact of specific nutrient deficiencies on the effectiveness of the immune system has been demonstrated, the functional significance in increased morbidity is less well established. The largest body of scientific evidence concerns the relationship between PEM and diarrhea. While virtually all studies show a strong association between these two widespread health problems of childhood, the direction of causality has been more difficult to establish. Careful longitudinal studies suggest that preexisting PEM has a limited effect on the incidence of diarrhea, but significantly increases duration (Leslie, 1982; Tomkins and Watson, 1989). A study of over 300 children between the ages of 6 and 32 months in northern Nigeria at the end of the rainy season found that diarrhea lasted 37 percent longer in stunted children and 79 percent longer in wasted children; in this particular study, wasted children also had diarrhea more frequently (Tomkins, 1981).

A longitudinal study of the functional consequences of malnutrition in the Embu district of Kenya produced several important findings concerning the relationship between nutritional deficiency and subsequent morbidity, not only among preschool-age children, but also among reproductive-age women (Neumann et al., 1992). One of the most striking results of the research was the finding that morbidity rates for the study sample as a whole doubled during a drought-related food shortage in 1984 compared with 1985, when dietary intake had returned to more normal levels.

The same research found that stunting among toddlers (18 to 30 months) and, to a lesser extent, low weight-for-age significantly increased risk of acute lower respiratory tract infections (Neumann et al., 1992). The percentage of time that female infants and toddlers spent ill was somewhat higher than for boys (47 percent versus 42 percent), and girls were found to have a duration of severe illness that was, on average, twice as long as for boys. Girls also experienced an energy deficit during severe illness that was more than double that of boys, although this was somewhat balanced by a larger food intake during convalescence. Lagged analysis showed improved quality and quantity of food intake to be protective against severe illness among girls and boys, with both incidence and duration affected. Insight into the life span effects of malnutrition was offered by the particularly notable finding of the Embu study that lower rates of maternal illness and a higher fat intake among mothers were both significant predictors of less morbidity among their toddlers. The researchers interpreted both factors as indicative of higher levels of energy among mothers, who would then be better able to prevent or treat their children's illness.

Morbidity rates among Embu women were significantly higher among pregnant women than among nonpregnant women of reproductive age (Neumann et al., 1992). In addition to the well-established negative effects of pregnancy on the immune system, the researchers attributed the greater morbidity among pregnant women to their lower food intake. As with toddlers, among both pregnant and nonpregnant women, higher levels of food intake (particularly total energy, fat, and animal protein) were found to be protective against severe illness. Overall, women in this study had higher illness rates than men, a difference that persisted even when pregnant women were excluded from the comparison. The authors caution, however, that because women were the main informants, male illness may have been underreported.

Cognitive Development and School Performance

One of the clearest intergenerational effects of female malnutrition is the significant level of cretinism, deafness, and other congenital abnormalities among infants born to mothers who are severely iodine-deficient. Endemic cretinism is estimated to affect up to 10 percent of the population living in severely iodine-deficient areas (Hetzel, 1988). There are pockets of severe iodine deficiency in the majority of Sub-Saharan African countries; in the region as a whole, there are estimated to be at least 500,000 overt cretins whose condition is ascribed to maternal iodine deficiency during pregnancy (UN, 1992). In addition to congenital cretinism, children who suffer from iodine deficiency during their preschool or school years also show delayed mental development—although unlike cretinism, these cognitive impairments can be reduced with appropriate nutritional intervention.

PEM in children is also strongly associated with impaired motor and mental development (Pinstrup-Andersen et al., in press; Pollitt, 1990). The effects appear to be both direct and indirect. A child who is malnourished is often apathetic or irritable, and thus tends to receive less attention and positive stimulation than a better-nourished child in a similar environment. PEM is negatively associated both with the likelihood that children will go to school and with how well they are able to learn there (Leslie and Jamison, 1990).

The study of the functional consequences of malnutrition among the Embu in Kenya discussed above found negative effects of malnutrition on cognitive development among both toddlers and school-age children (Neumann et al., 1992). In both age groups, stunted children were found to do less well on cognitive tests than children with normal height for age, controlling for other factors. Better dietary quality, particularly increased intake of animal-source protein, fat, and several micronutrients (including but not limited to iodine), was found to have a significant positive effect on cognitive development. In addition, current activity level was strongly related to concurrent energy intake, and activity level and exploratory behavior were found to be positively linked to learning among school-age children.

There are very few studies—in Sub-Saharan Africa or elsewhere—of the effect of malnutrition on attendance, repetition, or drop-out rates among school-age children, although it is virtually inevitable that a high prevalence of malnutrition or other health problems among school-age children will make them "inefficient" users of educational resources. A detailed study of health and nutrition problems among school-age Yoruba children in Nigeria documents a high proportion of children who go to school without breakfast and a high prevalence of growth retardation and micronutrient deficiencies. The study concludes that these lead to a high drop-out rate, poor intellectual performance, and low educational attainment that must represent a serious economic loss to the government of Nigeria, which spends a quarter of its annual recurrent budget on primary school education (Oduntan, 1975).

The life span consequences of malnutrition are also well illustrated by the linkages between malnutrition and schooling. Malnutrition during the preschool and school years has negative effects on girls' (as well as boys') school participation and performance. Low levels of maternal education are, in turn, significantly associated with poor child nutritional status, as well as higher levels of child mortality (Cochrane et al., 1982).

Reproductive Function

The functional impact of childhood malnutrition discussed above is felt by both males and females, although the long-term consequences may be different, and in some cases more severe, among females. The detrimental effect of malnutrition on reproductive function, however, is specific to females (with the possible exception of the effects of severe malnutrition on male fertility) and has grave life span and intergenerational consequences.

Significant declines in fertility during famine, as well as a predictable return to previous levels of fertility once the famine is over, have been well documented (Stein and Susser, 1978). Frisch (1978) has developed a comprehensive model that relates female malnutrition to a shorter and less efficient reproductive span through delayed menarche; reduced fecundity; lengthened postpartum amenorrhea; and, perhaps, earlier menopause. Nonetheless, there remains considerable debate about the magnitude of any effects of female malnutrition on fertility in the context of the chronically mildly to moderately malnourished populations of Sub-Saharan Africa. An analysis of data from unrelated nutrition and fertility surveys in Senegal, for example, found evidence of, at most, a minor negative effect of malnutrition on fertility (Cantrelle and Ferry, 1978). Two studies from Zaire, however, reached conclusions that suggest a much more significant effect of nutritional status on fertility. Caräel's (1978) analysis of data on lactation status and duration of postpartum amenorrhea among women from two different ecological zones of Zaire finds a strong relationship between birth intervals and nutritional patterns. Although the study did not have dietary intake data at the individual level, the researchers conclude that, controlling for duration of lactation, severe seasonal inadequacies of protein and lipids among rural highland women prolong postpartum amenorrhea by seven to nine months. Even more compelling evidence comes from a more recent study in Zaire. Again, women living in different ecological zones were compared, but in this case the researchers were able to relate longitudinal anthropometric data and salivary measures of steroids (indicating ovarian function) to seasonal variations in conception. They conclude that "variability in the seasonal pattern of rainfall in the Ituri Forest causes variability in Lese garden size, which translates into significant changes in nutritional status. Declines in female nutritional status result in reduced ovarian function, which produces seasonal reductions in rates of conception and implantation" (Bailey et al., 1992, pp. 404–405).

Despite widespread mild to moderate malnutrition, women in Sub-Saharan Africa achieve quite high levels of overall fertility. Even more surprising, perhaps, is that most Sub-Saharan African women also produce reasonably adequate birthweight infants and successfully breastfeed in spite of low energy intakes during pregnancy and lactation (in the range of 1,300 to 1,700 kilocalories) and a much lower weight gain during pregnancy (seven to eight kilos) than is recommended or observed among pregnant women in industrialized countries (Kennedy and Bentley, 1993; McGuire and Popkin, 1989). Part of the explanation for this is the high rate of fetal wastage and maternal and infant mortality—in Sub-Saharan Africa the most malnourished fetuses, infants, and mothers simply do not survive.

Some researchers have also hypothesized an unusual capacity on the part of pregnant and lactating African women to adjust to or compensate for low food intake, but findings are not consistent. A series of studies in The Gambia, for example, led to the conclusion that women are able to produce adequate birthweight infants and adequate amounts of breastmilk by mobilizing rather than building up fat stores during pregnancy, particularly during the wet season, and by achieving considerably greater metabolic efficiency than women in industrialized countries (Lawrence et al., 1987b; Prentice et al., 1987). Researchers in The Gambia report that women in their studies raise their BMR so little during pregnancy that the net extra cost of basal metabolism is only 1,000 kilocalories rather than the usual estimate of 36,000 kilocalories over the course of a pregnancy (Lawrence et al., 1980). These findings are not entirely supported by the results of a longitudinal study of reproduction among Embu women in Kenya (Neumann et al., 1992). The Kenya research also reports surprisingly good infant birthweight outcomes, in spite of low energy intake during pregnancy and a weight gain only half that recommended. In contrast with the reported findings from The Gambia, however, the Kenya study found no compensatory lowering of resting energy expenditure among pregnant women. Instead, the researchers found a compensatory behavioral adaptation: late in pregnancy women doubled their inactive time (at the expense of household care, child care, economic and agricultural activities, and food preparation) in order to accommodate to their low energy intakes in relation to the energy requirements at this stage of pregnancy. In addition, the study found that, as in industrialized countries, prepregnancy maternal size, energy intake during pregnancy, and pregnancy weight gain were all important determinants of infant birthweight and net postpartum maternal weight and fat gain.

Physical Work Capacity

Both the long-term consequences of childhood malnutrition and current nutritional deficiencies may have significant effects on women's capacity for physical work. Given the strenuous nature of the major tasks of rural women in Sub-Saharan Africa—pounding grain, carrying water and fuel, carrying out nonmechanized agricultural work, and undertaking long walks to and from markets—a woman's physical capacity for work may be one of the most important determinants of her own and her family's nutritional well-being.

In attempting to assess the effects of female malnutrition on physical work capacity, considerable extrapolation must be done from studies of males, because surprisingly little research has been done on females in this area. The long-term effects of childhood malnutrition, acting through short stature and reduced muscle mass, was found to have a reasonably clear negative effect on the productivity of Guatemalan men engaged in strenuous activities such as cutting cane or moving earth (Martorell and Arroyave, 1988). In addition, deficiencies of several micronutrients, particularly iron, but also vitamin C and the B-complex vitamins, have been found to have a negative effect on physical work capacity (Buzina et al., 1989). Intervention studies in which anemic female tea pickers in Asia were given supplemental iron showed that those who were supplemented were significantly more productive than unsupplemented controls (Leslie, 1991).

There is less consistency in studies that have tried to assess the association between energy status and physical work capacity, in part because a frequent initial response to inadequate energy intake is to mobilize fat stores rather than to reduce work (Pinstrup-Andersen et al., in press). One study from Kenya did find a positive association between nutritional status and work capacity among women in sugarcane farming households (Kennedy and Garcia, 1993). Women with higher BMI were able to spend more time in work-related activities, including home production, and at a given level of BMI, taller women appeared to engage in more energy-intensive work activities. In addition, the frequently cited report from researchers in The Gambia of women who received a dietary supplement and then sang while they worked in the fields (which they had not done previously) supports the importance of looking beyond physical capacity for work or labor productivity when assessing the functional consequences of adult malnutrition (Beaton, 1983).

CONCLUSIONS

The main cause of malnutrition among females in Sub-Saharan Africa is the same as it is for males— household food insecurity stemming from unreliable food availability, compounded by extremely low, and for the most part falling, incomes. Individual nutritional status of both males and females in Sub-Saharan Africa is further undermined by the continuing high burden of infectious disease in this region, which is particularly significant as a determinant of child nutritional status. Additional important causes of poor nutritional status among adult women in Sub-Saharan Africa are the high physiological burden of reproduction and the long hours of energy-intensive work common for rural women in the region.

As in other parts of the developing world, the two most prevalent nutritional deficiencies among females in Sub-Saharan Africa are PEM and iron-deficiency anemia. As Table 3-6 indicates, PEM adversely affects female health status across most age categories, although for different reasons. PEM in the early years can lead to stunting, which is associated with increased risk of obstructed labor. PEM during the childbearing years is associated with elevated morbidity and mortality because of the increased nutritional demands of pregnancy. Iron-deficiency anemia is most commonly observed in women ages 15 to 40 years, and is itself a risk factor for maternal mortality. PEM and iron-deficiency anemia during the childbearing years are also major risk factors for low birthweight. In childhood, PEM and iron-deficiency anemia are important risk factors for poor learning.

Evidence concerning other micronutrient deficiencies among girls and women in the region is limited, but it appears that iodine-deficiency disorders are a major problem in many inland areas of Sub-Saharan Africa. As seen in Table 3-6, goiter has been observed in girls as young as age 10. IDD is also a cause of poor learning in childhood and adolescence. During the childbearing years, IDD is of concern because of the severe negative reproductive outcomes for both mothers and infants (cretinism).

Vitamin A deficiency is quite prevalent in rural Sahelian communities, where there are significant seasonal fluctuations in the quantity and quality of the diet. There are no data, however, indicating that either prevalence or sequelae (for example, blindness) of vitamin A deficiency are worse in females than in males. Instead, vitamin A deficiency seems to be somewhat more prevalent among preschool-age boys than preschool-age girls.

In comparison with other regions of the world, Sub-Saharan African females seem to be nutritionally better-off than females in South Asia, but are equally or more malnourished than females in most other parts of the developing world. In contrast with South Asia, there is no consistent pattern of a higher prevalence of PEM among females than among males, despite a generally higher work burden among adult women compared with men in

TABLE 3-6   Nutritional Disorders and their Adverse Health Effects in Sub-Saharan African Females, by Age

In Utero	Infancy/ Early Childhood (birth through age 4)	Childhood (Ages 5–14)	Adolescence (Ages 15–19)	Adulthood (Ages 20–44)	Post-menopause (Age 45+)
IDD[a] (congenital birth defects)	IDD (poor learning)	IDD (poor learning, goiter)	IDD (goiter)		
Iron-deficiency anemia (low birthweight)	Iron-deficiency anemia (poor growth)	Iron-deficiency anemia (poor learning)	Iron-deficiency anemia (poor learning, hemorrhage during childbirth)	Iron-deficiency anemia (hemorrhage during childbirth)	Iron-deficiency anemia (fatigue)
PEM[b] (low birthweight)	PEM (poor growth/ stunting, increased risk of infection)	PEM (poor growth/ stunting, poor learning)	PEM (obstructed labor)	PEM (obstructed labor)	

[a]IDD = Iodine-deficiency disorders.
[b]PEM = Protein-energy malnutrition.

Sub-Saharan Africa. Small-scale studies from a few countries have found evidence of discrimination or disadvantage experienced by Sub-Saharan females in food consumption. The lack of attention to gender differences in much of the work done on the nutritional problems of Sub-Saharan Africa, however, allows no firm overall conclusion to be reached about the relative nutritional status of males and females. Beyond that, there is also probably considerable variability from one community to another.

Female malnutrition in Sub-Saharan Africa is responsible for a broad range of both short-term and long-term negative consequences. As a result of malnutrition, girls (like boys) suffer high levels of mortality and stunting in early childhood and poor school performance in later childhood. Malnutrition among adult women poses severe risks both to these women and to their infants. Although stunting is not as widespread among women in most Sub-Saharan African countries as in the rest of the developing world, the lack of access to timely medical intervention for cephalopelvic disproportion and prolonged labor puts women with inadequate pelvic development (whether because of size, age, or both) at extremely high risk. In addition, the high proportion of low-birthweight infants in many Sub-Saharan African countries is substantially attributable to maternal malnutrition, both prior to and during pregnancy.

Although some researchers have suggested that Sub-Saharan African females seem to "accommodate" remarkably well to inadequate food intakes, multiple pregnancies, long duration of breastfeeding, and long hours of energy-intensive domestic and market work, appearances can be deceiving. On the one hand, the extremely high infant, child, and maternal mortality rates and the short life expectancy in Sub-Saharan Africa suggest that women and children who are severely malnourished in this region simply fail to survive, perhaps because they are thus predisposed to greater vulnerability to highly prevalent infectious diseases and lack access to medical care. Even among those who survive, it seems almost certain that their marginal nutritional status severely restricts the energy that they have for any activities beyond those essential for survival. It may turn out that it is this restriction on discretionary activities that is most responsible for the perpetuation of malnutrition from one generation to the next.

RESEARCH NEEDS

Considerably more information exists about the extent, causes, and consequences of malnutrition among Sub-Saharan African females than about many of the other causes of morbidity and mortality reviewed in this report.

Nonetheless, inconsistencies in the findings from available studies and the lack of data on particular subgroups—such as adolescent girls; nonpregnant, nonlactating women of reproductive age; and older women—suggest important areas for future research. Available data on nutrition in Sub-Saharan Africa have been generally biased toward preschool children and women of reproductive age. Thus, our analysis, despite an emphasis on the life span perspective, has been limited by the scarcity of reliable data on the female population outside these age groups. In addition, only rarely are the available data nationally representative or comparable over time.

  • Research effort should, therefore, be directed to collection of data on the nutritional status of females beyond those of preschool children and women of reproductive age. Surveys should be designed to ensure that data collected are nationally representative and comparable over time.

Although it is useful to compare the regional information on child nutritional status from the *Second Report on the World Nutrition Situation* with the information on women's nutritional status, the ACC/SCN does not report child nutritional status disaggregated by gender. Similarly, although a substantial amount of research has been carried out to investigate the nutritional situation in Sub-Saharan Africa during the postcolonial period, the number, scope, and quality of nutrition studies varies substantially from one country to another, and many otherwise excellent studies (particularly of child malnutrition) do not report gender-disaggregated results.

  • Future surveys for the *Report on the World Nutrition Situation* and other studies of nutritional status in Sub-Saharan Africa should make every effort to collect and report data that are disaggregated by gender (including data on child nutritional status).

Studies indicate that, in comparison with other Sub-Saharan African regions, female nutritional status in eastern Africa tends to be protected, even in the context of low household food availability.

  • Further research is needed to determine if there are specific dietary or behavioral factors that contribute to the protection of nutritional status in eastern Africa, or the extent to which nondietary factors—for example, better access to health care—compensate for the negative effect of food insecurity.

The prevalence of obesity is an issue that has received little attention from researchers concerned with nutrition in Sub-Saharan Africa; relevant data are thus extremely limited.

  • Surveys of the prevalence of obesity in Sub-Saharan African populations are needed, particularly given the evidence of increasing obesity-related chronic diseases in the region (see Chapter 8, Chronic Diseases). Survey data should be disaggregated by age and gender and collected on representative populations.

A higher prevalence of iodine-deficiency diseases among adult women and a higher prevalence of vitamin A deficiency among preschool-age boys (and perhaps among older males) is documented by studies carried out in many different cultural settings. It appears to be primarily physiological, although the specific mechanisms are less well understood than in the case of iron-deficiency anemia.

  • Further research is needed to determine if there may be local dietary practices that enhance or reduce the biological gender differences.
  • Evidence concerning other micronutrient deficiencies among girls and women in the region is quite limited and requires further evaluation.

In attempting to assess the effects of female malnutrition on physical work capacity, considerable extrapolation must be done from studies of males, because surprisingly little research has been done on women.

  • Studies of the long-term effects of childhood malnutrition on female work capacity are needed. Studies of the effects of adult malnutrition should look at gender-specific effects beyond those associated with reproduction.

NOTES

1. The ACC/SCN data base was compiled from about 340 small- and medium-scale studies of the nutritional status of women between the ages of 15 and 49 years carried out since the late 1970s (UN, 1992).

2. Table 3-2 (and all other tables in this chapter) is organized alphabetically by subregion, and then alphabetically by country within each subregion. The four subregions—eastern, middle, southern, and western Africa—and the countries within them are listed according to WHO usage (WHO, 1992). For Table 3-2, two World Bank sources were consulted (World Bank, 1992a,b); where conflicting numbers were encountered, both are presented in Table 3-2. In most cases the numbers were close, but in a few cases they were so different as to make one, or both, suspect.

3. It should be noted that while 18.5 seems to be an appropriate cutoff in obstetrical risk, a lower cutoff, perhaps as low as 16, is more predictive of increased morbidity risk (Kennedy and Garcia, 1993).

4. In addition to diets that are deficient in iron, folate, and/or B12, hemolysis because of malaria and hemorrhage from hookworm or schistosomiasis are important causes of anemia. In many African countries genetic disease such as sickle-cell anemia and HIV infection can also lead to severe anemia.

5. Cutoffs used by WHO were less than 120g/L hemoglobin for nonpregnant adult women and less than 110g/L for pregnant women. Almost all studies in the review by WHO included only women of reproductive age.

REFERENCES

Alderman, H. 1990. Nutritional Status in Ghana and Its Determinants. Social Dimensions of Adjustment in Sub-Saharan Africa. World Bank Working Paper 3. Washington, D.C.: The World Bank.

Bailey, R. C., M. R. Jenike, P. T. Ellison, G. R. Bentley, A. M. Harrigan, and N. R. Peacock. 1992. The ecology of birth seasonality among agriculturalists in central Africa. J. Biosoc. Sci. 24:393–412.

Beaton, G. H. 1983. Energy in human nutrition: Perspectives and problems. Nutr. Rev. 41(11):325–340.

Bleiberg, F. M., T. A. Brun, and S. Goihman. 1980. Duration of activities and energy expenditure of female farmers in dry and rainy seasons in Upper Volta. Br. J. Nutr. 43:71–82.

Buzina, R., C. J. Bates, J. van der Beek, G. Brubacher, R. K. Chandra, L. Hallberg, J. Heseker, W. Mertz, K. Pretrazik, E. Pollitt, A. Pradilla, K. Suboticanec, H. H. Sandstend, W. Schalch, G. B. Spurr, and J. Westennofer. 1989. Workshop on Functional Significance of Mild-to-Moderate Malnutrition. Am. J. Clin. Nutr. 50:172–176.

Cantrelle, P., and B. Ferry. 1978. The influence of nutrition on fertility: The case of Senegal. In Nutrition and Human Reproduction, W. H. Mosley, ed. New York: Plenum.

Caplan, P. 1989. Perceptions of gender stratification. Africa 59(2):196–208.

Caräel, M. 1978. Relations between birth intervals and nutrition in three central African populations (Zaire). In Nutrition and Human Reproduction, W. H. Mosley, ed. New York: Plenum.

Cochrane, S. H., J. Leslie, and D. O'Hara. 1982. Parental education and child health: Intracountry evidence. Hlth. Pol. Ed. 2:213–250.

Dettwyler, K. A. 1992. Nutritional status of adults in rural Mali. Am. J. Phys. Anthropol. 88:309–321.

Dey, J. 1992. Gender asymmetries in intrahousehold resource allocation in Sub-Saharan Africa: Some policy implications for land and labour productivity. Paper presented at the International Food Policy Research Institute, World Bank Conference on Intrahousehold Resource Allocation, Washington, D.C., February 12–14, 1992.

Elegbe, I., E. O. Ojofeitimi, and I. A. Elegbe. 1984. Traditional treatment of pregnancy and anemia in Nigeria. Trop. Doctor 14(4):175–177.

Eveleth, P. B., and J. M. Tanner. 1976. Worldwide Variation in Human Growth. Cambridge, U.K.: Cambridge University Press.

Fakambi, L. K. 1990. Factors Affecting the Nutritional Status of Mothers. The Food and Nutrition Program of the Ouando Horticulture and Nutrition Center in the People's Republic of Benin. Washington, D.C.: International Center for Research on Women.

FAO and WHO (Food and Agriculture Organization and World Health Organization). 1992. Improving Household Food Security. International Conference on Nutrition, PREPCOM/ICN/92/INF/6. Rome.

Feachem, R. G., and D. T. Jamison, eds. 1991. Disease and Mortality in Sub-Saharan Africa. New York: Oxford University Press for the World Bank.

Feachem, R. G., D. T. Jamison, and E. R. Bos. 1991. Changing patterns of disease and mortality in Sub-Saharan Africa. In Disease and Mortality in Sub-Saharan Africa, R. G. Feachem and D. T. Jamison, eds. New York: Oxford University Press for the World Bank.

Ferguson, A. 1986. Women's health in a marginal area of Kenya. Soc. Sci. Med. 23(1):17–29.

Ferro-Luzzi, A., S. Sette, M. Franklin, and W. P. T. James. 1992. A simplified approach to assessing adult chronic energy deficiency. Eur. J. Clin. Nutr. 46:173–186.

Frisch, R. 1978. Nutrition, fatness, and fertility: The effect of food intake on reproductive ability. In Nutrition and Human Reproduction, W. H. Mosley, ed. New York: Plenum.

Habicht, J. P. 1992. Mortality, malnutrition, and synergies: Determinants and interventions: A discussion. In Child Health Priorities for the 1990s, K. Hill, ed. Baltimore, Md.: The Johns Hopkins University Institute for International Programs.

Harrison, K. A., C. E. Rossiter, and H. Chong. 1985. Relations between maternal height, fetal birthweight, and cephalopelvic disproportion suggest that young Nigerian primigravidae grow during pregnancy. Br. J. Obstet. Gynaecol. (Suppl.) 5:40–48.

Heini, A., Y. Schutz, E. Diaz, A. M. Prentice, R. G. Whitehead, and E. Jequier. 1991. Freeliving energy expenditure measured by two independent techniques in pregnant and nonpregnant Gambian women. J. Am. Physiol. Soc. 261(1 Pt. 1):E9–17.

Hetzel, B. S. 1988. The Prevention and Control of Iodine Deficiency Disorders. ACC/SCN State-of-the-Art Series, Nutrition Policy Discussion Paper, No. 3. Geneva: ACC/SCN.

Holmboe-Ottesen, G., O. Mascarenhas, and M. Wandel. 1989. Women's Role in Food Chain Activities and the Implications for Nutrition. ACC/SCN State-of-the- Art Series. Nutrition Policy Discussion Paper No. 4. Geneva: WHO.

Hussain, M. A., and I. O. Akinyele. 1980. Skinfold thickness of a group of Nigerian village women during pregnancy. Nutr. Rep. Int. 21(1):87–92.

IOM (Institute of Medicine), Subcommittee on Diet, Physical Activity, and Pregnancy Outcome. 1992. Nutrition Issues in Developing Countries. Washington, D.C.: National Academy Press.

Juster, F. T., and F. P. Stafford. 1991. The allocation of time: Empirical findings, behavioral models, and problems of measurement. J. Econ. Lit. 29:471-522.

Kennedy, E., and M. Bentley. 1993. Women's health and nutrition in Sub-Saharan Africa: A review and case study from Kenya. In Research in Human Capital and Development: Health and Nutrition in a Changing Economic Environment, A. Sorkin and I. Sirageldin, eds. Greenwich, Conn.: JAI.

Kennedy, E. T., and B. Cogill. 1987. Income and Nutritional Effects of the Commercialization of Agriculture in Southwestern Kenya. Washington, D.C.: International Food Policy Research Institute.

Kennedy, E., and M. Garcia. 1993. Effects of Selected Policies and Programs on Women's Health and Nutritional Status. Washington, D.C.: International Food Policy Research Institute.

Kennedy, E., H. Bouis, and J. von Braun. 1992. Health and nutrition effects of cash crop production in developing countries: A comparative analysis. Soc. Sci. Med. 35(5):689-697.

Kusin, J. A., W. M. van Steenbergen, S. A. Lakhani, A. A. J. Jansen, and U. Renquist. 1984. Food consumption in pregnancy and lactation. In Maternal and Child Health in Rural Kenya, J. K. van Ginneken and A. S. Muller, eds. London: Croom Helm.

Lado, C. 1992. Female labour participation in agricultural production and the implications for nutrition and health in rural Africa. Soc. Sci. Med. 34(7):789–807.

Lamba, C., and K. L. Tucker. 1990. Work Patterns, Prenatal Care, and Nutritional Status of Pregnant Subsistence Farmers in Central Malawi. Washington, D.C.: International Center for Research on Women.

Lawrence, M., and R. G. Whitehead. 1988. Physical activity and total energy expenditure of child-bearing Gambian village women. Eur. J. Clin. Nutr. 42:145–160.

Lawrence, M., M. A. Hussain, and I. O. Akinyele. 1980. Fat gain during pregnancy in rural African women. Skinfolds thickness of a group of Nigerian village women during pregnancy. Nutr. Rep. Int. 21:1.

Lawrence, M., J. Singh, F. Lawrence, and R. G. Whitehead. 1985. The energy cost of common daily activities in African women; increased expenditure in pregnancy? Am. J. Clin. Nutr. 42:753–763.

Lawrence, M., W. A. Coward, T. J. Cole, and R. G. Whitehead. 1987a. Energy requirements of pregnancy in The Gambia. Lancet 2(8567):1072–1075.

Lawrence, M., W. A. Coward, F. Lawrence, T. J. Cole, and R. G. Whitehead. 1987b. Fat gain during pregnancy in rural African women: The effect of season and dietary status. Am. J. Clin. Nutr. 45:1442–1150.

Leslie, J. 1982. Child Malnutrition and Diarrhea: A Longitudinal Study from Northeast Brazil. Baltimore, Md.: The Johns Hopkins School of Hygiene and Public Health.

Leslie, J. 1989. Women's time: A factor in the use of child survival technologies? Hlth Pol. Plan. 4:1–16.

Leslie, J. 1991. Women's nutrition: The key to improving family health in developing countries? Hlth Pol. Plan. 6:1–19.

Leslie, J., and D. T. Jamison. 1990. Health and nutrition considerations in education planning. 1. Educational consequences of health problems among school-age children. Food Nutr. Bull. 12(3):191–203.

Levin, H. M., E. Pollitt, R. Galloway, and J. McGuire. 1993. Micronutrient deficiency disorders. Pp. 421–451 in Disease Control Priorities in Developing Countries, D. T. Jamison, W. H. Mosley, A. Meashan, and J. L. Bobadilla, eds. New York: Oxford University Press for the World Bank.

Loutan, L., and J. M. Lamotte. 1984. Seasonal variations in nutrition among a group of nomadic pasteralists in Niger. Lancet 1 (8383):945–947.

Martorell, R., and G. Arroyave. 1988. Malnutrition, work output, and energy needs. In Capacity for Work in the Tropics, K. J. Collins and D. F. Roberts, eds. Cambridge, U.K.: Cambridge University Press.

May, J. M., and D. L. McLellan. 1965. The ecology of malnutrition in Middle Africa. Stud. Med. Geogr. 8.

May, J. M., and D. L. McLellan. 1970. The ecology of malnutrition in Eastern Africa and four countries of Western Africa. Stud. Med. Geog. 9.

May, J. M., and D. L. McLellan. 1971. The ecology of malnutrition in seven countries of Southern Africa and in Portuguese Guinea. Stud. Med. Geog. 10.

McGuire, J., and B. M. Popkin. 1989. Beating the zero-sum game: Women and nutrition in the Third World. Part 1. Food Nutr. Bull. 11(4):38–63.

Merchant, K. M., and K. M. Kurz. 1993. Women's nutrition through the life cycle: Social and biological vulnerabilities. Pp. 63–90 in The Health of Women: A Global Perspective, M. Koblinsky, J. Timyan, and J. Gay, eds. Boulder, Colo.: Westview.

Mock, N. B., and M. K. Konde. 1991. Correlates of maternal nutritional status in the Republic of Guinea. Paper presented at NCIH Annual Meeting, Washington, D.C.

Neumann, C., N. O. Bwibo, and M. Sigman. 1992. Functional Implications of Malnutrition: Kenya Project Final Report, Human Nutrition Collaborative Research Support Program. Los Angeles: UCLA School of Public Health.

Oduntan, S. O. 1975. The Health of Nigerian Children of School Age. Brazzaville: WHO.

Parker, L. N., G. R. Gupta, K. M. Kurz, and K. M. Merchant. 1990. Better Health for Women: Research Results from the Maternal Nutrition and Health Care Program. Washington, D.C.: International Center for Research on Women.

Peacock, N. 1992. Nutrition, reproductive status, and work effort in rural African women. Paper presented at the American Anthropological Association Meeting, San Francisco, December 1992.

Pinstrup-Andersen, P., S. Burger, J. P. Habicht, and K. Peterson. In press. Protein-energy malnutrition. Disease Control Priorities in Developing Countries, D. T. Jamison and W. H. Mosley, eds. New York: Oxford University Press for the World Bank.

Pollitt, E. 1990. Malnutrition and Infection in the Classroom. Paris: UNESCO.

Prentice, A. M. 1980. Variations in maternal dietary intake, birthweight, and breastmilk output in The Gambia. In Maternal Nutrition During Pregnancy and Lactation, H. Aebi and R. Whitehead, eds. Bern, Switzerland: Hans Huber.

Prentice, A. M., T. J. Cole, F. A. Foord, W. H. Lamb, and R. G. Whitehead. 1987. Increased birthweight after prenatal dietary supplementation of rural African women. Am. J. Clin. Nutr. 46:912–925.

Raikes, A. 1989. Women's health in East Africa. Soc. Sci. Med. 28(5):447–459.

Ravindran, S. 1986. Health Implications of Sex Discrimination in Childhood: A Review Paper and an Annotated Bibliography. Geneva: WHO.

Rose, D., and R. Martorell. 1992. The impact of protein-energy supplementation interventions on child morbidity and mortality. In Child Health Priorities for the 1990s, K. Hill, ed. Baltimore, Md.: The Johns Hopkins University Institute for International Programs.

Royston, E., and S. Armstrong, eds. 1989. Preventing Maternal Deaths. Geneva: WHO.

Simon, P. A., D. T. Jamison, and M. A. Manning. 1990. Gender differences in goiter prevalence: A review. Los Angeles: UCLA Graduate School of Education. Photocopy.

Slater, T. F., and G. Block, eds. 1991. Antioxidant vitamins and B-carotene in disease prevention. Am. J. Clin. Nutr. 53(Suppl.)(1):189S–396S.

Stein, Z., and M. Susser. 1978. Famine and fertility. In Nutrition and Human Reproduction, W. H. Mosley, ed. New York: Plenum.

Straus, J. 1990. Households, communities, and preschool children's nutrition outcomes: Evidence from rural Côte d'Ivoire. Econ. Devel. Cultu. Change 36(2):231–262.

Svedberg, P. 1990. Undernutrition in Sub-Saharan Africa: Is there a gender bias? J. Devel. Stud. 26(3):469–486.

Swimmer, K. 1990. Final report: Field research on traditional knowledge and practices related to child care and child feeding. The Zinder Child Health Project of CARE International/Niger. Interim Report. CARE, Niamey. Photocopy.

Thomas, D. 1991. Gender Differences in Household Resource Allocations. Living Standards Measurement Study Working Paper 79. Washington D.C.: World Bank.

Thomas, D., V. Lavy, and J. Strauss. 1992. Public Policy and Anthropometric Outcomes in Côte d'Ivoire. Living Standards Measurement Study Working Paper 89. Washington D.C.: World Bank.

Tomkins, A. 1981. Nutritional status and severity of diarrhea among preschool children in rural Nigeria. Lancet 1:860–862.

Tomkins, A., and F. Watson. 1989. Malnutrition and Infection: A Review. ACC/SCN State-of-the-Art Series, Nutrition Policy Discussion Paper No. 5. Geneva: ACC/SCN.

Tsu, V. D. 1992. Maternal height and age: Risk factors for cephalopelvic disproportion in Zimbabwe. Int. J. Epidemiol. 21(5):941–946.

UN (United Nations). 1991. The World's Women, 1970–1990: Trends and Statistics. Social Statistics and Indicators, Series K, No. 8. New York.

UN, ACC/SCN(Administrative Committee on Coordination/A System of National Accounts). 1992. Second Report on the World Nutrition Situation, Vol. 1, Global and Regional Results. Geneva: ACC/SCN.

Vesti, S. A., and J. Witcover. 1993. Gender differences in levels, fluctuations and determinants of nutritional status: Evidence from South Central Ethiopia. In Effects of Selected Policies and Programs on Women's Health and Nutritional Status, E. Kennedy and M. Garcia, eds. Washington, D.C.: International Food Policy Research Institute.

WHO (World Health Organization). 1990. Nutritional status of Somalia refugees in Eastern Ethiopia, September 1988–May 1989. Week. Epidemiol. Rec. 65:93–100.

WHO (World Health Organization). 1992. The Prevalence of Anemia in Women: A Tabulation of Available Information. WHO/MCH/MSM/92.2. Geneva: WHO.

World Bank. 1992a. Better health in Africa. World Bank, Africa Technical Department, Washington, D.C. Photocopy.

World Bank. 1992b. World Development Report 1992: Development and the Environment. New York: Oxford University Press for the World Bank.

Zumrawi, F. Y. 1988. Local influences and customs on diets in Sudan village community. Ahfad J. 5(2):27–32.

4

Obstetric Morbidity and Mortality

This section addresses the health risks of pregnancy and childbearing faced by women in Sub-Saharan Africa, and the factors that exacerbate or mitigate those risks. Maternal mortality and morbidity are reviewed as public health problems, and their causes, prediction, prevention, and cure are examined.

The likelihood that a woman will experience a maternal death is directly related to the number of times she is pregnant. Because contraceptives permit couples to plan their pregnancies and elect when to have children, the role of family planning in maternal health is discussed, as is the role of unsafe abortion.

The chapter also reviews breastfeeding and its implications for maternal health. While the benefits of breastfeeding for infants are well established, it places considerable demands on their mothers, consuming substantial proportions of their protein, caloric, and mineral intake. Since many African women are nutritionally compromised, the question of whether lactation has a detrimental effect on their overall health status is not trivial. The risk of transmitting HIV infections from mother to infant through breast milk compounds the dilemma.

Another dilemma addressed in this chapter is the tension between the beneficial aspects of traditional medical practices and those that are physiologically detrimental. Significant among the latter is the category of traditional practice that includes female circumcision.

The chapter closes with a section on menopause, a topic that should command increasing attention as more and more African women survive to enter this phase of their lives.

The specific focus of this chapter is obstetric health. The powerfully related and equally important topic of the sexually transmitted diseases is covered in Chapter 11. Because this chapter emphasizes the reproductive period of the female life span, no separate attention is given to that period in the following discussion of the life span approach.

GENDER BURDEN

Chapters 3 through 11 of this report all begin with a summary table that compares the relative burden of a given health problem or set of health problems by gender. At first thought, such a table in this chapter, which deals with the fundamental topic of female reproductive function, would seem neither appropriate nor necessary. Nevertheless, Table 4-1 presents a list of conditions and events that females actually do share with males, in many cases at roughly equal prevalence rates, that are of consequence for females precisely *because* they are female and *because* they reproduce. These conditions and events are rarely considered in any unitary way. For that reason,

TABLE 4-1   Obstetric Health Problems in Sub-Saharan Africa: Gender-Related Burden

Problem	Exclusive to Females	Greater for Females	Burden for Females and Males Comparable, but of Particular Significance for Females
Anemia		X	
Cardiomyopathies			X
Diabetes			X
Dracunculiasis			X
Genital mutilation, sequelae	X		
HIV/AIDS			X
Hypertension			X
Iodine deficiency/goiter		X	
Leprosy			X
Malaria			X
Onchocerciasis			X
Protein-energy malnutrition			X(?)
Schistosomiasis			X
Sexually transmitted diseases			X
Sickle-cell disease			X
Trypanosomiasis			X

NOTE: Males obviously do not have obstetric and gynecologic problems. There is, however, a gender difference. While all the health problems listed occur in both males and females, they may be exacerbated by the processes of pregnancy and parturition. This aspect of gender differences needs to be taken into account, both in clinical research and in application.

they are listed in Table 4-1 as preexisting or concurrent conditions that, with the exception of genital mutilation, also affect males, but are exclusively female in the way they either exacerbate risk during pregnancy and child-birth, or are exacerbated by those events.

The length of this list is impressive. It includes six highly prevalent and burdensome tropical infectious diseases (dracunculiasis, or Guinea worm disease; leprosy; malaria; onchocerciasis; schistosomiasis; and trypanosomiasis); five chronic diseases, one of which is clearly genetic (cardiomyopathies, diabetes, hypertension, rheumatic heart disease, and sickle-cell disease); three nutrition-related conditions (anemia, iodine deficiency, and protein-energy malnutrition); and three conditions related to female sexual identity (HIV/AIDS, the sequelae of female genital mutilation, and the entire group of sexually transmitted diseases).

In addition to their sometimes deleterious interactions with the gravid state and the act of parturition, a number of the health problems on this list have vigorous relationships with one another, a dynamic that reappears through-out this chapter and is summarized in the chapter's final table, Table 4-15.

THE LIFE SPAN: AN APPROACH TO MATERNAL MORBIDITY AND MORTALITY

The basic premise of the life span approach is that the morbidity and mortality associated with reproduction are not haphazard phenomena, but a culmination of events that begin much earlier, even before a woman's own birth. These may include her mother's poor nutritional and health status, intrauterine events, and perhaps lack of adequate prenatal care; her own diet; insult from infectious diseases; injuries and accidents; poor access to health, education, and other resources as she grew up; her work burden; gender discrimination; and the general conditions of poverty. From the time she is conceived to the time she herself conceives, the course of a woman's pregnancy and its outcome will both be affected by a variety of clinical, economic, social, and cultural factors and affect her health and well-being for the rest of her life.

Childhood

Episodes of infectious disease in childhood—notably tuberculosis; hepatic infections; rheumatic heart disease; and parasitic infections, especially malaria—often produce long-term sequelae and become chronic conditions (Elo and Preston, 1992). Certain infectious diseases may be more common among females than they are among males, if only because female domestic and productive activities increase exposures in distinctive ways (see Chapter 10). Malnutrition and childhood diarrhea further compromise the female immune system and contribute to recurrent infections during adulthood (Martinez et al., 1990). Poor childhood nutrition has special impact on females: stunting, and correspondingly small pelvic size, places them at risk for obstructed labor (Harrison, 1983; Mosley and Chen, 1984), the most important reported cause of maternal death in Sub-Saharan Africa (WHO, 1991b).

Adolescence

Adolescence is a period when differences between male and female health status can become striking. At a time when a woman's dietary demands expand because of rapid changes in her physiology, greater energy is required for meeting the mounting volume of taxing adult chores she is expected to assume, chores females are more likely to perform than males (Merchant and Kurz, 1992).

Foremost among these new stresses is childbearing. The evidence from the Demographic and Health Surveys (DHS) is that age at marriage in Africa is the lowest among all the world's regions. In Mali, Niger, Nigeria, Senegal, and Uganda, median age at first marriage among women aged 20–24 years at the time of the survey was under 18 years (Robey et al., 1992); the range is from a mean age at marriage of 16–17 in Mali and Niger to a mean of 25–26 in Botswana and Namibia (Guttmacher Institute, 1995).

The result of this early marriage is high proportions of teenage pregnancies in most African countries, as well as a larger absolute number of pregnancies simply because a longer period of time is spent in childbearing. That young women are single does not mean they are not having sexual intercourse, and in some cases, that they are not having babies. In the large majority of the Sub-Saharan African countries, a large proportion (37 to 78 percent) of single women ages 15–24 have already had a sexual relationship, and 2 to 42 percent have already had a child. Overall, women are almost as likely to have their first birth before age 20 as they are to marry before age 20. In Botswana, as one instance of what may be a regional phenomenon, the percentage of teenage mothers increased from 15.4 percent in 1971 to 22.6 percent in 1984 (Guttmacher Institute, 1995).

It is well known that a number of obstetric conditions are more common and more severe in the adolescent female because of her physiologic immaturity and her overall lack of social and economic resources (Harrison et al., 1985a; Liskin et al., 1985; UN, 1989). These include pregnancy-induced hypertension, anemia, malnutrition, cephalopelvic disproportion, vesico-vaginal and recto-vaginal fistulae, difficult delivery, retardation of fetal growth, premature birth, low birthweight, and perinatal mortality (UN, 1989). In a Nigerian study, for example, 17 percent of 14-year-olds developed hypertensive disease, compared with 3 percent of women aged 20–34 (WHO, 1989). In a hospital study in Cameroon, Leke (1989) reported that although adolescents represented only 28 percent of the obstetric population, they accounted for over 70 percent of obstetric complications. The number of young women with these problems can only be expected to grow because of the absolute increase in the size of the adolescent population (Gyepi-Garbrah, 1988). Persistently high birthrates and, even in Sub-Saharan Africa, declining death rates, especially with improving child survival, have led to dramatic growth in the number of adolescent and young-adult Third World males and females in their most sexually active years. The momentum of population growth created by the large numbers of individuals who are currently infants means that this trend will continue for several decades, even if fertility were to drop to replacement levels tomorrow (Germain and Dixon-Mueller, 1992).

Although many more girls now attend school than ever before, which serves to extend the premarital period, many still begin sexual relations early and are particularly vulnerable to problems they are singularly ill-equipped to handle, notably abortions and sexually transmitted diseases. Rates of abortion among adolescents are high. Studies of hospital records in Congo, Kenya, Liberia, Mali, Nigeria, and Zaire found that between 38 and 68 percent of women seeking care for complications of abortion were under 20 years of age (Tinker et al., 1994). At Kenyatta National Hospital, women aged 14 to 25 years, half of the reproductive age group, accounted for 84 percent of all septic abortions (Gyepi-Garbrah, 1988); a Benin City study found that almost 60 percent of maternal deaths from abortion occurred in teenagers, who accounted for over 72 percent of maternal deaths.

Rates of sexually transmitted diseases (STDs) are also high among adolescents, and rising dramatically: in Uganda, the highest incidence of STDs is among women aged 15–19 years (WHO, 1989). A study in Nigeria reported that 16 percent of the female patients presenting for treatment for STDs were children under age 5, and another 6 percent were aged 6 to 15 (Kisekka and Otesanya, 1988). Together, earlier sexual activity, longer periods of fertility, and growing prevalence of STDs among adolescent females mean that more and younger women are also at greater risk of HIV infection (Over and Piot, 1993). If, as anecdotal reports suggest, older men increasingly target younger women as sexual partners in the belief that they are less likely to be HIV-infected, the level and extent of this particular hazard are even greater.

Adolescence for many African women is, then, riskier than it used to be, and it is shorter. The period of adulthood arrives swiftly, and it is almost inevitably the most taxing time of a Sub-Saharan African female's life. An African mother is, more and more, the adult with the primary responsibility for her family, financially and otherwise. At the same time, she is in the peak years of her reproductive potential and will spend approximately half of those years either pregnant or breastfeeding (Raikes, 1989).

Menopause and Postmenopause

As their life expectancy has lengthened, African women complete their reproductive years only to face both the chronic diseases associated with longevity and possible morbidity accrued from infectious diseases survived in childhood. Respiratory infections, tuberculosis, and diarrhea may once again become significant, as well as other age-related diseases such as arthritis, and trauma-related diseases such as lower-back pain. The ever-larger numbers of African women experiencing menopause are also likely to confront the same or similar reproductive diseases as their agemates in the West, notably the gynecologic neoplasms, most of which reach their statistical peaks in women ages 45 to 60. Data are limited in this area because the study of women's health in all developing countries has been focused on reproductive function and pregnancy outcomes almost exclusively (Baumslag, 1985).

THE MAGNITUDE OF PREGNANCY-RELATED MORTALITY AND MORBIDITY

Quantification of Maternal Mortality

The adequacy of the assessment of maternal mortality depends on the data available. The three principal sources of such data are vital registration, health service statistics, and population-based inquiries. The countries of Sub-Saharan Africa do not differ significantly from other developing nations in this range of sources; the difficulty lies in generally lower levels of coverage, completeness, and reliability (Graham, 1991).

Vital Statistics

Vital statistics—in particular, death certificates—that could conceivably provide reliable information on cause of death cover less than one-tenth of national populations (Tietze, 1977), predominantly in the more privileged urban areas. They are especially constrained in the region's rural areas, where over 70 percent of African women live and where reports of deaths are typically obtained from next of kin, village chiefs, imams, funeral caretakers, or other untrained individuals (Boerma and Mati, 1989; Rosenfield, 1989; Toure et al., 1992). Many national ministries of health lack the wherewithal to maintain vital registries and may not see such efforts as pressing, given the larger hierarchy of problems they face. These low levels of overall coverage, together with the incompleteness that derives from underreporting and misclassification, seriously limit the value of data from vital registration for studying maternal deaths (Graham, 1991). The only exception in the region is Mauritius, notable for the completeness and coverage of its vital statistics and the long history of their accumulation (Graham, 1991).

It is only fair to note that, even when they exist and are highly developed, civil records tend to be error-prone. In assessing incidence of maternal mortality in the United States, in 1984 Smith and colleagues estimated that it has been as much as 20 to 30 percent higher than vital statistics indicated. When compared with death certificates, actual levels of maternal mortality were found to be 27 percent higher within the 42-day period after delivery, and 50 percent higher when that postpartum period was not limited to 42 days (Rubin et al., 1981). Benedetti and colleagues (1985) estimated that over the year of their study in the U.S. state of Washington, maternal mortality had been underreported by 112 percent. A conservative statement would be that estimates of maternal mortality are generally highly variable.

Health Services Statistics

Despite its significance, pregnancy-related mortality is still an event of limited occurrence in comparison, for instance, with infant mortality (Kwast et al., 1986). Thus, adequate assessment has traditionally been understood to require large sample sizes, ideally followed over an extended period of time. Because this approach is difficult and costly, many estimates of maternal mortality have been based on records of deaths at fixed health facilities.

In the case of Sub-Saharan Africa, this method is problematic. Although deaths that occur at lower-level facilities, such as clinics or health posts, should and could be included under health services statistics, they tend to be omitted because of general inefficiencies in health information systems—and, perhaps, concern about who might get blamed for a death. While a number of developing countries have had satisfactory experience with health information gathered by primary health workers, this is still a relatively rare practice among the Sub-Saharan African countries (Graham, 1991; Hill and Graham, 1988).

This means that estimates of maternal mortality in the region are principally hospital-based, a major source of bias because only a small proportion of women have access to, and use, hospitals (Boerma, 1987; Graham, 1991). In addition, relatively few women deliver in hospital, so that hospital-based figures are only reflective of the women who die there; they exclude the many women who deliver or die at home and never come to the attention of health care providers. Baumslag (1985) reports that only 2 percent of deliveries are attended by a physician or take place in hospitals; 52 percent are attended by an indigenous practitioner, 40 percent by a family member. In Niger, 84 percent of deliveries are at home (Niger Ministry of Finance and Planning, 1993), as are 62 percent of those in Nigeria (Nigeria Federal Office of Statistics, 1992).

Furthermore, those who can afford to go to a hospital may be of higher socioeconomic status, more educated, and more likely to have had access to health care during pregnancy. They are thus at lower risk than women without access to these services. This difference may lead to underestimating community mortality or morbidity levels. At the same time, women who deliver in hospital may also be those at high risk of complications, so that hospital-based estimates may overestimate the true population experience. It is difficult to calculate the combined impact of these opposing biases. In sum, the figures on pregnancy-related mortality presented in much of the literature may not even approximate the true situation (Boerma, 1987).

Population-Based Data

The third source of information on maternal mortality in Sub-Saharan Africa is the population-based inquiry; it is also the rarest (Graham, 1991). The gathering of such data anywhere presents conceptual and practical difficulties because the classical approaches used—prospective, retrospective, direct, and indirect, independently or in combination—all have methodological drawbacks (Timaeus, 1991). They also must take into account issues of comparability, sustainability, and cost. The number of longitudinal, population-based studies in Sub-Saharan Africa has been small, and the number that gathered maternal mortality data even smaller (cf. Ghana [Danfa Project]; Kenya [Machakos Project]; The Gambia [Keneba Project]). They have not been analyzed systematically as a group in terms of relevance and expense (Tarimo, 1991), but it is hard to imagine their replication in today's financial and political environments.

Furthermore, there are other considerations peculiar to estimating maternal mortality (Graham, 1991). First, as noted above, the event itself is rare. Second is the problem of the simple omission of events. For example, there may be no reliable informant to provide information on the deceased because of the household breakup that may follow a maternal death (Boerma, 1987; Timaeus, 1991). As also noted above, respondents may withhold information on maternal deaths for social, cultural, religious, or emotional reasons (Graham, 1991).

Third, reporting at the household or community level may suffer from the same variation in the definition of maternal death that complicates all assessment, particularly comparative assessment (Graham, 1991; Graham and Airey, 1987; Graham and Brass, 1988; Royston and Armstrong, 1989; WHO, 1987b). According to the World Health Organization's (1977) *International Classification of Diseases* (ICD-9), "A maternal death is defined as the death of a woman while pregnant or within 42 days of termination of pregnancy, irrespective of the duration and the site of the pregnancy, from any cause related to or aggravated by the pregnancy or its management, but not from accidental or incidental causes" (WHO, 1987b). The more recent definition of maternal mortality in the *International Classification of Diseases*, Volume 10 (ICD-10), has been revised to include deaths within one full year after termination of pregnancy (Fortney, 1990).

Another important definitional issue is related to terminology: although much of the literature refers to maternal mortality *rate*, very often what it is meant is the *ratio* of maternal deaths to live births (Fortney, 1987; Winikoff and Sullivan, 1987). The maternal mortality *ratio* is the number of maternal deaths per 100,000 live births. The numerator is "maternal deaths"; "live births" is the denominator because birth records are the only widely available data that can be used as a proxy for the number of pregnancies in the population. The maternal mortality *rate* is the number of maternal deaths in one year per 100,000 women of reproductive age (usually defined as 15 to 49). This chapter distinguishes between rates and ratios whenever possible.

Alternative Approaches

The "sisterhood method," a recent development in the population-based estimation of maternal mortality, overcomes some of the problems raised above (Graham and Brass, 1988). A comparatively simple and low-cost technique, it is particularly suited to situations in which conventional information sources are inadequate and unlikely to improve greatly in the near future. Still in evolution, the method is predicated on surveys that ask adult respondents whether any of their adult sisters have died from pregnancy-related causes. Because it maximizes the number of reported woman-years of exposure to risk, reasonably stable estimates may be calculated based on relatively small samples of respondents. Results from initial field trials and the plausibility of the technical modifications being made suggest real promise for the method in the future (Graham, 1991).

A government can opt for gathering information through the sisterhood method or any other data-gathering approach—for instance, retrospective and longitudinal analysis of facility records or perinatal audits (Mbaruku and Bergstrom, 1995) in "sentinel sites" in a number of districts or smaller geographic areas that have been selected as representative of nationwide socioeconomic and ecological realities (Tarimo, 1991).

The Burden of Maternal Mortality and Morbidity

Significant gains have been made in infant and child survival; less progress has been made in maternal survival. Every year, over half a million women worldwide still die as a result of complications associated with pregnancy or childbirth—about one woman a minute. Nearly 99 percent of these deaths occur in developing countries (WHO, 1991b). Maternal mortality rates in Africa are higher than anywhere else in the world. In Sub-Saharan Africa, 150,000 women a year die of maternal causes, about one every 3.5 minutes. If, on average, a woman in Africa has six children during her lifetime (World Bank, 1992), and women who die in their reproductive years leave an average of two or more children (Herz and Measham, 1987), such mortality probably leaves nearly one million children motherless each year.

These losses occur even though pregnancy and childbearing constitute a natural biological process, and the knowledge and means exist to remove or attenuate the hazards associated with that process. Yet women continue to die from hemorrhage, infection, obstructed labor, hypertensive disorders, and abortion, primarily because of lack of proper care, especially during delivery (Rosenfield, 1989; Royston and Armstrong, 1989). While the average number of maternal deaths in developed countries is between 10 and 15 per 100,000 live births, women in less-developed countries record rates of over 100 times this number. This is a much greater discrepancy than that observed in infant mortality rates, and it is the widest disparity in health statistics between developed and developing countries (Mahler, 1987; Rosenfield, 1989). If one considers that documentation of maternal deaths in developing countries is invariably incomplete, then the high figures reported undoubtedly underestimate the magnitude of the problem (Baumslag, 1985; Lettenmaier et al., 1988).

Table 4-2 and Figure 4-1 present a summary of maternal mortality ratios in a number of African countries and reveal significant variability among those ratios, with a high of 2,900 deaths per 100,000 live births in Mali and a low of 77 deaths per 100,000 live births in Zimbabwe. Five of the 32 countries for which data are available have ratios of over 1,000 deaths per 100,000 live births, over a hundred times the mortality ratio in the United States (Rosenfield, 1989), and only 12 have ratios under 200 deaths per 100,000 live births.

These summary figures do not tell the whole story. Within countries, certain categories of females are at greater risk than others. A very early first birth increases a woman's risk of dying from pregnancy-related causes. Women ages 15–19 face a 20 to 200 percent greater risk of pregnancy-related death than older women, and the younger the adolescent, the higher the risk (WHO, 1989). In Nigeria, for example, women under 15 were found to be 4 to 8 times more likely to die of pregnancy-related conditions than those aged 15–19 (Harrison and Rossiter, 1985); data from Ethiopia indicated that teenage women were twice as likely to die from pregnancy-related conditions as were women ages 20–24 (UN, 1989). In sum, pregnant adolescents have a higher likelihood of pregnancy-related complications and consequent risk of pregnancy-related mortality than women further along in their reproductive years; the risk rises again toward the end of those years.

Percent of Pregnancy-Related Deaths and Lifetime Risk of Dying

An illustrative measure of the level of maternal mortality is the percent of deaths among women of reproductive age that are pregnancy-related, as well as the lifetime risk of dying from maternal causes. In Asia and Africa, 21 to 46 percent of deaths among women ages 15–49 can be traced to pregnancy, compared with less than 1 percent in the United States (WHO, 1991b). In The Gambia, for example, Billewicsz and McGregor (1981) documented that 29 percent of all deaths of women aged 15–49 between 1951 and 1975 were caused by pregnancy. In a follow-up study in the same country, Greenwood and colleagues (1987) found that the percentage was still high: one out of every eight rural women was still dying in pregnancy or childbirth.

The likelihood that a woman will die in pregnancy or childbirth depends on how many times she is pregnant. The lifetime risk of maternal mortality is many times greater than ratios indicate, because the ratio ignores the effect of repeated pregnancies; each pregnancy adds to total lifetime risk (Walsh et al., 1993). Because women in Africa have many pregnancies, their lifetime risk of dying is elevated. WHO (1991b) estimates that, given a maternal mortality ratio of 640/100,000 live births and an average of 6.4 children per woman, the average lifetime risk for a woman is 1 in 21. It can rise as high as 1 in 15, especially in rural areas, where women have more children and many more pregnancies. In comparison, the lifetime chance of a maternal death in North America is 1 in 6,366 (Merchant and Kurz, 1992), and in Bangladesh, it is 1 in 25 to 1 in 49 (Figure 4-2). Overall, pregnancy in Africa is a more hazardous experience than it is in other parts of the world.

Estimates of Maternal Morbidity

Despite all the difficulties associated with the study of mortality, the study of morbidity is still more complicated. In the context of pregnancy, childbirth, or the puerperium, a death is an unmistakable event. In contrast, an illness associated with those periods of female reproductive life can progress slowly, sometimes imperceptibly; the reproductive origins of long-term or delayed morbidity (such as prolapse) can be tricky to ascertain, and misclassifications are frequent (Liskin, 1992). It is also the case that an illness may not be defined as such because of prevailing views of what is normative (for example, goiter). Many women require some convalescence even after an uncomplicated delivery; postpartum ailments, such as stress incontinence, are seen as unavoidable (Liskin,

TABLE 4-2 Maternal Mortality in Sub-Saharan Africa

Country	Female Population Ages 15–49 (1,000s), 1990	Maternal Mortality/ 100,000 Live Births		
		Ratio	Year	Source
Angola	2,273	113	1973	a
Benin	1,068	160	1981	b
Botswana	294	200–300	1981–85	a
Burkina Faso	2,065	810	1986	a
Burundi	1,237	—	—	—
Cameroon	2,526	430	1980s	b
Cape Verde	94	107	1980	a
Central African Rep	721	—	—	—
Chad	1,323	858	1972	a
Comoros	104	500	1980	a
Congo, PR of	506	1,000	1971	b
Cote d'Ivoire	2,527	—	—	—
Djibouti	92	700	1980s	b
Equatorial Guinea	84	430	1987	b
Ethiopia	10,839	2,000	1972	a
Gabon	269	—	—	—
Gambia, The	200	1,500	1984	b
Ghana	3,287	500–1,500	1984	a
Guinea	1,315	—	—	—
Guinea-Bissau	233	—	—	—
Kenya	4,980	168	1977	a
Lesotho	410	—	—	—
Liberia	553	—	—	—
Madagascar	2,542	403	1984	a
Malawi	1,946	167	1987	b
Mali	1,959	1,750–2,900	1987	a
Mauritania	455			
Mauritius	306	99	1987	a
Mozambique	3,653	300	1981	a
Namibia	1,818[c]	—	—	—
Niger	1,704	700	1988	b
Nigeria	25,726	800	1988	b
Reunion	580[c]	31	1985	a
Rwanda	1,558	210	1982	a
Senegal	1,645	600	1981–85	b
Sierra Leone	945	450	1980	b
Somalia	1,393	1,100	1981	b
South Africa	34,492[c]	—	—	—
Sudan	5,562	—	—	—
Swaziland	172	120	1982	—
Tanzania	5,855	185	1979–89	a
Togo	823	87	1977	—
Uganda	3,789	300	1984	b
Zaire	8,077	—	—	—
Zambia	1,814	151	1983	b
Zimbabwe	2,282	77	1988	a

[a]Civil registration data, government estimates.
[b]Other national estimates.
[c]UN Demographic Yearbook, 1991.

SOURCES: Population estimates are from the World Bank, 1992. Maternal mortality ratios are from WHO, 1991b.

88

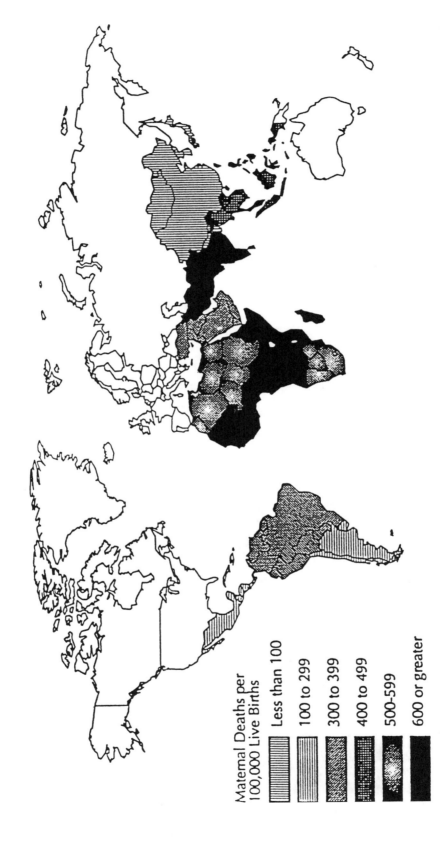

Maternal Deaths per
100,000 Live Births

Less than 100

100 to 299

300 to 399

400 to 499

500-599

600 or greater

FIGURE 4-1 Maternal mortality in Sub-Saharan Africa. SOURCE: WHO, 1991b.

89

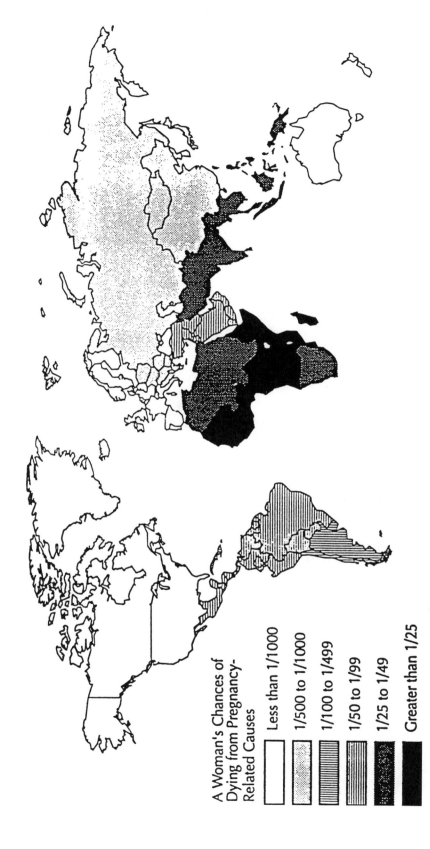

FIGURE 4-2 A woman's lifetime risk of maternal death, by region. Around the world, women's lifetime risk of dying from pregnancy-related causes varies 500-fold—from 1 in 20 in tropical Africa to 1 in 10,000 in Northern Europe. Lifetime risk (R) is calculated using the maternal mortality ratio (MMR) and the total fertility rate (TFR). $R = 1 - (1 - MMR)^{(1.2TFR)}$ SOURCE: Lettenmaier et al., 1988.

1992; Tahzib, 1989; WHO, 1991a); and health care providers and their clients may define illness in divergent, and sometimes dangerous, ways. Nausea, vomiting, swollen hands, and fatigue are usually considered minor complaints and are rarely addressed (Lettenmaier et al., 1988; Liskin, 1992). Composite conditions, such as "maternal depletion syndrome"—a term that describes the cumulative effects of multiple and frequent pregnancies, overlapping periods of lactation and pregnancy, the burdens of work, and maternal nutritional deficiencies (Herz and Measham, 1987; Merchant et al., 1990)—are hard to quantify and may not be regarded as "maternal" *per se.*

Another issue has to do with attribution. Pregnancy-associated illnesses may be either caused or aggravated by pregnancy. For instance, hypertension found during the course of pregnancy or puerperium may stem from preeclampsia, essential (preexisting) hypertension, or chronic renal disease, and the relative proportions of those etiologies in African women do not seem to follow the patterns found in Americans of African origin (Shaper et al., 1974). In addition, when women are reluctant to seek treatment or supply accurate information, as in the case of clandestine abortion, the nature and level of morbidity is, once more, significantly underestimated.

For every maternal death worldwide, it is thought that another 16 women suffer serious health consequences from either pregnancy or childbirth (Mahler, 1987; Royston and Armstrong, 1989). If a similar ratio holds true in Africa, then for the 150,000 women who die each year from those causes, another 2.4 million women incur some morbidity or disability.

As in the case of maternal mortality, estimates of maternal morbidity are typically derived from hospital studies. Many women in Sub-Saharan Africa do not present at hospital, for a variety of reasons. Women who do present at hospital tend to do so because of an acute condition, even though they may have longer-term problems that may or may not be related to the current pregnancy. This further affects the representativeness and completeness of pregnancy-related morbidity data (Liskin, 1992).

Trends

Knowledge about trends in maternal morbidity and mortality in Africa is limited, partly because it is difficult and costly to conduct the necessary research once, much less several times. Given the underlying problems of data, the lack of plausible baseline information, and the issues of definition discussed above, it is not surprising that the studies that are available are inconclusive. Only Mauritius reliably demonstrated a downward trend in maternal mortality between 1972 and 1987 (WHO, 1991b). This is a function of the country's pattern of social and economic development, which has fostered such improvements in maternal health (UNDP, 1994) and, as noted earlier, a good system of vital statistics that permit its documentation. In a study of ten hospitals between 1973 and 1985, Chukudebelu and Ozumba (1988) found no consistent pattern of decline in maternal mortality and attributed that finding primarily to data deficiencies. Greenwood and colleagues (1987) encountered no observable improvement in pregnancy outcomes in rural areas of The Gambia during their approximately 20 years of work there. WHO reports that, while there seems to be little evidence of an overall decline in maternal mortality in Africa (WHO, 1987b), maternal mortality declined an average of 4 to 9 percent between 1960 and 1975 in the Americas, Europe, Japan, and selected Asian countries (Petros-Barvazian, 1984). Decline was greatest in countries that had the lowest levels at the start of the study.

Part of the lack of significant change in Africa is in some part the result of larger dynamics: political upheaval, civil war, a variety of economic traumas, health system strikes, famine, and disease outbreaks, each of which can do its part to quickly erase any previous health gains. Getting a clear picture of what has actually happened in real epidemiologic terms is also confounded by fertility dynamics and socioeconomic variability. A fall in fertility will automatically "translate" into a fall in the number of maternal deaths, because fewer women will be exposed to the risks of pregnancy in a given period; this does not necessarily mean that the level of obstetric risk has fallen as well, and may vary significantly by socioeconomic subgroup. It is also possible that maternal mortality will fall because of other factors, even when overall fertility rates remain high (Graham, 1991; Winikoff and Sullivan, 1987).

THE NATURE OF MATERNAL MORTALITY AS A PUBLIC HEALTH PROBLEM

Maternal mortality is unlike other public health problems in several ways. First, although mortality is an ever-present threat, most women wish to be pregnant and to deliver a child at least once in their lives. Thus, although primary prevention is not entirely relevant, the prevention of *unwanted* pregnancy is not simply crucial, it is the single most important preventive intervention.

Second, maternal mortality has multiple clinical causes. In this, it is similar to infant mortality and, like infant mortality, it is an event defined by time rather than by cause. But unlike infant mortality, there are no magic bullets—no Expanded Programme of Immunization (EPI) or oral rehydration therapy (ORT)—with which to respond.

Third, cure plays a central role in reducing maternal mortality. Once a woman is pregnant, only a few of the conditions that lead to maternal mortality can be prevented; the actual saving of lives, or cure, is generally dependent on appropriate response.

Prediction, Prevention, and Cure

Prevention is a fundamental principle of public health. Its core strategies are to target high-risk groups and to apply interventions of known effectiveness—routine immunizations, breastfeeding, family planning, nutrition education, and food supplements are classic examples, together with early detection of disease through interview, screening procedures, physical examination, and early intervention. It is uncommon for curative measures to be a focus of public health interventions; oral rehydration therapy in the treatment of childhood diarrhea is a notable exception. For reasons discussed below, strategies that address maternal mortality and morbidity are another—and important—exception.

Prediction: Risk Factors and the Utility of Risk Scores

The risks of maternal mortality and morbidity can be assigned to two major categories: (1) maternal, or "host," characteristics, including age, parity, stature, and underlying or concurrent disease; and (2) community characteristics, primarily location and isolation, whose main effects have to do with the availability and quality of health care. Not all the traditionally accepted risk factors are of equal predictive value, and some of the traditional wisdom that has accumulated around them is questionable; a classic study in Kasongo, Zaire, catalogs some of the difficulties in risk-factor scoring systems for maternal mortality and inspires caution (Kasongo Project Team, 1983). At the same time, there are risk factors that can be useful in identifying women who require special attention. Of course, this does not mean that women with no risk factors will have uncomplicated deliveries.

Maternal Characteristics

Age and Parity Women who are too old, too young, or have had too many pregnancies are at higher risk of obstetric complications; birth interval is an additional and confounding factor (Graham, 1991). The definitions of "old," "young," and "many" are, of course, debated. Regardless of the precise definitions, adolescents (< 16), older women (> 40), primiparae ($P = 0$), and grandmultiparae ($P > 4$) are all more likely to experience a complication during pregnancy or delivery, and their infants are more likely to die before, during, or soon after birth. Very young women, whose pelvic bone growth is still not completed, are more likely to have a narrow birth canal, the leading cause of difficult deliveries that prolong labor and increase the risk of obstetric fistulae. Young women and primiparae are more likely to develop hypertension and eclampsia. Both young unmarried women and older mothers with several children are more likely to seek abortions because of unwanted pregnancies.

At the same time, there are subsets of risk where attribution is less clear. For instance, it is widely believed that grandmultiparae are at increased risk of postpartum hemorrhage. Yet a recent analysis of 9,598 vaginal births in the United States (3.9 percent of which involved a postpartum hemorrhage) found that risk of hemorrhage was

TABLE 4-3   The Value of Height as a Predictor of Cesarean Section (CS) for Cephalopelvic Disproportion (CPD), Ouagadougou, Burkina Faso (percent)

Height (cm)	At Each Cut-off Point CS for CPD	Sensitivity	Specificity
< 150	48.8 (2/41)	8	98
150–154	46.7 (10/214)	46	86
155–159	17.2 (8/466)	77	59
160–164	10.8 (6/553)	100	26
165–169	0 (0/342)	170+	0(0/98)

NOTE: *Sensitivity* is defined as the percentage of women with a problem (CS for CPD) who were identified as high-risk (2/26 = 8 percent at 150 centimeters; 12/26 = 46 percent at 155 centimeters). *Specificity* is defined as the percentage identified as low-risk who had no problem (no CS for CPD [1,649/1,673 = 98 percent at 150 centimeters; 1,459/1,688 = 86 percent at 155 centimeters]).

SOURCE: Adapted from Sokal et al., 1991.

not correlated with greater parity. The most robust risk factor in this study was primiparity *per se*; preeclampsia was also (independently) strongly associated with hemorrhage (Combs et al., 1991). The vast majority of primiparae deliver safely, and the proportion of postpartum hemorrhages that occur to primiparae will depend simply on the proportion of births to women having their first births, a proportion that is lower in Africa than elsewhere in the world because absolute parity in the region is so high.

Stature   In general, very short women are more likely to have obstructed labors; as a group they can thus be expected to account for more cesarean sections (CS) (Sokal et al., 1991; see Table 4-3), both because they require them and because there is some predilection among physicians to section small women as a matter of course.

There are some methodologic questions about maternal height as a predictor for obstructed labor. Although the measure is commonly utilized as a risk factor for that obstetric event, most often with a maternal height of 150 cm used as the critical cutoff point, Table 4-3 suggests that it is a poor measure. Of 26 women who had a cesarean section for cephalopelvic disproportion (CPD), only 8 percent would have been correctly predicted with a cutoff of 150 cm; that figure rises to 46 percent if the cutoff is raised to 155 cm. Looked at another way, of women defined as "at risk"—that is, under 150 cm in height—95 percent did not have a cesarean section. As a consequence, the study authors (Sokal et al., 1991) recommend a 155-cm cutoff as a more sensitive and specific predictor. It is important to call attention to the risks of drawing conclusions from such a small sample; this is a point of general relevance for health policy recommendations in Sub-Saharan Africa, because there are still so few studies of the size and scientific rigor required to permit comfortable inferences (W. Graham, personal communication, 1994)

Underlying, Latent, and Concurrent Disease   A number of conditions and health events can coincide with pregnancy and childbirth and conspire to elevate the degree of risk to fetus, mother, and infant. These can be divided into: (1) those that do not affect pregnancy and are not exacerbated by it and (2) those that either affect or are affected by pregnancy and delivery. Of the latter group, the most important for Sub-Saharan African women at present are HIV/AIDS, sexually transmitted diseases and other genital infections, tuberculosis, hepatitis, malaria and other parasitic diseases, iodine deficiency, genetic diseases (sickle-cell anemia, thalassemia), and certain chronic diseases (some cardiovascular diseases, diabetes, hypertension, renal disease, and cervical cancers). The majority of these are addressed in detail in the relevant chapters of this report. Women with any of these conditions require special vigilance during pregnancy and delivery, although an appropriate course of management is not always available. They must all be considered as possible clinical causes in the multiple causality of maternal death, which is taken up below. That African women continue heavy work late into pregnancy further compounds these risks (Feachem et al., 1989; Raikes, 1989).

Community Characteristics

Women who live in communities far from health facilities are not only more likely to experience complications of pregnancy and delivery, but are also less likely to receive adequate treatment for those complications (Thaddeus and Maine, 1990). They are also at risk if they live in communities that are isolated for other reasons—such as weather that makes roads impassable in the rainy season or geographic factors such as water barriers—risk that is compounded in remote or isolated villages that lack telecommunications, as most do. Finally, women and their communities can be isolated for cultural reasons: nomads, refugees, and members of particular religious or ethnic groups are notable examples. Women who are directly isolated by culturally rooted seclusion, or *purdah*, or indirectly by illiteracy or age, may also be less likely to receive adequate care during pregnancy and delivery. It is absolutely crucial to keep in mind that the usual co-variates of remoteness in Sub-Saharan Africa are poverty, poor nutritional status and short stature, and illiteracy, which have their own strong and independent influence on all aspects of the reproductive process.

It was for these reasons that a seminal multidisciplinary review (Thaddeus and Maine, 1990) was keyed to the "three phases of delay" that block the effective treatment of an obstetric complication in many developing countries: (1) delay in the decision to seek care (lack of information about complications, lack of women's autonomy), (2) delay in reaching appropriate care (bad roads, no affordable transportation), and (3) delay in the provision of adequate care (shortages of qualified staff, clinical mismanagement, lack of essential drugs and supplies, and the like). The "three delays" provided the theoretical and structural underpinnings of the Prevention of Maternal Mortality Network, which has been established as a major component of the Safe Motherhood Initiative (Carnegie Corporation, 1993). This focus does not in any way imply a disregard for the very fundamental problems of large numbers of early teenage primigravidae, high parity, and lack of antenatal care (Harrison and Rossiter, 1985).

Calculations of Risk

High-risk pregnancies are usually defined as those occurring before age 18 and after age 35, those among women with more than four births, and those less than two years apart (Herz and Measham, 1987; Royston and Armstrong, 1989).

The use of a risk-scoring system has intuitive appeal, and many physicians instinctively do their own informal calculations. A formal risk-scoring system assigns a score to each risk factor and then totals them to get a combined risk score; women with multiple risk factors obviously get higher scores. Such approaches can be helpful, but all systems developed so far have a large number of false positives (women with high scores who have uncomplicated deliveries), false negatives (women with low scores who experience a complication), poor sensitivity (women with complications who received a low score), and poor specificity (women with no complication who received a high score). Furthermore, in some populations nearly all women have at least one risk factor (Fortney and Whitehorne, 1982). Although there are indubitable risk factors for maternal mortality and morbidity, applying them rigidly to predict those events and conditions has its own hazards, the most important among them the sense of false security concerning women with low scores. Overall, previous obstetric history is probably the most valuable predictor of obstetric difficulties in a current pregnancy. It is useless for application to the prospects for primiparae, however, since they have no history to call upon. In sum, a major challenge in achieving "safe motherhood" is the great difficulty of predicting which women will develop complications based on easily measurable characteristics. With few exceptions, it is hard to identify "proneness" to obstetric complications (W. Graham, personal communication, 1994), so that the risk approach to maternity care may not be the best option for reducing maternal deaths in developing countries. By virtue of the greater representation of "low-risk" and "no-risk" women in the female population, more actual cases of obstetric complication occur in these groups in absolute numbers than among women identified as being at high risk (Ekwempu, 1993; Maine, 1991).

TABLE 4-4 A Paradigm for Prevention of Maternal Mortality

Condition	Before Pregnancy	During Pregnancy	During Delivery	Response Only
Postpartum hemorrhage	No	Yes; raising hemoglobin to enhance tolerance of blood loss prevents some deaths.	Yes; active management of 3rd stage of labor prevents some postpartum hemorrhage	Blood transfusion, oxytocics
Obstruction	Yes; adequate nutrition in childhood and adolescence prevents some obstruction. Delaying pregnancy until full growth is attained will have a comparable effect. No	No	Yes; use of partogram	Prompt cesarean section if appropriate
Eclampsia	No	Yes; monitoring blood pressure	Yes; monitoring blood pressure	Drug therapy, bed rest
Sepsis	No	No; except possibly reducing anemia	Yes, clean delivery technique	Antibiotics
Abortion	Yes; access to family planning	No	No	Appropriate management of complications

Prevention

As suggested by the discussion of the risk approach, application of the term "prevention" to maternal mortality and morbidity is ambiguous. The most common clinical causes of maternal death—hemorrhage, obstructed labor, eclampsia, sepsis, and abortion—cannot be prevented in the strict, proximate sense of the term, because so many of these problems are rooted in conditions and events beginning with the mother's own conception. At the same time, mortality and prolonged morbidity from virtually all those causes can be prevented by appropriate and timely medical response. Table 4-4 presents a paradigm for the "prevention" of maternal mortality that displays the spectrum of possibilities for intervention across the female life span.

Cure

The appropriate medical responses to the complications of pregnancy have, for the most part, been known for decades. In the developed world, maternal mortality from hemorrhage and sepsis declined dramatically in the 1940s and 1950s, when cross-matching of blood became possible and the sulfa drugs and antibiotics were developed. Mortality from obstructed labor had declined still earlier, when surgical skills for cesarean section improved and anesthetic techniques were refined. There was no comparable breakthrough in reducing mortality from eclampsia, although case-fatality rates started to decline in the 1950s as sedatives came into use in the clinical management of the condition. Mortality from complications of abortion was also reduced through blood transfusion and antibiotics. None of these medical responses is especially "high tech," and all should be within the skills of general physicians (and some nonphysicians) with basic surgical skills.

Reviews of maternal deaths often reveal that clinical management of the cases under analysis, even when technically correct, was sadly delayed or delivered by a practitioner with too little experience. Appropriate medical response involves knowing not just what to do and how to do it, but having the resources (drugs, operating rooms, blood supply, and the like) to respond, having the suitable personnel, and responding soon enough. These issues are addressed below in the context of health services as crucial variables in the multiple causality of maternal death, and deficits in these areas belong at the top of the list of factors that should be considered "avoidable."

THE MULTIPLE CAUSALITY OF MATERNAL DEATH

At the 1987 Safe Motherhood Conference in Nairobi, Kenya, Professor Mahmoud Fathalla described the death of "Mrs. X" (Fathalla, 1987; see Box 4-1). Clinical cause of death was hypovolemia from antepartum hemorrhage, but there were eight other nonclinical contributing factors. The cardinal point of this landmark presentation was that the probability of "safe motherhood" is enhanced by healthy, literate women having wanted pregnancies; focused and effective prenatal care; accessible, affordable, and appropriate attention for normal deliveries and obstetric emergencies; and physicians and other health care providers who are suitably trained and have adequate access to necessary drugs and services. Although these elements are of unequal importance, the failure of a society to provide any one of them should be considered a contributor to maternal mortality, as well as morbidity.

For purposes of this analysis, the multiple causes of maternal death are sorted into three categories: clinical causes, health services issues, and sociocultural factors. These obviously overlap, but there is utility in considering them separately.

Clinical Causes

Distinguishing among individual causes for diagnostic and reporting purposes is not straightforward. Immediate and underlying causes may be confused—for example, cardiac failure and toxic shock. Different data sources are more likely to reveal some causes rather than others. For example, hemorrhage may be recorded either as hemorrhage or as retained placenta. Hospital reports are more likely to be deficient in recording deaths of a sudden nature, such as a massive postpartum hemorrhage, compared with deaths from causes with a less rapid progression, such as sepsis. Complications from induced abortion may be coded as such, or without any reference to abortion. Indirect causes of maternal mortality such as pneumonia, tuberculosis, cerebral malaria, and diarrheal diseases may be completely masked under some category called "Other" (Graham, 1991).

BOX 4-1
Why Did Mrs. X Die?

* Hypovolemia, due to antepartum hemorrhage.
* Lack of blood for transfusion.
* Delay in seeking treatment. Failure to recognize significance of antenatal bleeding.
* Anemia due to parasites and poor diet.
* No antenatal care which might have recognized significance of bleeding, and treated the anemia and the parasites.
* High age and parity (Mrs X was 39 and had 7 babies). She wanted no more children.
* No access to family planning.
* Mrs X lived in a remote village with no access to transportation.
* Mrs X was illiterate and poor.

SOURCE: Fathalla, 1987.

Anemia

The World Health Organization has estimated that 52 percent of pregnant women in Africa—56 percent in West Africa, 47 percent in Central Africa, and 54 percent in Middle Africa—have substandard hemoglobin levels (below 100g/L) (WHO, 1982). Severe anemia can contribute to maternal mortality by impairing a woman's ability to resist infection or to survive hemorrhage. A hospital-based study of maternal deaths in Malawi estimated that anemia contributed to 23 percent of those deaths (Keller, 1987). Very young mothers present a special situation: pregnant adolescents (< age 16) in Nigeria who received iron and folic acid supplements and antimalarials grew as much as 16 centimeters during pregnancy, thereby reducing their risk of obstructed births (Harrison et al., 1985a). Parasitic infestations also contribute to anemia; of the parasitic infestations, malaria seems to produce the most egregious insults; in females of reproductive age, mean hemoglobin values tend to be consistently lower in the presence of parasitemia, an association most marked in primiparas (McGregor, 1991; see also Chapter 10). Unfortunately, many of the currently preferred antiparasitic therapies, primarily those in the benzimidazole group, are counterindicated during pregnancy because of their presumed teratogenic effects.

Complications of Pregnancy and Delivery

The most common clinical causes of maternal death and chronic morbidity during pregnancy and delivery are anemia, eclampsia (convulsions resulting from hypertensive disease during pregnancy), hemorrhage, obstructed labor, sepsis, ruptured uterus, and unsafe induced abortion. Three-quarters of all maternal deaths can be attributed to hemorrhage, sepsis, or eclampsia (Graham, 1991). Conditions that can constitute an obstetric emergency include ectopic pregnancy, anesthetic accidents, embolisms from blood clots or amniotic fluid that may result from oxytocin induction, trauma, or medical emergencies associated with such underlying conditions as those discussed earlier.

Hemorrhage and Retained Placenta Bleeding during pregnancy may indicate several conditions, including, in early pregnancy, threatened abortion. Later in pregnancy, it suggests problems in placentation; ideally, women who bleed should receive careful follow-up and deliver in a facility with an operating room. Because bleeding is an easily recognized condition, it is, in principle, more likely to receive medical attention than less apparent conditions. Nonetheless, its significance is often underestimated by pregnant women, and even by many health care providers. The gravity of postpartum hemorrhage can be difficult to define: "excessive" bleeding is a subjective assessment and actual blood loss is rarely accurately measured. Yet in anemic women, even a small amount of blood loss is poorly tolerated.

Retained placenta is defined as a placenta, or placental part, that is not delivered within two hours after delivery of the infant. It has several possible causes, including uterine atony, anomalies of placentation such as *placenta accreta*, or even a full bladder. Retained placenta or too rapid separation of the placenta (for example, by pulling too hard on the cord) may also cause uterine bleeding.

Interventions to prevent postpartum hemorrhage include careful management of the third stage of labor—that is, appropriate delivery of the placenta—and maintaining an empty bladder. Interventions to treat postpartum hemorrhage include use of oxytocins after delivery of the infant, nipple stimulation after delivery (although this practice is controversial), massage of the uterus, bimanual pressure, packing (also controversial and a last resort), and transfusion of whole blood or other fluids. Occasionally, hysterectomy is necessary.

Postpartum hemorrhage is one of the most common reasons for blood transfusion, an intervention that may be overused in some settings and, since the advent of AIDS, bears additional risks. Although postpartum hemorrhage is potentially fatal, women who survive it rarely suffer long-term consequences.

Sepsis Infection can occur when aseptic procedures are not followed, when the amniotic sac ruptures long before delivery occurs, when vaginal examinations are too frequent, or when prolonged or obstructed labor occurs. Long-term consequences of puerperal sepsis include pelvic inflammatory disease (PID), secondary infertility, and, although uncommon, maternal tetanus.

Infection is the most preventable of the obstetric emergencies. Training of traditional birth attendants in "the three cleans" (clean hands, clean surface for delivery, clean cord care), attention to antisepsis in hospitals and maternity homes, judicious use of antibiotics and fluid support in case of prolonged rupture of membranes, and treatment of anemia to enhance resistance to infection are all solid, low-cost preventive interventions.

Obstructed Labor Obstruction occurs when an infant cannot readily pass through the birth canal because of disproportion between its size and the size of its mother's pelvis, because of a pelvic distortion, because of a transverse lie, or because of severe scarring from female genital mutilation (FGM). Unattended, obstruction characteristically leads to prolonged labor (variously defined as more than 18 or more than 24 hours), and sometimes to rupture of the uterus. Obstructed labor can also result in other complications, including necrosing of tissue in the vagina or uterus that can lead to death or, at a minimum, produce highly burdensome morbidity, including secondary infertility or obstruction in subsequent births. Obstruction can also increase the risk of obstetric fistulae, a tearing of the walls between the vagina and bladder or rectum. Women with unrepaired fistulae constantly drip urine or feces and may frequently be ostracized by both their husbands and the community (Tahzib, 1983). Often, such women are quite young: in Nigeria, 33 percent of fistulae cases involved women under age 16; in Niger, 80 percent were between the ages of 15 and 19.

No other complication of delivery is associated with as much chronic morbidity as obstructed labor. While it cannot be prevented, its most severe consequences can be avoided or attenuated by intervention. Use of the partogram during labor leads to early detection of problems, permitting timely intervention, generally cesarean section. While symphysiotomy has some advocates, its use remains controversial (van Roosmalen, 1987). Operative delivery usually requires antibiotics, rehydration, and blood transfusion or plasma expanders.

Hypertensive Disorders Hypertensive disease of pregnancy appears to be most common among primigravidas. The pattern of increased risk for younger primigravidas, below age 20, may be less a reflection of increased physiologic risk than of other differences between this group and women who have their first child at ages 20 to 24 (Zimicki, 1989). These are the most difficult of the obstetric emergencies to prevent and manage, as well as the least understood, yet they are an important cause of maternal death in many areas of Africa. Prevention includes monitoring blood pressure during pregnancy and watching for edema, especially of the hands and face. Clinical trials are underway to determine whether daily administration of low-dose aspirin reduces the incidence of preeclamptic toxemia and eclampsia. Unfortunately for predictive purposes, not all episodes of eclampsia are preceded by preeclamptic toxemia, or even by hypertension.

Treatment of eclampsia includes rapid delivery of the infant, by cesarean section if necessary, and administration of either magnesium sulfate or diazepam. While diazepam is widely available, magnesium sulfate is rarely available below the level of tertiary hospitals. Although eclampsia is potentially fatal, women who recover usually suffer no long-lasting effects, although hypertension may prove persistent.

Abortion The emergencies associated with the complications of clandestine abortion are the same as those related to delivery: that is, infection and bleeding. Treatment is therefore similar. More serious complications can be avoided by prompt aspiration of the uterus to remove remaining products of conception. This can be done in many health centers if staff are appropriately trained and equipment is available. Primary prevention through family planning is preferred.

Response Times The most common obstetric complications vary in their demands for speed. Maine and colleagues (1987) have estimated the average interval from onset to death for the major obstetric complications, absent medical intervention (Table 4-5).

Sociocultural Factors: Traditional Medical Practices

There is a large body of traditional medical practice in Sub-Saharan Africa that is highly pertinent to obstetric

TABLE 4-5   Estimated Average Interval from Onset to Death

Complication	Hours	Days
Hemorrhage: postpartum	2	
Hemorrhage: antepartum	12	
Ruptured uterus		1
Eclampsia		2
Obstructed labor		3
Infection		6

SOURCE: Maine et al., 1987.

mortality and morbidity, either because of the positive contributions those practices make to female health, or because they may be deleterious. These comprise the traditional management of pregnancy, labor, and delivery, customarily a responsibility of traditional birth attendants (TBAs); food prescriptions and proscriptions associated with the pre- and postpartum periods of a woman's life, which are addressed in Chapter 3; and the traditional procedures that have been customarily termed "female circumcision," but are increasingly referred to as "female genital mutilation." This latter group is discussed, from different perspectives, in this chapter and in Chapter 2.

Of all geographic regions, Africa has the lowest percentage of births attended by trained personnel (Starrs, 1987) and the highest maternal mortality rates (Walsh et al., 1993). The degree to which that mortality and related morbidity can be attributed to harmful traditional practices is almost impossible to measure. A recent study in Nigeria determined that 4 percent of reported maternal deaths were attributable to such practices (WHO, 1991b). The authors' view, however, is that such attributions are highly tenuous, and that it is more useful to look at what is known about the practices in themselves, and to ask which among them are objectively harmful. It is equally important to be clear about what practices are beneficial, so that those can be encouraged and preserved.

The Traditional Birth Attendant

Throughout the developing world, there is a large arsenal of customary behavior employed to deal with the period from pregnancy through the puerperium. The prime custodian of this arsenal is the TBA, who dominates the obstetric and gynecologic picture in Sub-Saharan Africa. TBAs cover 40 percent of deliveries in Lesotho, 45 percent in Malawi, 50 percent in Swaziland, 60 percent in Tanzania, 70 percent in Zimbabwe, and 77 percent in Botswana (Kaiser Family Foundation, 1993). Their numbers appear to be declining in some areas; in Tanzania, for example, the midwife/live-birth ratio has declined by 50 percent in the last ten years (Kwast, 1991).

Generally a highly esteemed, local older woman, the TBA is considered an authority on the traditional medical practices associated with childbearing, as well as childrearing, traditional methods of family planning, and the treatment of infertility. Birth attendants or other traditional healers are from the community, speak the local language, charge modest fees or accept payment in kind, and, patients insist, can handle the common exertions of childbirth. Equally important, they provide strong emotional support during and following labor. Thus, in some African countries, such as Ghana, TBAs, already highly regarded by local populations, have been given medical and paramedical training and have proven to be valuable adjuncts to the government health care system and to other community and traditional practitioners. Success is not inevitable: in Nigeria, relationships between TBAs and untrained traditional midwives were strained enough to require remedial attention (Okafor, 1991). It is also possible that the indigenous setting does not offer a solid basis for such training: in some ethnic groups, women are expected to experience labor in stoic solitude, and the birth attendant is called in only to cut the umbilical cord, wash the baby, and ritually bury the placenta.

The initial focus of many TBA training programs worldwide has been on practices that are important to the well-being of the neonate, primarily prevention of tetanus and ocular hygiene. The second area of training deals with practices related to potentially life-threatening situations for the mother: hemorrhage, obstructed labor, and maternal sepsis.

Treatment of hemorrhage relies on locally available herbal medicines; while these may not in themselves do harm, the delay involved before more appropriate care can be reached may prove fatal. Somewhat analogous is utilization of oxytocin-containing medicines and equivalent substances, often ergot derivatives, to induce or accelerate labor (Zimicki, 1989). These are available in pharmacies or in traditional forms and can be beneficial in the postpartum period for restoring uterine tonus. At the same time, because they produce quick, strong, and sustained contractions, they can produce uterine rupture when employed during labor itself. When oxytocins in herbal form are inserted directly into the vagina, there is a high risk of intrauterine infection and tetanus. A study in Kenya reported rates of upper reproductive tract infections that were approximately 10 times the rates in developed countries; one cause of such infection was the introduction of foreign objects such as leaves, earth, or cow dung into the birth canal by untrained birth attendants for purposes of inducing or hastening labor or halting hemorrhage (Plummer et al., 1987). Whether pharmaceutical or herbal, the misuse of uterine stimulants has been implicated in deaths from obstructed labor and ruptured uterus, and many of the herbal medicines used to facilitate labor in East and West Africa seem to contain ingredients with definite oxytocic action (Egwuatu, 1986).

Another source of infection cited in the same study was the entry of germs into the genital tract by use of unsterilized instruments and by insertion of unwashed hands during vaginal examination by the untrained midwife, usually to ascertain the degree of cervical dilation. A TBA must also confront such emergency situations as fetal malpresentation. An understandable but regrettable response is vaginal manipulation, forcible internal version of the fetus, and vigorous handling of the parturient herself, all behaviors with high risks of infection, excessive blood loss, or both (Beddada, 1982; Modawi, 1982). Expulsion of the placenta, particularly in the case of retained placenta, may evoke such forcible and deleterious interventions as pulling the umbilical cord out, reaching into the birth canal to extract it, or forcing a gagging reflex (Otoo, 1973), rather than relying on natural contractions or gentle abdominal massage to effect expulsion. The longer and more difficult the labor, the more likely it is that a TBA will resort to extreme measures, the longer those may last, and the higher the risks.

As is the case in recent evaluations of the impact of training community health workers (CHW) on community health status, assessment of the effectiveness of TBAs has been largely focused on their effect on child survival, because TBA training has placed considerable emphasis on such relevant practices as antisepsis to prevent neonatal tetanus through anti-tetanus immunization and hygienic management of the umbilicus. In these respects, TBA training programs in Burkina Faso, Liberia, Malawi, Mozambique, Senegal, Sierra Leone, and Zaire have produced real decreases in neonatal mortality attributable to tetanus (Ewbank, 1993). In The Gambia, however, a mortality survey to assess the impact of a TBA program on maternal mortality showed no effect (Knippenberg et al., 1990), although, as suggested at the outset of this chapter, the relative infrequency of maternal deaths is a problem for any evaluative exercise.

The value of TBAs to their communities in general, and to women in particular, could be substantial; an especially useful and supportive body of evidence for this effect is the comprehensive ethnographic work of Sargent in Benin (Sargent, 1977, 1982, 1985). When access to nondomiciliary birthing facilities is severely limited, as it is in much of Sub-Saharan Africa, having someone who is experienced and nearby is, in itself, highly positive. The traditional practices of massage, motivation for breastfeeding, and an attitude of support for the parturient are absolutely desirable. In Ghana, the general sense is that even when good-quality maternity care is accessible, by custom women prefer to deliver at home, assisted by a traditional midwife or relative (Carnegie Corporation, 1993).

Trained for appropriate management of pregnancy and perinatal risk, for recognition of warning signs, and stabilization and referral as appropriate, the traditional midwife has the potential to be a crucial ally in resource-constrained environments. At the same time, there is ample evidence that where there has been no clearly mandated and well-defined connection to an existing health system, where supervision and support have been inconsistent, and where necessary logistical support has failed, the involvement of community workers, including TBAs, in health care delivery inevitably crumbles (Herz and Measham, 1987; World Bank, 1994).

Gishiri Cuts

The *Gishiri* cut is a traditional procedure among the Hausa in northern Nigeria in which the vagina is cut, usually by a traditional healer, typically an older woman, for the purpose of treating a number of gynecologic and obstetric conditions (Harrison and Rossiter, 1985). These include amenorrhea, urinary dysfunction (dysuria), backache, infertility, painful intercourse (dyspareunia), and prolonged labor. The intervention consists of cuts in the anterior and, sometimes, posterior area of the vagina. Hemorrhage, reproductive tract infections, and vesico-vaginal fistula are common complications. Tahzib (1983) found that 13 percent of all fistula diagnoses in his sample of 1,443 women were directly attributable to *gishiri* cuts, particularly in older females. It is sometimes the case that *gishiri* incisions are superficial, and therefore less potentially deleterious, but the percentages of cases, where, and under what circumstances this more superficial intervention occurs are completely unknown. There also appears to be little systematic knowledge of how extensively the practice is employed by TBAs during childbirth as a form of episiotomy.

Female Genital Mutilation (FGM)

Three types of FGM are practiced: *sunna* circumcision, which involves removal of the prepuce of the clitoris, with the clitoris itself preserved; excision or clitoridectomy, which involves removal of the prepuce and glans of the clitoris and the *labia minora*, with no intentional closure of the vulva; and infibulation or "Pharaonic circumcision," which involves removal of the clitoris, *labia minora*, and at least the anterior two-thirds, and often the entire medial part, of the labia majora, with the vulva sewn shut and a small opening left for urine and menstrual flow. The differences among the types of intervention reside in the extent of the procedure and the portions of the genitalia excised (see Table 4-6).

The intervention is practiced in some form, with varying prevalence, in a band that crosses Sub-Saharan Africa north of the equator, in a total of 26 Sub-Saharan African countries with an "affected population" of 114,296,900 (Table 4-7) (Toubia, 1993). Prevalence of each procedure varies not only geographically but, to some degree, by level of education (see Table 4-8). In a sample of over 3,000 women and 1,500 men, a major study in northern Sudan between 1977 and 1981 found level of education to be a powerful predictor: 75 percent of infibulated women were from illiterate families (El Dareer, 1982b), which suggests that they were also from poor families (World Bank, 1993). At the same time, the practice is not limited to females from the lower socioeconomic strata: for example, government-trained TBAs and nurse-midwives in northern Sudan are reported to provide the service to elite, educated women (Kheir et al., 1991).

The Procedure   Most excisions are performed by TBAs, trained midwives, or men and women identified within a group as having special skills, notably heads of secret societies (Lightfoot-Klein, 1989). The practice generally enhances the income of the practitioner, which some commentators (e.g., Hosken, 1982) perceive as an important

TABLE 4-6   Types of Female Circumcision

Type of Surgery	Description
Sunna circumcision (Type I)	Removal of the prepuce of the clitoris, while the clitoris itself is preserved. Recovery is approximately 7 days.
Excision (Type II)	Removal of prepuce and glans of the clitoris, and part or all of the labia minora. No (intended) closure of the vulva. Recovery is between 7 and 15 days.
Infibulation (Type III)	Removal of the clitoris, labia minora, and at least the anterior two-thirds and often the entire medial part of the labia majora. The vulva is sewn shut, leaving a small opening for urine and menstrual flow. Recovery is approximately 40 days.

consideration in its maintenance. Razor blades, scissors, kitchen knives, or sharp pieces of glass are among the tools used; in parts of Sierra Leone and a number of other countries, surgical scalpels are now in use. No general anesthetic is administered in most cases; local anesthesia may be administered and various indigenous herbs and medicines employed to stop bleeding and promote healing (Kheir et al., 1991). Antibiotics and tetanus toxoid are frequently unavailable. In urban areas, particularly among the elite, the procedure is likely to be performed by trained nursing persons or physicians in clinic or hospital settings under sterile conditions, suturing is done with catgut or silk, and anesthesia and antibiotics are used (Gordon, 1991).

Age at Time of Procedure   The age range of child and adolescent genital excision varies from a few days after birth into adulthood. In Sudan, it is performed at age 10, before puberty (Kheir, 1991); in most countries of West Africa, it is usually performed on adolescents between 11 and 15 years, less frequently at ages 5 to 6. In some areas it had not been uncommon in the past for the procedure to be performed directly prior to the marriage ceremony, but there now seems to be a tendency to perform the procedure at earlier ages (Lightfoot-Klein, 1989; Slack, 1988). Younger girls can be more easily restrained, so that excision tends to be more precise, and there is some feeling that the intervention is less traumatic for younger girls because their genitalia are less developed (Koso-Thomas, 1985).

Like circumcision for Sub-Saharan African males, FGM for females in many African societies is viewed as a rite of passage—that is, it marks movement from one major life stage to another—and is characteristically managed by secret societies. This explains some of the attitudinal context for the practice, and perhaps at least some of its persistence and prevalence.

Complications and Sequelae   Because even the most minimal forms of FGM are invasive, complications are frequent. Since so many of these complications can become chronic, they are usefully categorized by duration—immediate and long-term—and by their obstetric implications (Tables 4-9 and 4-10). The sequelae of infibulation are the most serious. For example, pelvic inflammatory diseases (PID) are three times more common in women who have been infibulated than in those who have not (Cook, 1982). In turn, recurrent PIDs are identified as one of the major causes of high infertility, even when antibiotic therapies are available; this is a very consequential side-effect in societies that place a high value on fecundity.

Immediate complications range from injury to adjacent structures, such as the urethra and anus, to severe hemorrhage and shock. There may also be acute site infection, beginning a recurring cycle of infection, and even minor infections can prove fatal in the absence of antibiotics. The practice of infibulation requires that the patient's legs be tied together from thighs to ankles to permit healing, but drainage is also impaired even with light bandaging, and the spread of infection into vagina and uterus is promoted (Verzin 1975, in Cook, 1982).

Long-term complications begin for girls when the passage of menstrual flow is impeded at the onset of menarche. The result is, at a minimum, discomfort; if the impedance (cryptomenorrhea) is substantial, pain is considerable and the risk of pelvic infection increases, which may lead to infertility (see Chapter 11, Sexually Transmitted Diseases). Attempts at penetration upon first intercourse may be effected through use of a knife or other sharp object; sepsis leading to PID is possible, and severe pain would seem to be inevitable. In the case of the *sunna* procedure, complete penetration requires three to seven days; if the woman has been excised, two to five weeks are required; and, after infibulation, complete penetration can take between two and twelve weeks to be effected (El Dareer, 1982b). Forcible penetration can cause development of a "false vagina" or lacerations of the perineum, rectum, and urethra. Long-term dyspareunia (painful intercourse) is common, and the sequelae of that condition may not only be felt physiologically, but also in interpersonal relations between spouses.

The very limited research into the effects of FGM on sexual arousal is inconclusive. Because the operation destroys sensitive nerve endings in the clitoris and *labia minora*, leaving only scar tissue, sexual arousal in excised women can be impaired or delayed (Bakr, 1982). Nevertheless, available published research is limited and contradictory. In a study of Nigerian women, Megafu (1983) found that the sexual urge in her sample was not impaired by removal of the clitoris; Koso-Thomas (1985) found that excised women were less likely to experience orgasm than unexcised women. El Dareer (1982b) reports that 75 percent of the women in her survey sample of 3,210 never experienced sexual pleasure or were indifferent.

TABLE 4-7　Female Genital Mutilation in Africa[a]

Country	Prevalence (%)	Actual Number	Notes
Benin*	50	1,200,000	
Burkina Faso*	70	3,290,000	
Cameroon*	—	—	Information on prevalence not available.
Central African Republic*	50	750,000	
Chad	60	1,530,000	Prevalence based upon 1990 and 1991 studies in three regions.
Côte d'Ivoire*	60	3,750,000	
Djibouti	98	196,000	Infibulation almost universally practiced. The Union Nationale des Femmes de Djibouti (UNFD) runs a clinic where a milder form of infibulation is performed under local anesthesia.
Egypt	50	13,625,000	Practiced throughout the country by both Muslims and Christians. Infibulation reported in areas of south Egypt closer to Sudan.
Ethiopia and Eritrea	90	23,940,000	Common among Muslims and Christians and practiced by Ethiopian Jews (Falashas), most of whom now live in Israel. Clitoridectomy is more common, except in areas bordering Sudan and Somalia, where infibulation seems to have spread.
Gambia*	60	270,000	
Ghana	30	2,325,000	A 1987 pilot survey in one community showed that 97% of interviewed women above age 47 were circumcised, while 48% of those under 20 were not.
Guinea*	50	1,875,000	
Guinea Bissau*	50	250,000	
Kenya	50	6,300,000	Decreasing in urban areas, but remains strong in rural areas, primarily around the Rift Valley. 1992 studies in four regions found that the age for circumcision ranged from eight to 13 years, and traditional practitioners usually operated on a group of girls at one time without much cleaning of the knife between procedures.
Liberia*	60	810,000	
Mali*	75	3,112,500	
Mauritania*	25	262,500	
Niger*	20	800,000	
Nigeria	50	30,625,000	Two national studies conducted, but not released. A study of Bendel state reported widespread clitoridectomy among all ethnic groups, including Christians, Muslims, and animists.
Senegal	20	750,000	Predominantly in the north and southeast. Only a minority of Muslims, who constitute 95% of the population, practice FGM.
Sierra Leone	90	1,935,000	All ethnic groups practice FGM except for Christian Krios in the western region and in the capital, Freetown.
Somalia	98	3,773,000	FGM is universal; approximately 80% of the operations are infibulation.
Sudan (North)	89	9,220,400	A very high prevalence, predominantly infibulation, throughout most of the northern, eastern and western regions. Along with a small overall decline in the 1980s, there is a clear shift from infibulation to clitoridectomy.
Tanzania	10	1,345,000	Clitoridectomy reported only among the Chagga groups near Mount Kilimanjaro.

TABLE 4-7   Continued

Country	Prevalence (%)	Actual Number	Notes
Togo*	50	950,000	
Uganda*	5	467,500	
Zaire*	5	945,000	
Total		114,296,900	

*Anecdotal information only; no published studies.

[a]Estimated prevalence rates have been developed from reviews of national surveys, small studies, and country reports and from F. Hosken, WIN News 18(4), Autumn 1992.

SOURCE: Toubia, 1993.

TABLE 4-8   Type of Female Circumcision, by Country, Sub-Saharan Africa

Type of Surgery	Country
Sunna circumcision and excision	Benin, Burkina Faso, Central African Republic, Chad, Djibouti, Ghana, Côte d'Ivoire, Kenya, Liberia, Mali, Mauritania, Niger, Nigeria, Senegal, Sierra Leone, Sudan, Tanzania, Togo
Infibulation	Central African Republic, Djibouti, Eritrea, Ethiopia, Kenya, Mali, Nigeria, Somalia, Sudan
Unknown (or published information unavailable)	The Gambia, Guinea, Guinea Bissau, Uganda, Zaire

Recently, the possibility that the most extreme surgical forms produce limits on overall physical agility has been raised (Walker and Parmar, 1993). This is not implausible, but it is contemplated in a fictional context that, while compelling, can only suggest a direction for more systematic investigation.

A natural expectation is that obstetric complications would be almost inevitable for women who have been infibulated (Table 4-11). Anterior episiotomy is generally an essential part of childbirth for these women; where this is effected with unsterile instruments, not only is infection probable, but scar formation is enhanced. In each successive birth, then, the small size of the residual vaginal aperture continues to be a problem, one that is exacerbated by the inflexibility of accumulated scar tissue. Vesico-vaginal and recto-vaginal fistulae, which produce their own sequelae as noted earlier in this chapter, are common.

Reinfibulation   Following delivery, it is not uncommon for the vulva to be resutured and reinfibulated (Hosken, 1982). El Dareer (1982b) found that 80 percent of her sample of 3,210 married women had been reinfibulated following delivery, citing "custom" as their rationale. Husbands who pay for the additional surgery may be considered as lending at least tacit approval. There are also cases of widows, divorced women, and married women requesting reinfibulation (El Dareer, 1982b).

Mortality and Morbidity   The discussion has so far emphasized morbidity. There is also cause to suspect some burden of mortality deriving from FGM sequelae (Tables 4-3 and 4-4), but its dimensions are unknown. The highest maternal mortality rates have been reported from areas that practice female circumcision (Hosken, 1982), but whether this relationship is causal or coincidental is simply not known, since there is ample latitude for confounding. Degrees of morbidity and occurrence of fatality not only relate to the extent of the intervention itself,

TABLE 4-9 Immediate Complications and Sequelae of Female Circumcision

Complication	Description	Sequelae
Hemorrhage	Severe bleeding resulting from severing of the dorsal artery of the clitoris, or from the labial branches of the pudendal artery	Anemia; shock; possible death
Trauma to adjacent structures	Particularly to the urethra, urinary meatus, vaginal opening, or anus; in extreme cases, the entire urinary meatus is excised	Damage to the urethra can lead to permanent incontinence; acute and chronic urinary retention; damage to the vaginal walls can lead to total occlusion of the vaginal opening
Acute urinary retention	Can occur if the urethra is covered with a flap of skin and dried blood, sometimes requiring reopening	Urinary tract infection(s)
Acute site infection	Infection at excision site	Infection can spread upward into the vagina and uterus, contributing to infertility; lack of antibiotics can lead to death
Tetanus	An infection that releases tetanus toxoid which causes severe and painful muscle spasms	Tetanic convulsions, usually fatal
Septicemia	Blood infection	Hypotension, vascular collapse, renal failure, death
Behavioral disturbances	Irritability, disturbed sleep, restlessness	May develop into confusional state with clinical manifestations

SOURCES: Tables 4-9 through 4-11 are original constructions using many published sources, including, but not limited to: Aziz, 1980; Bakr, 1982; Cook, 1982; Cutner, 1985; Dorkenoo and Elworthy, 1992; El Dareer, 1982; Gordon, 1991; Harrison, 1983; Hosken, 1982; Ismail, 1982; Ladjali and Toubia, 1990; Kheir, 1991; McLean and Graham, 1985; Modawi, 1982; Slack, 1988; Tahzib, 1983; Verzin, 1975; Williams, 1993; and WHO Chronicle, 1986.

but also to the abilities and knowledge of the practitioner, cleanliness of surgical instruments and environment, accessibility of medical facilities, and cultural acceptance of those facilities. Female circumcision may be ostensibly discouraged by authorities, and even be illegal in some regions, so that children and adolescents residing near a hospital often may not be brought in for attention to immediate complications. In addition, because of strong cultural prohibitions, women in general may be reluctant to deliver themselves to the care of a male physician; they may actually be prevented from doing so, either by habit or by the realities of seclusion (El Dareer, 1982b).

Psychological Sequelae   As is the case everywhere, the psychological impact of a given condition or event is difficult to measure and attribute. Several researchers over the past decade have taken up this elusive aspect of FGM (Armstrong, 1991; Baasher, 1982; Koso-Thomas, 1985; Lightfoot-Klein, 1989). Psychological sequelae of these traditional interventions may begin at the time of the intervention itself or accumulate and emerge in subsequent periods of stress in a woman's life: at menarche, marriage, childbirth, and even in later life. Timing and degree of impact will depend on the type of intervention, the severity and durability of any physical sequelae, and the existence and quality of social support. Marriage may be the most vulnerable period: the long, painful processes of penetration and the potentially grievous repercussions of infertility would appear to lead the list of risks to female health and well-being.

Correlation with HIV Infection   Despite speculation, there is no evidence in the published literature of a causal relationship between FGM and HIV infection. Because the procedure is not usually performed under sterile conditions, and because the instrument(s) employed are used in multiple operations during the same ritual event, young women undergoing the surgery could conceivably be at some risk of transmission. A more likely mode of transmission is from an HIV-infected sexual partner, because the possibility of transmission of the infection during intercourse exists when the scarred vagina is subjected to unremitting trauma or lesions through the use of a sharp instrument. This possibility, however, remains at the level of conjecture.

TABLE 4-10 Long-Term Complications and Sequelae of Female Circumcision

Complication	Description	Sequelae
Dysuria	Painful or difficult urination	Difficulty increases over time
Chronic urinary retention	Can occur if the urethra is covered, sometimes requiring more surgery	Urinary tract infection(s); formation of calculi, pyelonephritis
Recurrent urinary tract infection	Bridge of skin hiding urinary meatus results in a distorted stream and in the area being constantly wet	Chronic bacterial infection; can ascend to bladder and kidneys, leading to renal failure, septicemia, and death
Chronic infection of the uterus and fallopian tubes	Due to retention of urine and menstrual blood	Severe pain; contributes to primary infertility
Dysmenorrhea	Painful menstruation	If the vagina is too tightly sewn and anal intercourse takes place by choice or by accident, can cause anal fissures and incompetent sphincter
Stenosis	Narrowing of the vagina	Vaginal intercourse difficult; can cause dyspareunia; forcible penetration may cause lacerations of perineum, rectum, and urethra and, possibly, produce formation of a "false vagina"
Hematocolpos and cryptomenorrhea	Complete obstruction of the vagina results in accumulation of menstrual blood in the vagina due to damage to the vaginal walls	Contributes to pelvic infections
Dyspareunia	Painful intercourse	
Vaginismus	Painful spasm of the vagina	Can prevent or impede intercourse
Implantation dermoid cysts	Very common complication in which a cyst resembling skin grows very large	Cyst can become infected
Keloid formation	Leads to excessive scar tissue	Inability to wash inner epithelial surface of this area, so that skin remains irritated by urine and prone to local bacterial infection; can make later surgery difficult
Calculus formations found in the posterior vaginal fornix (the recess formed between the vaginal wall and the vaginal part of the cervix) or under the bridge of skin that covers the urinary meatus	An abnormal concretion, generally composed of calcium	Can cause obstruction and secondary infection
Retention cyst	Sebaceous substance composed of fat and epithelial debris	Cyst can become infected
Neuroma	Tumor on the nerve to the clitoris	Can cause severe dyspareunia
Disfiguration of external genitalia		No physical sequelae

SOURCES: Tables 4-9 through 4-11 are original constructions using many published sources, including but not limited to: Aziz, 1980; Bakr, 1982; Cook, 1982; Cutner, 1985; Dorkenoo and Elworthy, 1992; El Dareer, 1982a,b; Gordon, 1991; Harrison, 1983; Hosken, 1982; Ismail, 1982; Ladjali and Toubia, 1990; Kheir, 1991; McLean and Graham, 1985; Modawi, 1982; Slack, 1988; Tahzib, 1983; Verzin, 1975; Williams, personal communication, 1993; and WHO, 1986.

In sum, these traditional procedures produce morbidity in Sub-Saharan African females and may also contribute to their mortality. At the same time, the practices encode central values about gender, male-female relationships, maturity, and community. The resolution of this tension will require a deeper, more comprehensive, and better-quantified understanding than is now the case, in order to develop innovative and constructive solutions to address the negative effects of these practices on Sub-Saharan female health.

TABLE 4-11 Obstetric Complications and Sequelae of Circumcision

Complication	Description	Possible Sequelae
Failure to expel fetus during miscarriage or abortion		Acute infection, may result in PID and contribute to infertility
Deinfibulation	Cut along the original scar to permit passage of the baby	Infection
Vaginal stenosis	Very small vaginal opening	Vaginal examination during labor very difficult; difficult to assess progress of labor; episiotomy is often necessary for childbirth, including a postero-lateral episiotomy in primigravidae
Episiotomy	Cutting of the skin to prevent tearing	Increased scar tissue; bladder and urethral fistulae injury to anus; late uterine prolapse
Obstructed labor and prolonged second stage of labor, vaginal rupture	Fibrous vulvar tissue fails to dilate during contractions; labor is impeded due to obstruction in the birth canal	Hemorrhage resulting from tearing of scar tissue through cervix or perineum; danger to infant; vesico-vaginal and recto-vaginal fistulae; fistulae can result in incontinence, infection, infertility; bad odor can cause social ostracization

SOURCES: Tables 4-9 through 4-11 are original constructions using many published sources, including, but not limited to: Aziz, 1980; Bakr, 1982; Cook, 1982; Cutner, 1985; Dorkenoo and Elworthy, 1992; El Dareer, 1982; Gordon, 1991; Harrison, 1983; Hosken, 1982; Ismail, 1982; Ladjali and Toubia, 1990; Kheir, 1991; McLean and Graham, 1985; Modawi, 1982; Slack, 1988; Tahzib, 1983; Verzin, 1975; Williams, personal communication, 1993; and WHO Chronicle, 1986.

Health Services

Access to Antenatal and Intrapartum Care

As initially discussed in the section on "Community Characteristics" above, the barriers to maternity care that can affect maternal mortality and morbidity fall into three categories: (1) geographic and convenience factors, (2) acceptability factors, and (3) factors related to quality of care. Although these same barriers exist for both antenatal and intrapartum care, clients are willing to overcome more barriers in the presence of an obstetric complication than they are for routine antenatal care or uncomplicated delivery.

Geographic and Convenience Factors   These include distance from the health facility, in miles, time, and cost; weather; terrain; and the availability of transportation. Convenience factors include clinic hours—many clinics are open only in the morning, when women must do their work—and waiting times. Single-purpose clinics are another impediment: a health center may offer a well-baby clinic on two days of the week and antenatal care on the other three days, so that a woman bringing an infant for immunizations must make a separate trip for her own antenatal care. Maternal and child health (MCH) centers or primary health care clinics are usually open only a few hours a day, and women experiencing complications may be forced to bypass those facilities and go directly to a hospital, even when the basic facility has the capability to manage the complication.

Acceptability Factors   These include the way women are treated when they present for care. Sometimes they are berated for missing appointments, for presenting late in pregnancy, or for not complying with treatment. The social distance between physician and patient is great, even when both are from upper-socioeconomic levels. Patients may not understand instructions, their concerns and traditional practices may be belittled, and they may be given instructions they are unable to follow, such as recommendations to eat nutritious meals and rest more. Women may also be apprehensive about operative deliveries, clinical insistence on an unfamiliar or unacceptable delivery position, isolation from family, and their inability to observe such traditional practices as ritual disposal of the placenta.

Quality of Care Quality of care may be, correctly or incorrectly, perceived as poor. Antenatal care may offer no more than weighing and nutritional information, and the importance of effective measures such as STD screening and measurement of blood pressure and hemoglobin may not be understood. A self-fulfilling prophecy ensures that hospitals are often seen as a place where people die, so women wait far too long to make the journey. People may believe, often justifiably, that the hospital has limited resources and is therefore ineffective. This fuels their reluctance.

Medical facilities in Sub-Saharan Africa do have fewer resources than they need; shortages are acute and tend to worsen when economies decline (Ekwempu et al., 1990). This means that the quality of care in antenatal clinics and obstetric wards is generally low. Much of the antenatal care that is available contributes little to the primary objective of preventing life-threatening complications (Rooney, 1992). The interventions that are effective—blood pressure measurement, management of hypertension, screening and treatment of sexually transmitted and parasitic diseases, supplemental iron and folic acid, and patient education in the significance and management of symptoms of impending complications—are sometimes unavailable. Some hospitals are often unprepared to manage the most extreme complications, and sometimes lack the human and material resources to manage the common obstetric emergencies. This leads to documented higher case-fatality rates and the failure to command community confidence.

This lack of response capacity is exacerbated by medical inflexibility. Formally trained providers are not always prepared to adapt maternity care to the special needs of poor and illiterate women, and the traditional organization of medical training around treatments of first choice means that providers are not prepared to make do with second and third treatment options. Maternal death case reviews suggest that when first-line pharmaceuticals are not available, many physicians are unaware of alternatives or unprepared to innovate when the resource base is less than ideal. While it seems far-fetched to count lack of imagination as yet another cause of maternal death, this may sometimes be the case.

Still, some highly innovative and workable alternatives have been developed in the region. In Zaire, nursing persons have been trained to do cesarean deliveries, laparotomies, and hysterectomies, and their case-fatality rates have been about the same as those for physicians (White et al., 1987). In Mozambique, "surgical technicians" are trained to perform surgical procedures, including obstetric procedures. In both situations, physicians are on call if needed. As one more example, there is the role-expanding approach used by the Ghana Registered Midwives Association that focuses on "Life-Saving Skills" for midwives. The idea of assigning greater responsibilities to midwives, however, has generally been resisted by the larger medical community (Carnegie Corporation, 1993).

MATERNAL HEALTH AND FAMILY PLANNING

Broadly speaking, maternal mortality and morbidity can be reduced by decreasing the absolute number of times all women become pregnant, the number of pregnancies among high-risk women, the number of unwanted pregnancies that might otherwise end in abortion, and by making pregnancy and childbirth safer.

Women not contracepting are likely to have more pregnancies, each of which adds to overall risk, a risk further increased by the growing likelihood that women whose pregnancies are unwanted will resort to clandestine abortion. Women with unwanted pregnancies are also more likely to be at the extremes of the reproductive period (too old or too young), of high parity, and are less likely to seek prenatal care, all of which further jeopardizes their health and elevates their risk status (Royston and Armstrong, 1989; WHO, 1987b). They may also be less economically, socially, or psychologically prepared for pregnancy, further compounding their existing health problems.

The Demographic and Health Surveys (DHS) show that African women continue having children even when they do not wish to do so (see Table 4-12). In Burundi, over half of all women respondents noted that they wanted to delay their next pregnancy, and 18 percent wanted no more children, but only 9 percent were currently using family planning. In Mauritius, 70 percent of the women responded that they did not want any more children, and

TABLE 4-12 Fertility Desires Among Currently Married Women Aged 15–44, DHS and Family Planning Surveys, 1985–1991 (percent)

Country and Year	Pregnant	Want More Children Now[a]	Want More Children Later[b]	Want No More Children	Are Using Family Planning[c]
Botswana, 1988	10	25	33	32	35
Burundi, 1987	15	15	52	18	9
Ghana, 1988	14	20	47	19	13
Kenya, 1988–1989	13	13	28	46	27
Liberia, 1986	17	33	36	14	6
Mali, 1987	16	34	36	13	5
Mauritius, 1985[d]	8	22	22	70	75
Nigeria, 1990	16	34	37	13	6
Senegal, 1986	22	14	44	21	12
Sudan, 1989–1990	16	32	32	21	9
Togo, 1988	14	19	48	20	12
Uganda, 1988–1989	27	36	32	15	5
Zimbabwe, 1988–1989	14	22	37	28	45

[a]Want more children within 2 years.

[b]Want more children after 2 years or longer.

[c]Currently using any method of family planning.

[d]The Mauritius Survey asked pregnant women whether they wanted another child, but not when they wanted one.

SOURCE: Robey et al., 1992.

75 percent were using family planning. Women in Burundi were obviously at greater risk of an unwanted pregnancy than their Mauritian counterparts.

If African women were to have only the number of children they say they want, there would be 4 million fewer births, a 17 percent decrease (Maine et al., 1987). Maternal deaths would fall in comparable proportion, simply by diminishing the numerical risk of dying as a result of pregnancy (Royston and Armstrong, 1989).

In Africa, family planning could lower maternal mortality risk by changing the profile of parity history (Maine et al., 1987; Winikoff and Sullivan, 1987). In a reanalysis of Harrison and Rossiter's (1985) hospital-based data from Zaria, Northern Nigeria, Winikoff and Sullivan (1987) show that preventing births above para four would have resulted in a 52 percent reduction in mortality among the patients; preventing births below age 20, over age 30, and above para 4 would have reduced maternal mortality by 66 percent. These data suggest that appreciable gains in maternal survival could be realized by concentrating childbearing during the safest years of female reproductive life.

A review of abortion data leads to similar conclusions. Results from a community-based study in Addis Ababa by Kwast and colleagues (1986) suggest that if all pregnancies that ended in abortion had been prevented by contraception, direct obstetrical deaths would have been reduced by 54 percent. In Cameroon, where abortion-related mortality at a local hospital was 56 times higher than mortality from all other causes in the same unit (Leke, 1989), and in Benin City, Nigeria, where a hospital-based study reported that abortions accounted for one-fifth of all maternal deaths (Unuigbe et al., 1988a,b), prevention of those pregnancies alone would have significantly reduced maternal mortality. In addition to mortality reduction, there would have been substantial reduction in morbidity and liberation of hospital beds and resources for other pressing needs.

Although statistically it seems to make more sense to target family planning programs at all high-risk groups, Winikoff and Sullivan (1987) demonstrate that it is more efficient to tighten the focus of family planning programs to the at-risk groups that are most likely to be receptive. Even though prevention of births among women under 20 years would eliminate 42 percent of maternal deaths (Harrison and Rossiter, 1985), acceptance of family planning among this group would be low because its members are under great pressure to commence childbearing immediately.

TABLE 4-13 Reproductive Risk: Mortality Rates Associated with Childbearing, Compared with Mortality Rates Associated with Contraceptive Use

| | Estimated Annual Deaths per 100,000 Women | | | |
| | Developed Countries | | Developing Countries | |
	Age<35	Age 35+	Age <35	Age 35+
Maternal deaths with no contraception	10	27	60	160
Deaths from side-effects of oral contraceptives among nonsmokers	1	23	1	23
Deaths from side-effects of IUDs	1	2	2	4
Deaths from side-effects of condoms	0	0	0	0

SOURCE: Adapted from Rinehart, 1987.

Although contraceptive use remains low in most of Sub-Saharan Africa, it has risen appreciably. In Zimbabwe, Botswana, and Kenya, use of modern methods has risen sharply since the 1980s, and fertility has shown a corresponding decline (Robey et al., 1992). The dangers of contraceptives are often cited as reasons for nonuse, yet when the safety of contraceptives is compared with the risks associated with pregnancy, especially as those risks accumulate, contraceptive use proves to be far safer than childbearing (see Table 4-13).

Provision of Family Planning Services

Family planning service provision is a complicated process, entangled in social, political, moral, and cultural debate in many African countries. Services to teenagers, who would benefit with significant mortality reduction, are often tightly restricted. Immediate childbearing is expected after marriage, and often after an infant death to replace the lost child. Where marriage comes early and infant mortality rates are high, family planning may not be the desired option for many women. Even if the social and political debates were resolved, there remain many reasons for nonuse: side-effects are a significant concern; method failure is not uncommon; and refusal on religious grounds remains salient. To be successful, family planning programs must be sensitive to these reservations and to the community being served, and services must be delivered in a manner that meets users' needs.

Access to family planning services is restricted for many of the same reasons that affect access to health care services overall: insufficient governmental commitment, lack of knowledge about services, distance, and logistics. There are also social barriers, such as requirements for spousal permission or proof of a given number of living children, and encounters with the medical establishment can be intimidating for women. If family planning is not integrated into other services that have some logical affinity (MCH, STD screening, infertility management, and activities for enhancing women's skills), it is marginated, theoretically and practically, in ways that constrain both access and effectiveness (Herz and Measham, 1987; Raikes, 1989; Royston and Armstrong, 1989). This limitation also affects women's ability to gain sufficient knowledge about family planning, as well as an adequate understanding of their options, to make informed decisions. According to the DHS, fewer than 40 percent of women in Burundi, Ghana, Liberia, Mali, Niger, Senegal, and Uganda are able to name any modern family planning method (Robey et al., 1992).

Cost is another impediment. Although contraceptives are provided free by many government-based sources, private outlets continue to be crucial for women who place a premium on confidentiality. In Nigeria, over half the family planning outlets are private pharmacists and chemists, and less than 40 percent of current users of modern methods obtain their contraceptives from hospitals (Johns Hopkins University, 1992). Recent efforts in some Sub-

Saharan countries to require clients to pay part of the cost of family planning methods will inevitably have some effect on utilization.

It is not unreasonable to argue that because of the clear relationship between childbearing and female health, women will be able to improve their health status significantly when they have made significant gains in reproductive freedom, and family planning programs are conceptually and practically integrated into health programs and overall thinking about the meaning of development.

Abortion

Part of societal reaction to voluntary termination of pregnancy in Sub-Saharan Africa is rooted in strong traditional and religious sentiments. A large portion of the population adheres to pronatalist beliefs deriving from a Christian-Islamic cultural heritage. This, in turn, affects the way abortion and contraceptive services are delivered. In Kenya, maternal and child health services were initially provided by missionaries, contraception was not promoted, and abortion was illegal. Little of this was changed in most African countries after independence (Raikes, 1989). Even in Zambia, where abortion is legal, 25 incomplete abortions are treated for every abortion that is performed legally (Bradley et al., 1991).

Assertions that abortion is relatively rare in Sub-Saharan Africa are not supported by the evidence (Coeytaux, 1988). Because it is so restricted and services are poor even where laws are liberal, most abortions are clandestine or occur out of hospital, and prevalence data therefore present far from the real picture. A growing body of evidence indicates that abortions may account for at least half the maternal mortality in the entire region (Kwast et al., 1986; Rosenfield, 1989).

The large majority of clandestine abortions end up in a hospital as incomplete—and usually septic—abortions. Major hospitals in Nairobi and Kinshasa, which reported 2,000 to 3,000 admissions a year for abortion complications in the late 1970s and early 1980s (Aggarwal and Mati, 1982), were treating 30 to 60 a day by the end of the decade (Rogo et al., 1987), or about 10,000 a year, a fivefold increase (Coeytaux, 1988).

Because it is clandestine, abortion is characteristically performed under unsanitary conditions, and is thus a significant contributor to infection, infertility, and mortality among women of all ages. In Kenya, Aggarwal and Mati (1982) report that only 11 percent of the abortions they reviewed had been performed by qualified personnel. In Cameroon, the abortion-related mortality rate at a local hospital was 56 times higher than mortality from other causes in the same maternity unit (Leke, 1989). In Addis Ababa, Kwast and colleagues (1986) found that the main cause of maternal mortality was septic abortion, which accounted for 54 percent of the direct obstetric deaths. In Benin City, Nigeria, abortions—only 10 percent of which were spontaneous—accounted for one-fifth of all maternal deaths (Unuigbe et al., 1988a,b), and Odejide (1986) reports illegal abortion as the leading cause of death among unmarried women aged 15–24, particularly those in school. At the University of Calabar Teaching Hospital, Archibong (1991) estimated that 20 percent of the maternal deaths and 40 percent of all gynecological admissions were abortion-related. In Cameroon, Leke (1989) reported that abortion was responsible for one-third of the emergency hospital admissions to a principal maternity hospital. In a review of 123 maternal deaths in Guinea (Conakry), Toure and colleagues (1992) found that abortion was the third leading cause of mortality, after hypertension and postpartum bleeding. Rogo (Rogo et al., 1987) estimated that 20 percent of all maternal deaths in East and Central Africa were the result of complications of induced abortion. Most of this research, however, is hospital-based, revealing nothing about those unable to obtain medical services, and it provides only a hint of the magnitude of the problem (Coeytaux, 1988).

Abortion is a major health problem for women of all ages, marital status, and socioeconomic strata in Sub-Saharan Africa. Crowther (1986) reports that, of 99 patients who had an abortion at Harare Hospital in Zimbabwe, 76 percent were married, more than half were over 30, and nearly 35 percent had more than four children. In Addis Ababa, Kwast and colleagues (1986) found that of 13 women who died of direct obstetric complications of abortion, over half were married and nearly 70 percent were over 20. In Nigeria, Odejide (1986) found abortion to be the course of action among 90 percent of unmarried and working women with unwanted pregnancies. In their study of 1,800 never-married Nigerian adolescents and young women aged 14–25, Nichols and colleagues (1986) reported that almost half the female students and two-thirds of the female nonstudents had been pregnant, and nearly all had terminated their pregnancies with an induced abortion.

In general, abortion predominates among younger, single, educated women in the higher social classes. Education, employment, and urbanization have contributed to delays in family formation, and many women with these characteristics who find themselves pregnant will resort to abortion (Boerma, 1987). Abortions, however, are not restricted to urban areas, as popular wisdom would have it. A Kenya study shows that rural women are just as likely to have an abortion as urban women (Lema et al., 1989; Mbizvo et al., 1993).

The infections that so often accompany illicit abortions have their own sequelae. In addition to immediate complications, such infections may spread throughout the reproductive tract and produce PID, with tubal damage, secondary infertility, and predisposition to ectopic pregnancy (Meheus, 1992). The procedure itself may cause mechanical damage to the vagina, cervix, or uterus, and chemicals introduced into the vagina may destroy tissue, which can also contribute to infection; cervical lacerations may be responsible for subsequent miscarriage or premature births (Aggarwal and Mati, 1982). In Nigeria, Oronsaye and Odiase (1981) found that 22 percent of women who presented with ectopic pregnancies had histories of abortion, nearly three times the number of those who had experienced "normal" pregnancies.

Illegal abortion also makes great demands upon health systems. Complicated abortion uses scarce hospital resources that would otherwise be available to other patients. At Kenyatta National Hospital during one six-month period, 60 percent of the beds in the Acute Gynecological Ward were occupied by abortion patients (Aggarwal and Mati, 1982). In 1968–1969, 41 percent of the blood supply of the major referral hospital in Ghana was used to treat the sequelae of such abortions (Gyepi-Gabrah, 1985). Current issues with the blood supply are somewhat different: women in Zambia who need transfusions for abortion-related hemorrhage refused them for fear of AIDS (Castle et al., 1990).

The question of who makes decisions about abortion is as critical in Sub-Saharan Africa as it is in many other parts of the world. In Zambia, where the laws, exemplified by the Termination of Pregnancy Act, are more liberal than elsewhere in Africa, a woman still must obtain written consent from three physicians who attest to the negative physical or mental consequences to her or her children of a continued pregnancy (Castle et al., 1990). A similar law, the Abortion and Sterilization Act, is in force in South Africa, but only one-third of those who filed for abortion for mental reasons under this act were granted permission; some of the remainder turned to illegal means and, in 1987 alone, nearly 15,000 operations were performed in South Africa to remove the residues of incomplete abortion (Nash, 1990). As elsewhere in the world, ambivalence remains; a study in Nigeria found that 35 percent of women seeking abortions were opposed to legalization (Ujah, 1991).

Lactation

The benefits of breastfeeding are well established and breast milk is recognized as the best form of nutrition for infants. It contains all the nutrients needed in the first few months of life, meets those needs at no economic cost, confers some immunity against infection on the infant through its mother's antibodies, and is preferable to bottle-feeding because the risk of contamination is reduced. Breastfeeding may also protect the mother against anemia and more general depletion by reducing postpartum hemorrhage, delaying return of menses, and contributing to the length of birth intervals. It also facilitates return of the uterus to its normal size and provides emotional bonding between mother and infant (McCann et al., 1984).

Although duration of breastfeeding is declining, particularly in urban areas, it is still almost universal in Africa. Table 4-14 shows that median duration of any breastfeeding in Sub-Saharan Africa ranges from 18 months in Botswana to 26 months in Burundi. Exclusive breastfeeding is brief, however, and most mothers begin supplementing breast milk between the baby's first and seventh month. Although overall duration of breastfeeding is longer in Sub-Saharan Africa than in most of other areas of the world, only in Burundi and Mali are over 50 percent of children under 4 months breastfed exclusively; this suggests that breast milk substitutes, such as water or formula, are introduced very early in most countries (Robey et al., 1992).

Nevertheless, while breastfeeding is good for infant health, the tradeoffs in maternal health may not be as advantageous, particularly in the presence of severe malnutrition and famine. Production of breast milk requires

TABLE 4-14 Median Duration of Breastfeeding in Months Among Married Women Aged 15–49

Country and Region	Breastfeeding	
	Any	Full[a]
AFRICA		
Botswana, 1988	18	3
Burundi, 1987	26	5
Ghana, 1988	22	3
Kenya, 1989	21	2
Liberia, 1986	16	1
Mali, 1987	20	7
Nigeria, 1990	20	2
Senegal, 1986	19	4
Togo, 1988	23	1
Uganda, 1988–1989	20	4
Zimbabwe, 1988–1989	19	2
ASIA AND PACIFIC		
Indonesia, 1987	26	1
Pakistan, 1990–1991	20	1
Sri Lanka, 1987	27	2
Thailand, 1987	15	1
LATIN AMERICA AND CARIBBEAN		
Bolivia, 1989	17	3
Brazil, 1986	5	<1
Columbia, 1990	9	2
Dominican Republic, 1990	6	1
Ecuador, 1987	14	1
Guatemala, 1987	22	NA
Mexico, 1987	8	1
Paraguay, 1990	11	1
Peru, 1991–1992	17	1
Trinidad and Tobago, 1987	6	1
NEAR EAST AND NORTH AFRICA		
Egypt, 1988–1989	20	2
Jordan, 1990	12	1
Morocco, 1987	16	3
Tunisia, 1988	17	3

[a]Includes both exclusive and infrequent and supplemented breastfeeding. <1 = less than 0.5 months.

NA = Not available.

SOURCE: Robey et al., 1992.

extra energy expenditure by the mother, energy she would not expend were she not lactating; the Food and Agriculture Organization of the World Health Organization (FAO/WHO) recommends that lactating women consume an extra 2,090 kJ/d more than nonlactating, nonpregnant women to meet those additional energy demands (FAO/WHO, 1985). Assuming a mother of adequate prepregnancy weight, this translates to roughly 500 kCal/day during the first three postpartum months (Hamilton et al., 1984; Parker et al., 1990).

These extra kCals are not easily acquired. Up to 45 percent of the women aged 15–44 in less-developed countries do not consume enough calories daily even in their nonpregnant state (Hamilton et al., 1984), and Sub-Saharan Africa is no exception (see Chapter 3). During times of marginal food availability, lactating mothers appear to adjust physiologically to lower caloric intake without compromising milk quality by mobilizing fat reserves accumulated during pregnancy or by developing other adaptive mechanisms (Hamilton et al., 1984; Jellife and Jellife, 1978). Some research (in The Gambia and Kenya) indicates that even among poorly nourished women, breast milk quality remains good and lactation performance is protected (Frigerio et al., 1991a; van Steenbergen et al., 1984). Other research documents cumulative negative effects of poor nutrition and high parity on milk quality and quantity (Funk et al., 1990; Neuman, et al., 1992; Prentice et al., 1987). This suggests that maternal adjustment does not always entirely accommodate lactational demands.

The main indicator of breastfeeding's impact on maternal health appears to be changes in the mother's weight, and there is limited evidence that lactating women lose weight at a higher rate than their nonlactating counterparts. In Kenya, Jansen and colleagues (1984) conducted a longitudinal study of 2,874 women and found that they had lost an average of 2.4 to 2.6 kilograms in weight to subsidize milk production. In Zaire, Pagezy (1983) found that weight loss among lactating women was almost a direct reflection of the baby's weight gain, and that the energy costs of nursing were highest during the first few months. Weight loss may be even more pronounced when there is an overlap between breastfeeding and pregnancy, a situation common in Africa. The results are not always in the same direction: lactating Gambian women lost weight, but only during the rainy seasons because of heavy agricultural work, as did nonlactating women (Paul et al., cited in Hamilton et al., 1984).

The effect of lactation on maternal health is difficult to study because of different kinds of resilience in response to stress. Frequent illness among children may result in lower demand for breast milk. Smaller infants demand less milk. Seasonal variation and changes in daily activities further confound the effects (Calloway et al., 1988). Finally, findings from studies conducted in stable environments may not apply in conditions of war or famine.

MENOPAUSE

Menopause is the cessation of menstruation for a year or more, in conjunction with loss of ovarian function, and normally occurs between ages 40 and 55. Its onset is often accompanied by climacteric symptoms such as hot flashes, excessive perspiration, and chills, and perimenopausal women may also be more prone to headaches, nervousness, agitation, or depression (Judd and Meldrum, 1981; WHO, 1981; Wynn, 1983). Manifestations of the condition can range from mild to severe: hot flashes, as one example, can be severe enough to impair sleep, leading to fatigue and decreased energy. In some women, symptoms last a short time (two years or less in half of menopausal women in the United States (Wentz, 1988); in others, symptoms recur periodically.

Loss of ovarian function leads to reduction of estrogen levels, which may be accompanied by vaginal atrophy and pruritus, and dryness and pain during intercourse. In some women, menopause may be associated with cardiovascular degeneration and osteoporosis; others may be have no symptoms because significant amounts of estrogens are still being produced (Judd and Meldrum, 1981; WHO, 1981).

The nature of menopause and women's response to its onset have generally not been matters of concern in developing countries. Sub-Saharan Africa is no exception. Nevertheless, because women aged 40 and above now comprise nearly 17 percent of the regional population (U.S. Bureau of the Census, 1995), and, as in other parts of the world, female life expectancy exceeds male life expectancy by several years, it is time to pay some attention to these age cohorts. Evidence in the very scanty literature that does exist is that average age of onset of menopause in Nigerian women is age 48 (Okonofua et al., 1990) and that, at least in parts of Nigeria, the health problems associated with menopause are similar to those experienced in the West. In Ghana, Kwawukume and colleagues (1993) estimated onset of menopause to be approximately 48 years of age as well. Characteristics included hot flashes, palpitations, anxiety, sleeplessness, headaches, frequent urination, depression, irritability, tiredness, weight gain, poor memory, and negative attitudes toward coitus. Circumstances that might make the African experience different, such as general undernutrition and repeated episodes of infectious disease, have not been explored.

The potential medical needs of a growing cohort of menopausal and postmenopausal women will at some point present an additional challenge to health budgets that customarily have been constrained, and are likely to remain so. For these systems, and for those who tend to think that African women characteristically die young, topics such as estrogen replacement will seem irrelevant, even effete. At the same time, the needs of this grandmother generation may be increasing or changing, not only because they are living longer, but because societal demands on them are mounting: war and the HIV infections have created a population of orphans who need the grandmothers' care, a requirement for new caretaking roles at the very time when they themselves may need new kinds of care.

A related issue is that of the chronic, noncommunicable diseases. For instance, very little is known about cancer in women in the postreproductive, or even late reproductive, years in Sub-Saharan Africa. Human papilloma virus (HPV) infections have strong epidemiological links with the genesis of cancer of the cervix, which is the most common female malignancy in Nigeria (Adekunle and Ladipo, 1992) and Zimbabwe (Kasule, 1988). Estimated crude incidence rates of cervical cancer range from 14.0 per 100,000 women in western Africa to 23.2 per 100,000 in eastern Africa, which also had the highest number of new cases in 1980 (Parkin et al., 1988). Harare Central Hospital data on gynecological malignancies between 1981 and 1983 indicated that 78 percent of all malignancies were the result of cervical cancer, almost 99 percent were rural, and 78 percent of cases presented were in the advanced stages (Kasule, 1988). High rates of cervical cancer have been reported from a number of other Sub-Saharan African countries as well. It may prove inappropriate to consider the disease as exclusive to the postreproductive period, because it has been reported in women in their twenties and thirties. Indeed, one of the mysteries of the disease is how an infection that is usually acquired in early adulthood leads to cervical cancer 10, 20, or 30 years later (WHO, 1987a).

CONCLUSIONS

Table 4-15 summarizes the unfolding of obstetric complications across the female life span in Sub-Saharan Africa. It does not reflect the numerous feedback loops and meshing of different factors and events throughout that span, during the years of active reproduction, and before and after that time. For example, an anemic mother is more likely to have a small baby; small babies often grow up to be small adults, and thus are at increased obstetric risk. Micronutrient deficiencies can affect size and intelligence of the offspring, with implications for their later obstetric performance. Nutrition during infancy affects adult stature, and frequent illness may cause "failure to thrive" and short stature, which in turn can affect the course of labor. During childhood, nutrition continues to be important and immunizations prevent some diseases. A number of childhood diseases—for example, polio, rheumatic fever, and rickets—may lead to chronic disability, with consequences for pregnancy.

As females enter fertile age, nutrition and underlying health persist in their importance, and social factors become more prominent. Marriage during adolescence is likely to result in too early and too frequent childbearing, and early sexual debut outside of marriage increases the risk of unwanted pregnancy and clandestine abortion. In contrast, education elevates self-esteem, delays marriage, and increases the likelihood of health-seeking behavior. As women move through adulthood and full reproductive activity, the many dimensions of male-female relationships, family life, and the character of work interact with cumulative biomedical history and concurrent disease exposures to influence fecundity and pregnancy outcomes; women with some of the long-term sequelae of obstructed labor and female genital mutilation may be divorced and possibly ostracized. When women reach and pass menopause, those with living children have enhanced status; women who do not lack social support. Again, some of the sequelae of childbearing, sexually transmitted disease, and FGM persist or worsen.

Ten years ago, this chapter would have concluded by pointing to the topic of childbearing and its implications as a virtual wasteland, at best patchily tended. At the height of the child survival campaigns of the 1980s, however, concerned researchers and professionals observed that the worthiest efforts to promote maternal and child health in developing countries were doing little to reduce mortality and morbidity among mothers (Rosenfield and Maine, 1985). In 1987, the World Bank, World Health Organization, and United Nations Fund for Population Activities sponsored a groundbreaking International Safe Motherhood Conference in Nairobi, Kenya. Out of that event grew collaboration among the Bank, UN organizations, and private institutions to foster operations research on maternal mortality and, in other ways, to advance the goal of cutting maternal deaths in half by the year 2000. Subsequently, the Prevention of Maternal Mortality Network (PMM) was established to engage the capabilities of leading physicians, midwives, and social scientists within Africa in research on the magnitude and causes of maternal mortality and morbidity in their region and to take responsibility for advocating or implementing pro-

TABLE 4-15 Ages at Which Obstetric Disorders, and Their Sequelae, Occur in Sub-Saharan African Females

CATEGORY	Infancy/ Early Childhood (birth through age 4)	Childhood (ages 5–14)	Adolescence (ages 15–19)	Adulthood (ages 20–44)	Postmenopause (age 45+)
Gestation	Birth trauma				
		Rape/economically-coerced sex/ Coerced pregnancy/ very early marriage	Very early first pregnancy Induced abortion Obstructed labor Structural damage	Fistula Urinary/fecal incontinence Divorce	
			Pelvic, other infection	Infertility	No children, status/loss of social support
		Genital mutilation/ structural trauma	Obstructed labor, fistula, incontinence, ostracism Urinary retention Stenosis	Recurrent/chronic urinary tract infection Dyspareunia/vaginismus Pain, divorce	Dysuria, renal infection
		Sepsis	Pelvic infection	Infertility	No children

grams to promote maternal health (Carnegie Corporation, 1993). Other results of these efforts have included smaller programmatic initiatives that are showing some success, such as the Essential Obstetric Functions at the First-Referral level, greater use of the partogram, and maternity waiting homes. Perhaps more important is that a wider awareness has been created around the sheer numbers involved and their human and economic costs.

This chapter has sought to expand the subject of maternal mortality and morbidity beyond the boundaries of customary demography to look at what happens before a female formally enters her reproductive years and after she leaves them. As a result, the research recommendations that follow include probes into aspects of those "pre-" and "post-" years that are important, but remain unexplored.

RESEARCH NEEDS

While the need for good, insightful, systematic research is constant, research in a resource-poor situation may be more useful if it is focused on design and evaluation of interventions to reduce morbidity and mortality.

• There is no longer a need for research to determine the clinical causes of maternal deaths or the characteristics of women who die; both are now well known. Research intended to determine the cause of death should focus instead on causes inherent in the health care system. Case analyses, or "audits," and "confidential inquiries" are an effective way to identify where improvements in care could have been made. Simple protocols for use by facilities managers, perhaps based on path analysis or decision-tree models, could reward investment.

• Because research to establish the level of maternal mortality is expensive and fraught with methodologic difficulty, other indicators of progress, such as those developed by UNICEF (Maine et al., 1992), should be used in country efforts to monitor progress. From a biomedical perspective, it might be possible to develop a few surrogate endpoints that could have large utility in both clinical practice and program evaluation.

• The manner in which education influences pregnancy outcome is not well understood and requires elucidation. Its correlation with income and residence would need to be inspected as well.

• Virtually all research into induced abortion and its complications is hospital-based, reveals nothing about girls and women who were unable to obtain medical services, and provides only a dim indication of the magnitude of the problem. Further characterization of the mortality, morbidity, and disability associated with induced abortion is essential.

• In countries where the prevalence and impact of traditional surgical procedures are not well understood, clinic-level recording of health problems that derive from these interventions could be helpful to policymakers. This recommendation takes into account the limitations of using presenting samples in general, as well as the limitation that, in many countries, large numbers of women do not present for clinical care at all, or certainly are not presenting to male physicians. In these situations, data-gathering would have to be designed for extra-clinical settings.

• Despite speculation, there is no published evidence of a causal relationship between female genital mutilation and HIV infection, yet transmission from an HIV-infected partner when a scarred vagina is subjected to repeated trauma or lesions is possible. Inclusion of this dimension in other studies of HIV transmission could be helpful in this respect.

• Imaginative approaches have been taken, in Sub-Saharan Africa and elsewhere, to resolving aspects of health care delivery services that are unresponsive to women's gynecologic and obstetric needs. These, however, have not been documented or catalogued in a practical way that might foster replication. The same can be said for the treatment guidelines and algorithms that have been developed in a number of settings for different levels of care. More of a compilation task than research, such catalogues, well distributed, could be extremely helpful.

• The degree to which lactation affects mothers in negative ways needs to be better understood and quantified, and means of improving nutrition for lactating mothers, as well as guiding them toward the wisest practice, should be developed and evaluated.

• Almost nothing is known about the sociocultural or biomedical impact of menopause on African women. Qualitative research is needed to determine the nature and magnitude of its effects, including ethnographic studies to determine the symptomatology and management of menopause-related conditions and to shed light on the options women currently have, or might find helpful. Research into the effects of nutrition and general well-being on the onset of the climacteric symptoms would assist those who would develop policies and programs geared toward their management.

REFERENCES

Adekunle, A. O., and O. A. Ladipo. 1992. Reproductive tract infections in Nigeria: challenges for a fragile health infrastructure. In Reproductive Tract Infections: Global Impact and Priorities for Women's Reproductive Health, A. Germain, K. K. Holmes, P. Piot, and J. N. Wasserheit, eds. New York: Plenum.

Adetunji, J. A. 1992. Church-based obstetric care in a Yoruba community in Nigeria. Soc. Sci. Med. 35(9):1171–1178.

Aggarwal, V. P., and J. K. G. Mati. 1982. Epidemiology of induced abortion in Nairobi, Kenya. J. Obstet. Gyn. East. Cent. Afr. 1:54-57.

Akingba, J. B. 1971. Abortion, maternity, and other health problems in Nigeria. Nigeria Med. J. 7(4):465–471.

Alemu, Z. 1988. Girl mothers. Future 24-25:6–7.

Archibong, E. 1991. Illegal induced abortion—a continuing problem in Nigeria. Int. J. Gynaecol. Obstet. 34(3): 261–265.

Armon, P. J. 1977. Rupture of the uterus in Malawi and Tanzania. E. Afr. Med. J. 54(9):462–471.

Armstrong S. 1991. Female circumcision: fighting a cruel tradition. New Sci.

Aziz F. A. 1980. Gynecological and obstetric complications of female circumcision. Intl. J. Gynaecol. Obstet.17:560.

Baasher, T. 1982. Psycho-social aspects of female circumcision. In Traditional Practices Affecting the Health of Women and Children, Background Papers for the WHO Seminar, T. Baasher et al., eds. WHO EMRO Technical Publication 2(2):163–180.

Bakr, S. A. 1982. Circumcision and infibulation in the Sudan. In Traditional Practices Affecting the Health of Women and Children, Background Papers for the WHO Seminar, T. Baasher et al., eds. WHO EMRO Technical Publication 2(2):138–144.

Baumslag, N. 1985. Women's status and health: world considerations. In Advances In International Maternal and Child Health, D. B. Jellife and E. F. Jellife, eds. Oxford: Clarendon.

Beddada, B. 1982. Traditional practices in relation to pregnancy and childbirth. In Traditional Practices Affecting the Health of Women and Children, Background Papers for the WHO Seminar, T. Baasher, et al., eds. WHO EMRO Technical Publication 2 (2).

Benedetti, T. J., P. Starzyk, and F. Frost. 1985. Maternal deaths in Washington State. Obstet. Gynecol. 66:99–101.

Bhatia, J. 1993. Levels and causes of maternal mortality in a southern state of India. Stud. Fam. Plan. 24(5)310–318.

Billewicz, W. Z., and I. A. McGregor. 1981. The demography of two West African (Gambia) villages (1951–1975). J. Biosoc. Sci. 13(1):219–240.

Blanc, A. 1991. Demographic and Health Surveys World Conference, August 5–7, 1991, Executive Summary. Columbia, Md.: IRD/Macro International.

Boerma, J. K. G. 1987. The magnitude of the maternal mortality problem in Sub-Saharan Africa. Soc. Sci. Med. 24(6):551–558.

Boerma, J. K. G., and J. K. T. Mati. 1989. Identifying maternal mortality through networking: Results from coastal Kenya. Stud. Fam. Plan. 20(5):245–252.

Bradley, J., N. Sikazwe, and J. Healy. 1991. Improving abortion care in Zambia. Stud. Fam. Plan. 22(6):391–394.

Buchanan, R. 1975. Effects of Childbearing on Maternal Health. Population Reports, Series J, No. 8. Washington, D.C.: George Washington University Medical Center, Population Information Program.

Calloway, D. H., S. P. Murphy, C. H. Beaton, et al. 1988. Food intake and human functions: a cross point project perspective of the Collaborative Research Support Program in Egypt, Kenya, and Mexico. University of California, Berkeley. Photocopy.

Carnegie Corporation of New York. 1993. Making pregnancy and childbearing safer for women in West Africa. Carnegie Quarterly 38(1).

Castle, M. A., R. Likwa, and M. Whittaker. 1990. Observations on abortion in Zambia. Stud. Fam. Plan. 21(4):231–235.

Chukudebelu, W. O., and B. C. Ozumba. 1988. Maternal mortality in Anambra State, Nigeria. Int. J. Gynaecol. Obstet. 27:365–370.

Coeytaux, F. M. 1988. Induced abortion in Sub-Saharan Africa: what we do and do not know. Stud. Fam. Plan. 19(3):186–190.

Combs, C. A., E. L. Murphy, and R. K. Laros. 1991. Factors associated with postpartum hemorrhage with vaginal birth. Obstet. Gynecol. 77:69–76.

Cook, J. D., M. Carriaga, S. G. Kahn, W. Schalch, and M. S. Skikne. 1990. Gastric delivery system for iron supplementation. Lancet 335:1136–1139.

Cook, R. 1982. Damage to physical health from pharonic circumcision (infibulation) of females. In Traditional Practices Affecting the Health of Women and Children, Background Papers for the WHO Seminar, T. Baasher et al., eds. WHO EMRO Technical Publication 2(2):145–154.

Crowther, C. 1986. The prevention of maternal deaths: A continuing challenge. Centr. Afr. J. Med. 32(1):11–14.

Cutner, L. P. 1985. Female genital mutilation. Obstet. Gynecol. Surv. 40(7):437–443.

Dahabo, A. M. 1989. Somalia poem on feminine pain. Inter-African Committee on Traditional Practices Newsletter 7.

Defense for Children International. 1991. The Effects of Maternal Mortality on Children in Africa: An Exploratory Report on Kenya, Namibia, Tanzania, Zambia, and Zimbabwe. New York.

Dorkenoo, E., and S. Elworthy. 1992. Female Genital Mutilation: Proposals for Change. London: Minority Rights Group International.

Dorland's Illustrated Medical Dictionary, 27th Edition. 1988. Philadelphia, Penn.: W. B. Saunders.

Egwuatu, V. E. 1986. Childbearing among the Igbos of Nigeria. Intl. J. Gynaecol. Obstet. 24(2):103–109.

Ekwempu, C. C. 1993. Editorial. Bull. Act. Intl. Med. January.

Ekwempu, C. C., D. Maine, M. B. Olorukoba, E. S. Essien, and M. N. Kisseka. 1990. Structural adjustment and health in Africa. Lancet 336:356.

El Dareer, A. 1982a. Woman, Why Do You Weep? London: Zed.

El Dareer, A. 1982b. A study of the prevalence and epidemiology of female circumcision in Sudan. In Traditional Practices Affecting the Health of Women and Children, Background Papers to the WHO Seminar, T. Baasher et al., eds. WHO EMRO Technical Publication 2(2):312–334.

El Dareer, A. 1983. Attitudes of Sudanese people to the practice of female circumcision. Intl. J. Epidemiol. 12(2):138–144.

Elo, I. T., and S. H. Preston. 1992. Effects of early life conditions on adult mortality: A review. Pop. Index. 58(2):186–212.

Ewbank, D. C. 1993. Impact of health programmes on child mortality in Africa: evidence from Zaire and Liberia. Intl. J. Epidemiol. 22(Suppl. 1):S64-S72.

Fathalla, M. F. 1987. The long road to maternal death. People 14:8–9.

FAO (Food and Agriculture Organization). 1985. Expert Consultation: Energy and Protein Requirements. Geneva: WHO Technical Report Series 724.

Feachem, R. G., W. J. Graham, and I. M. Timaeus. 1989. Identifying health problems and health research priorities in developing countries. J. Trop. Med. Hyg. 92:133–191.

Fortney, J. A. 1987. The importance of family planning in reducing maternal mortality. Stud. Fam. Plan. 18(2):109–115.

Fortney, J. A. 1990. Implication of the ICD-10 definition related to death in pregnancy, childbirth in the pueperium. World Health Stat. Q. 43:246–248.

Fortney, J. A., and E. W. Whitehorne. 1982. The development of an index of high-risk pregnancy. Am. J. Obstet. Gynecol. 43:501–508.

Frigerio, C., Y. Schutz, R. Whitehead, and E. Jequier. 1991a. A new procedure to assess the energy requirements of lactation in Gambian women. Am. J. Clin. Nutr. 54(3):526–533.

Frigerio, C., Y. Schutz, and A. Prentice. 1991b. Is human lactation a particularly efficient process? Eur. J. Clin. Nutr. 45(9):459–462.

Funk, M. A., L. Hamlin, and M. F. Picciano. 1990. Milk belenium in rural African women: the influence of maternal nutrition, parity, and length of lactation. Am. J. Clin. Nutr. 51:220–224.

Germain, A., and R. Dixon-Mueller. 1992. Stalking the elusive "unmet need" for family planning. Stud. Fam. Plan. 23:330–335.

Gordon D. 1991. Female circumcision and genital operations in Egypt and the Sudan: A dilemma for medical anthropology. Med. Anthropol. 5(1):3–14.

Graham, W. J. 1991. Maternal mortality: levels, trends, and data deficiencies. In Disease and Mortality in Sub-Saharan Africa, R. G. Feachem and D. T. Jamison, eds. New York: Oxford University Press.

Graham, W. J., and P. Airey. 1987. Measuring maternal mortality: sense and sensitivity. Hlth. Pol. Plan. 2(4):323–333.

Graham, W. J., and W. Brass. 1988. Field performance of the sisterhood method for measuring maternal mortality. Paper presented at the IUSSP/CELADE Seminar on the Collection and Processing of Demographic Data in Latin America, Santiago, 23–27 May.

Greenwood, A. M., B. M. Greenwood, and A. K. Bradley. 1987. A prospective study of the outcome of pregnancy in a rural area of The Gambia. Bull. WHO 65(5):635–643.

Greenwood, A. M., A. K. Bradley, P. Byass, et al. 1990. Evaluation of a primary health care programme in The Gambia. I. The impact of trained traditional birth attendants on the outcome of pregnancy. J. Trop. Med. Hyg. 93:58–66.

Guttmacher Institute. 1995. Women, Families and the Future: Sexual Relationships and Marriage Worldwide. New York: Alan Guttmacher Institute.

Gyepi-Garbrah, B. 1985. Adolescent fertility in Kenya. Boston, Mass.: Pathfinder Fund.

Gyepi-Garbrah, B. 1988. Fertility and marriage in adolescents in Africa. Paper presented at IUSSP African Population Conference, Dakar, Senegal, Nov. 7–12.

Hamilton, S., B. Popkin, and C. Spicer. 1984. Women and Nutrition in Third World Countries. New York: Praeger.

Harrison, K. A. 1983. Obstetric fistula: one social calamity too many. Br. J. Obstet. Gynaecol. 90:385–386.

Harrison, K. A. 1985. Child-bearing, health and social priorities: a survey of 22,774 consecutive hospital births in Zaria, Northern Nigeria. Br. J. Obstet. Gynaecol. (Suppl.5):110–115.

Harrison, K. A. 1986. Literacy, parity, family planning and maternal mortality in the Third World. Lancet 2(8511):865–866.

Harrison, K. A., and C. E. Rossiter. 1985. Maternal mortality. Br. J. Obstet. Gynaecol. (Suppl.5):110–115.

Harrison, K. A., A. F. Fleming, N. D. Briggs, and C. E. Rossiter. 1985a. Growth during pregnancy in Nigerian teenage primigravidae. Br. J. Obstet. Gyn. (Suppl.5):40–48.

Harrison, K. A., C. E. Rossiter, H. Chong, et al. 1985b. The influence of maternal age and child-bearing with special reference to primigravidae age 15 years and under. Br. J. Obstet. Gynaecol. (Suppl.5):25–31.

Herz, B., and A. R. Measham. 1987. The Safe Motherhood Initiative: Proposals for Action. World Bank Discussion Paper 9. Washington, D.C.: World Bank.

Hill, A. G., and W. J. Graham. 1988. West African Sources of Health and Mortality Information: A Comparative Review. Technical Study 58e. Ottawa: International Development Research Centre.

Hosken, F. P. 1982. Female circumcision in the world today: a global review. In Traditional Practices Affecting the Health of Women and Children, Background Papers to the WHO Seminar, T. Baasher et al., eds.. WHO EMRO Technical Publication 2(2):195–214.

Hurlich, S. 1986. Women in Zambia. Rural Science and Technology Institute, Canadian International Development Institute.

Ismail, E. A. 1982. Child marriage in Somalia. In Traditional Practices Affecting the Health of Women and Children, Background Papers to the WHO Seminar, T. Baasher et al., eds.. WHO EMRO Technical Publication 2(2):130–133.

Jacobson, J. C. 1990. The global politics of abortion. Worldwatch Paper 97. Washington, D.C.: Worldwatch.

Jamison, D. T., W. H. Mosley, A. R. Measham, and J. L. Bobadilla, eds. 1993. Disease Control Priorities in Developing Countries. New York: Oxford University Press.

Jansen, A. A., J. A. Kusin, B. Thiuri, et al. 1984. Anthropometric results in pregnancy and lactation. In Maternal and Child Health in Rural Kenya: An Epidemiological Study, J. K. Van Ginneken and A. S. Muller, eds. London: Croom Helm.

Jellife, D. B., and E. F. Jellife. 1978. The volume and composition of human milk in poorly nourished communities: A review. Am. J. Clin. Nutr. 31(3):492–515.

Johns Hopkins University. 1992. Logo materials, distribution survey report, Nigeria. Baltimore: Population Communication Service. Photocopy.

Judd, H. L., and D. R. Meldrum. 1981. Physiology and pathophysiology of menstruation and menopause. In Gynecology and Obstetrics: The Health Care of Women, 2d ed., S. L. Romney, M. J. Gray, A. B. Little, J. A. Merril, E. S. Quilligan, and R. W. Stander, eds. New York: McGraw-Hill.

Kaiser Family Foundation. 1993. Reproductive Health Policy and Programs: Reflections on the African Experience—A Conference Report. Harare.

Kasongo Project Team. 1983. The Kasongo Project. World Health Forum 4:41–45.

Kasule, J. 1988. The pattern of gynecological malignancy in Zimbabwe. Department of Obstetrics and Gynecology, University of Zimbabwe. Photocopy.

Kaunitz, A. M., C. Spence, T. S. Danielson, R. W. Rochat, and D. A. Grimes. 1984. Perinatal and maternal mortality in a religious group avoiding obstetric care. Am. J. Obstet. Gynecol. 150:826–831.

Keller, M. E. 1987. Maternal mortality in Kamazu Central Hospital for 1985. Med. Q. Malawi 4(1):13–16.

Kheir A-HHM, S. Kumar, and A. R. Cross. 1991. Female circumcision: Attitudes and practices in Sudan. Paper presented at the Demographic and Health Surveys World Conference, Washington, D.C.

Kisekka, M., and B. Otesanya. 1988. Sexually transmitted disease as a gender issue: Examples from Nigeria and Uganda. Paper presented at the AFARD/AAWORD Third General Assembly, Dakar, Senegal, August.

Knippenberg, R., S. Ofosu-Amaah, and D. Parker. 1990. Strengthening PHC Services in Africa: An Operations Research Agenda. New York: UNICEF.

Koso-Thomas, O. 1985. Female Circumcision: Strategies for Eradication. London: Zed.

Kwast, B. E. 1991. Midwives' role in safe motherhood. J. Nurse Midwif. 36(6):366–372.

Kwast, B. E., R. W. Rochat, and W. Kidane–Mariam. 1986. Maternal mortality in Addis Ababa, Ethiopia. Stud. Fam. Plan. 17:288–301.

Kwawukume, E. Y., T. S. Gosh, and J. B. Wilson. 1993. Menopausal age of Ghanaian women. Intl. J. Gynaecol. Obstet. 40(2):151–155.

Ladjali, M., and N. Toubia. 1990. Female circumcision: Desperately seeking a space for women. Intl. Plan. Parenthood Fed. Med. Bull. 24(2).

Leke, R. J. 1989. Commentary on unwanted pregnancy and abortion complications in Cameroon. Intl. J. Gynaecol. Obstet. (Suppl.) 3:33–35.

Lema, V. M. 1990. The determinants of sexuality among adolescent school girls in Kenya. E. Afr. Med. J. 67(3)191–200.

Lema, V. M., R. K. Kamau, and K. O. Rogo. 1989. Epidemiology of abortions in Kenya. The Center for the Study of Adolescence (CSA), Nairobi. Photocopy.

Leslie, J., and G. R. Gupta. 1989. Utilization of formal services for maternal nutrition and health care. International Center for Research on Women, Washington, D.C. Photocopy.

Lettenmaier, C. L., L. Liskin, C. Church, and J. Harris. 1988. Mothers' Lives Matter: Maternal Health in the Community. Population Reports, Series L, No. 7. Baltimore, Md.: Johns Hopkins University, Population Information Program.

Lightfoot-Klein, H. 1989. Prisoners of Ritual: An Odyssey into Female Genital Circumcision in Africa. New York: Harrington Park.

Likwa, R., and M. Whittaker. n.d. The characteristics of women presenting for abortion or for complications of illegal abortions at the University Teaching Hospital, Lusaka, Zambia—An exploratory study. The Population Council, New York. Photocopy.

Liskin, L. 1992. Maternal morbidity in developing countries: a review and comments. Int. J. Gynaecol. Obstet. 37(2):77–87.

Liskin, L., N. Kak, A. Rutledge, et al. 1985. Youth in the 1980's: Social and Health Concerns. Population Reports, Series M, No 9. Baltimore, Md.: Johns Hopkins University, Population Information Program.

Mahler, H. 1987. The safe motherhood initiative: a call to action. Lancet (March): 668–670.

Mahmood, T. A., D. M. Campbell, and A. W. Wilson. 1988. Maternal height, shoe size, and outcome of labour in white primigravidas: A prospective anthropometric study. Br. Med. J. 297(6647):515–517.

Maine, D. 1991. Safe Motherhood Programs: Options and Issues. New York: Center for Population and Family Health, School of Public Health, Columbia University.

Maine, D., A. Rosenfield, A. Wallace, A. M. Kimball, B. Kwast, E. Papiernik, and S. White. 1987. Prevention of maternal deaths in developing countries: Program options and practical considerations. Paper presented at the International Safe Motherhood Conference, Nairobi, February 10–13.

Maine, D. et al. 1992. Barriers to treatment of obstetric emergencies in rural communities of West Africa. Stud. Fam. Plan. 23(5):279–291.

Maine, D., J. McCarthy, and V. M. Ward. 1992. Guidelines for monitoring progress in the reduction of maternal mortality (a work in progress). UNICEF: New York.

Martinez, J. M., M. Phillips, and R. G. Feachem. 1990. Diarrheal Diseases: Health Section Priorities Review. Washington, D.C.: World Bank.

Mbaruku, G., and S. Bergstrom. 1995. Reducing maternal mortality in Kigoma, Tanzania. Hlth. Pol. Plan. 10(1):71–78.

Mbizvo, M. T., S. Fawcus, G. Lindmark, and L. Nystrom. 1993. Maternal mortality in rural and urban Zimbabwe: social and reproductive factors in an incident case-referent study. Soc. Sci. Med. 36(9):1197–1205.

McCann, M. F., L. S. Liskin, P. J. Piotrow, W. Rinehart, and G. Fox. 1984. Breastfeeding, Fertility and Family Planning. Population Reports, Series J, No. 24. Baltimore, Md.: Johns Hopkins University, Population Information Program.

McGregor, I. A. 1991. Morbidity and mortality at Kenneba, The Gambia, 1950–75. In Disease and Mortality in Sub-Saharan Africa, R. G. Feachem and D. T. Jamison, eds. New York: Oxford University Press.

McLean S., and S. E. Graham. 1985. Female Circumcision, Excision and Infibulation: The Facts and Proposals for Change. Report 47. London: The Minority Rights Group.

Megafu, U. 1983. Female circumcision in Africa: An investigation of the presumed benefits among Ibos of Nigeria. E. Afr. Med. J. 60(11)793–800.

Meheus, A. 1992. Women's health: importance of reproductive tract infections, pelvic inflammatory disease, and cervical cancer. In Reproductive Tract Infections: Global Impact and Priorities for Women's Reproductive Health, A. Germain, K. K. Holmes, P. Piot, and J. N. Wasserheit, eds. New York: Plenum.

Melrose, E. B. 1984. Maternal deaths at King Edward VIII Hospital, Durban. S. Afr. Med. J. 65(5):161–165.

Merchant, K., M. Reynaldo, and J. D. Haas. 1990. Consequences for maternal nutrition of reproductive stress across consecutive pregnancies. Am. J. Clin. Nutr. 52:616–20.

Merchant, K. M., and K. M. Kurz. 1992. Women's nutrition through the life cycle: Social and biological vulnerabilities. In Women's Health: A Global Perspective, M. A. Koblinsky, J. Timyan, and J. Gay, eds. Boulder, Colo.: Westview.

Miller, J. E., and R. Huss-Ashmore. 1989. Do reproductive patterns affect maternal nutritional status? An analysis of maternal depletion in Lesotho. Am. J. Human Biol. 1(4):409–419.

Modawi, O. 1982. Traditional practices in childbirth in Sudan. In Traditional Practices Affecting the Health of Women and Children, Background Papers for the WHO Seminar, T. Baasher et al., eds. WHO EMRO Technical Publication (2):75–87.

Mosley, W. H., and L. Chen. 1984. An analytical framework for the study of child survival in developing countries. Pop. Dev. Rev. 10 (Suppl.):25–45.

Muller, A. S. and J. K. van Ginneken. 1991. Morbidity and mortality in Machakos, Kenya, 1974-81. In Disease and Mortality in Sub-Saharan Africa, R. G. Feachem and D. T. Jamison, eds. New York: Oxford University Press.

Nash, E. S. 1990. Teenage preganacy—need a child bear a child? S. Afr. Med. J. 77(3): 147–151.

Neuman, C., N. O. Bwibo, and M. Jifman. 1992. Functional Implication of Malnutrition, Final Report. Office of Nutrition, United States Agency for International Development, Washington, D.C.

Nichols, D., O. A. Ladipo, J. M. Paxman, and E. O. Otolorin. 1986. Sexual behavior, contraceptive practice, and reproductive health among Nigerian adolescents. Stud. Fam. Plan. 17(2):100–106.

Niger Ministry of Finance and Planning. 1993. Niger Demographic and Health Survey, 1992. Niamey: General Division of Planning, Ministry of Finance and Planning.

Nigeria Federal Office of Statistics and Macro International. 1992. Nigeria Demographic and Health Survey. Lagos: Federal Office of Statistics.

Odejide, T. O. 1986. Offering an alternative to illegal abortion in Nigeria. New Era Nursing Image International 2(2):39–42.

Okafor, C. B. 1991. Availability and use of services for maternal and child health care in rural Nigeria. Int. J. Gynaecol. Obstet. 34(4):331–346.

Okonfua, F. E., A. Lawal, and J. K. Bamgvose. 1990. Features of menopause and menopausal age in Nigerian women. Intl. J. Gynaecol. Obstet. 31(4):341–345.

Okonofua, F. E., A. Abejide, and R. A. Makanjuola. 1992. Maternal mortality in Ile–Ife, Nigeria: A study of risk factors. Stud. Fam. Plan. 23(5):319–324.

Oronsaye, A. U., and G. I. Odiase. 1981. Incidence of ectopic pregnancy in Benin City, Nigeria. Trop. Doctor 11(4):160–163.

Otoo, S. N. 1973. The traditional management of pregnancy and childbirth among the Ga people, Ghana. Trop. Geog. Med. 25:88–94.

Over, M., and P. Piot. 1993. HIV infection and sexually transmitted diseases. In Disease Control Priorities in Developing Countries, D. T. Jamison, W. H. Mosley, A. R. Measham, and J. L. Bobadilla, eds. New York: Oxford University Press.

Pagezy, H. 1983. Attitudes of Ntomba society towards the primiparous woman and its biological effects. J. Biosoc. Sci. 15(4):421–431.

Parker, L. N., G. R. Gupta, K. M. Kurz, and K. M. Merchant. 1990. Better health for women: Research results from the Maternal Nutrition and Health Care Program. The International Center for Research on Women, Washington, D.C. Photocopy.

Parkin, D. M., E. Laara, and C. S. Muir. 1988. Estimates of the worldwide frequency of sixteen major cancers in 1980. Intl. J. Cancer 32:407–415.

Petros–Barvazian, A. 1984. World priorities and targets in maternal and child health in the year 2000. Intl. J. Gynaecol. Obstet. 22:439–448.

Plummer, F. A., M. Laga, R. C. Brunham, et al. 1987. Postpartum upper genital tract infections in Nairobi, Kenya: epidemiology, etiology and risk factors. J. Infect. Dis. 156:92–98.

Prema, K., R. Madhavapeddi, and B. A. Ramalakshmi. 1981. India. Indian Council of Medical Research, National Institute of Nutrition. Photocopy.

Prentice, A. M., A. Prentice, W. H. Lamb, and P. G. Lunn. 1983. Metabolic consequences of fasting during Ramadan in pregnant and lactating women. Human Nutr. Clin. Nutr. 37C(4):283–294.

Prentice, A., T. J. Cole, and R. G. Whitehead. 1987. Impaired growth in infants born to mothers of very high parity. Human Nutr. Clin. 41C:319–325.

Raikes, A. 1989. Women's health in East Africa. Soc. Sci. Med. 28(5):447–759.

Rinehart, W. 1987. Employment-based family planning programs. Pop. Rept. J. 34:J921–951.

Robey, B., S. O. Rutstein, L. Morris, and R. Blackburn. 1992. National Family Planning Surveys: What Women Say. Population Reports, Series M, No. 11. Baltimore, Md.: Johns Hopkins University, Population Information Program.

Rogo, K., and J. M. Nyamu. 1989. Legal termination of pregnancy at the Kenyatta National Hospital using prostaglandin F2 in mid–trimester. E. Afr. Med. J. 66(5):333–339.

Rogo, K., et al. 1987. Menarche in African secondary school girls in Kenya. E. Afr. Med. J. 64(8):511–515.

Rooney, C. 1992. Antenatal Care and Maternal Health: How Effective Is It? Geneva: WHO.

Rosenfield, A. 1989. Maternal mortality in developing countries: an ongoing but neglected epidemic. J. Am. Med. Soc. 262(3):376–379.

Rosenfield, A., and D. Maine. 1985. Maternal mortality—a neglected tragedy: where is the M in MCH? Lancet 2:83–85.

Royston, E., and S. Armstrong, eds. 1989. Preventing Maternal Deaths. Geneva: WHO.

Rubin, G., B. McCarthy, J. Shelton, et al. 1981. The risk of childbearing reevaluated. Am. J. Pub. Hlth. 71(7):712–716.

Rushwan, H. 1990. Female circumcision. World Health, April–May.

Sargent, C. 1977. The integration of the traditional midwife in a national health delivery system. Paper presented at the Ford Foundation Regional Family Health Management Workshop at Cotonou, Benin, December 2. Photocopy.

Sargent, C. 1982. The implications of role expectations for birth assistance among Bariba women. Soc. Sci. Med. 16:1483–1489.

Sargent, C. 1985. Obstetrical choice among urban women in Benin. Soc. Sci. Med. 20(3)287–292.

Shaper, A. G., M. S. R. Hutt, and Z. Fejfar. 1974. Cardiovascular Disease in the Tropics. London: British Medical Association.

Sherris, J., and G. Fox. 1983. Infertility and Sexually Transmitted Disease: A Public Health Challenge. Population Reports, Series L, No. 4. Baltimore, Md.: Johns Hopkins University, Population Information Program.

Slack, A. T. 1988. Female circumcision: A critical appraisal. Human Rights Q. 10:437–486.

Smith, J. B., N. F. Burton, G. Nelseon, J. A. Fortney, and S. Duale. 1986. Hospital deaths in a high risk obstetric population: Karawa, Zaire. Intl. J. Gynaecol. Obstet. 24:225–234.

Smith, J. C., J. M. Hughes, P. S. Pekow, et al. 1984. An assessment of the incidence of maternal mortality. Am. J. Pub. Hlth. 74(8):780–783.

Sokal, D., L. Swadogo, and A. Adjibade. 1991. Short stature and cephalopelvic disproportion in Burkina Faso, West Africa. Intl. J. Gynaecol. Obstet. 35:347–350.

Starrs, A. 1987. Preventing Maternal Deaths. A Report on the International Safe Motherhood Conference, Nairobi, Kenya, February 1987. New York: World Bank, WHO, and UNFPA.

Tahzib, F. 1983. Epidemiological determinants of vesicovaginal fistulas. Br. J. Obstet. Gynaecol. 90:387–391.

Tahzib, F. 1989. Searching for the M in MCH. Lancet 2(8666):795.

Tanner, J. M. 1962. Growth at Adolescence. London: Blackwell Scientific.

Tarimo, E. 1991. Community-based studies in Sub-Saharan Africa: an overview. In Disease and Mortality in Sub-Saharan Africa, R. G. Feachem and D. T. Jamison, eds. New York: Oxford University Press.

Thaddeus, S., and D. Maine. 1990. Too Far to Walk. New York: Center for Population and Family Health, School of Public Health, Columbia University.

Tietze, C. 1977. Maternal mortality, excluding abortion mortality. World Hlth. Stat. Rpt. 30:312–339.

Timaeus, I. M. 1991. Adult mortality: levels, trends, and data sources. In Disease and Mortality in Sub-Saharan Africa, R. G. Feachem and D. T. Jamison, eds. New York: Oxford University Press.

Tinker, A., P. Daly, C. Green, H. Saxenian, R. Lakshminarayanan, and K. Gill. 1994. Women's Health and Nutrition: Making a Difference. Washington, D.C.: The World Bank.

Toure, B., P. Thonneau, P. Cantrelle, T. M. Barry, T. Ngo-Khac, and E. Papiernick. 1992. Level and causes of maternal mortality in Guinea (West Africa). Intl. J. Gynecol. Obstet. 37:98–95.

Toubia, N. 1993. Female Genital Mutilation: A Call for Global Action. New York: Women Ink.

Uche, C. 1980. The context of mortality in Nigeria. Paper presented at the International Union for the Scientific Study of Population Seminar on Social Aspects of Mortality and the Length of Life, Fiuggi Terme, Italy, May 13–16.

Ujah, I. A. 1991. Sexual activity and attitudes toward contraception among women seeking termination of pregnancy in Zaria, northern Nigeria. Intl. J. Gynaecol. Obstet. 35(1):73–77.

Unuigbe, J. A., et al. 1988a. Abortion-related morbidity and mortality in Benin City, Nigeria: 1973–1986. Intl. J. Gynaecol. Obstet. 26(3):435–439.

Unuigbe, J. A., A. U. Oronsaye, and A. A. Orhue. 1988b. Preventable factors in abortion-related maternal mortality in Africa: Focus on abortion deaths in Benin City, Nigeria. Trop. J. Obstet. Gynecol. 1 (1 special ed. ser.):36–39.

UN (United Nations). 1989. Adolescent Reproductive Behavior: Evidence from Developing Countries, Volume 11, UN Population Studies 109. New York.

UNDP (United Nations Development Programme). 1994. Human Development Report. New York: Oxford University Press.

U.S. Bureau of the Census. 1995. International Database. Washington, D.C.: U.S. Bureau of the Census, Aging Studies Branch.

van Roosmalen, J. 1987. Symphysiotomy as an alternative to cesarean section. Intl. J. Gynaecol. Obstet. 25:451–458.

van Steenbergen, W. M., J. A. Kusin, M. Van Rens, et al. 1984. Lactation performance. Pp. 153–166 in Maternal and Child Health in Rural Kenya: An Epidemiological Study, J. K. van Ginneken and A. S. Muller, eds. London: Croon Helm.

Verzin, J. A. 1975. Sequelae of female circumcision. Sudan Med. J. 5:178–212.

Vis, H. L., and P. Hennart. 1987. Exclusive and partial breastfeeding and infant development in Central Africa. In Weaning: Why, What and When? A. Gallabriga and J. Veny, eds. Nevey, Switzerland: Nestle Nutrition.

Walker, A., and P. Parmar. 1993. Warrior Marks: Female Genital Mutilation and the Sexual Blinding of Women. New York: Harcourt Brace.

Walsh, J. A., C. M. Feifer, A. R. Measham, and P. J. Gertler. 1993. Maternal and perinatal health. In Disease Control Priorities in Developing Countries, D. T. Jamison, W. H. Mosley, A. R. Measham, and J. L. Bobadilla, eds. New York: Oxford University Press.

Wentz, A. C. 1988. Management of menopause. Pp. 397–442 in Novak's Textbook of Gynecology, 11th ed., H. W. Jones et al., eds. Baltimore: Williams and Wilkins.

White, S. M., et al. 1987. Emergency obstetric surgery performed by nurses in Zaire. Lancet 28:337–342.

Whitehead, R. G., M. Hutton, E. Muller, et al. 1978. Factors affecting lactation performance in rural Gambian mothers. Lancet 2(8082):178–181.

Winikoff, B., and M. Sullivan. 1987. Assessing the role of family planning in reducing maternal mortality. Stud. Fam. Plan. 18(3):128–143.

World Bank. 1992. Better Health in Africa. Washington D.C.: World Bank, Africa Technical Department.

World Bank. 1993. World Development Report 1993: Investing in Health. New York: Oxford University Press.

World Bank. 1994. Better Health in Africa. Washington, D.C.: World Bank.

WHO (World Health Organization). 1981. Research in Menopause. WHO Technical Report Series 670:1-120. Geneva.

WHO (World Health Organization). 1982. The Prevalence of Anaemia in Women. Geneva.

WHO (World Health Organization). 1986. A Traditional Practice that Threatens Health-Female Circumcision. WHO Chronicle 40(1):31–36.

WHO (World Health Organization). 1987a. Genital human papilloma virus infections and cancer: memorandum from a WHO meeting. WHO Bull. 65:817–827.

WHO (World Health Organization). 1987b. Maternal mortality dimensions of the problem. Paper presented at the Safe Motherhood Conference, Nairobi, February 10–13.

WHO (World Health Organization). 1989. The Health of Youth, Facts for Action. Youth and Sexually Transmitted Diseases. A42/Technical Discussions/10. Geneva.

WHO (World Health Organization). 1990. Maternal Health and Safe Motherhood Programme Progress Report, 1987–90. Geneva.

WHO (World Health Organization). 1991a. Essential Elements of Obstetric Care at First Referral Level, 1986. WHO Technical Report No. 3328E. Geneva.

WHO (World Health Organization). 1991b. Maternal Mortality: A Global Factbook. Geneva.

Wrinkrist, A., K. M. Rasmussen, and J. P. Habicht. 1992. A new definition of maternal depletion syndrome. Am. J. Pub. Health 82(5):691–694.

Wynn, R. M. 1983. Obstetrics and Gynecology: The Clinical Core, 3d Ed., Philadelphia: Lea and Febiger.

Zimicki, S. 1989. Fertility and maternal mortality. In Contraceptive Use and Controlled Fertility: Health Issues for Women and Children—Background Papers, A. M. Parnell, ed. Washington, D.C.: National Academy Press.

5

Nervous System Disorders

The evidence available for Sub-Saharan Africa suggests that the burden of nervous system disorders may be heavier in African communities than in comparable communities in other parts of the developing world (Osuntokun, 1970, 1971a; Spillane, 1973). There is also evidence that the burden of certain of these disorders may be heavier in females than in males. Because of their particular significance for females, it is these disorders, presented in Table 5-1, that are the focus of this chapter. They are: toxic and nutritional disorders, headache syndromes, cerebrovascular diseases associated with oral contraceptive use, epilepsies, demyelinating diseases, neurologic complications of collagen diseases, and impaired cognition and dementia. An exception to this picture of gender-distinctive burden is cerebral malaria, potentially a greater problem for females because of their heightened susceptibility during pregnancy. This condition is discussed in depth in Chapters 4 and 10.

LIFE SPAN PERSPECTIVE

The female, like the male, is at risk of suffering from specific disorders of the nervous system at certain stages of life, although disease onset for a number of these disorders occurs over a wide spectrum of age. Table 5-2 provides a listing of nervous system disorders, by age category, that affect both African males and females.

Because many of the nervous system disorders listed in Table 5-2 are believed to affect males and females equally over the life span, they are not discussed in this chapter. Other illnesses, such as tetanus and cerebral malaria, are reviewed elsewhere in this report (see Chapters 4 and 10, respectively). As noted above, this chapter focuses on the following nervous system disorders for which African females appear to be particularly susceptible or at risk: toxic and nutritional disorders, headache syndromes, cerebrovascular diseases associated with use of oral contraceptives, epilepsies, demyelinating diseases, neurologic complications of collagen diseases, and impaired cognition and dementia. The evidence for these disorders is presented below.

TOXIC AND NUTRITIONAL DISORDERS OF THE NERVOUS SYSTEM

Nutritional syndromes involving the nervous system are common in Sub-Saharan Africa. Protein-energy malnutrition may afflict 40 percent or more of preschool children at a stage when the maturation of the nervous system is still under way, and malnutrition can result in long-term or permanent damage to cognition and intellect

TABLE 5-1   Nervous System Disorders in Sub-Saharan Africa: Gender-Related Burden

Disorder	Exclusive to Females	Greater for Females than for Males	Burden for Females and Males Comparable, but of Particular Significance for Females
Cerebrovascular diseases associated with oral contraceptive use	X		
Demyelinating diseases		X	
Epilepsies		X	
Headache syndromes		X	
Impaired cognition and dementia			X
Neurologic complications of collagen diseases		X	
Toxic and nutritional disorders		X	

NOTE: Significance is defined here as having impact on health that, for any reason—biological, reproductive, sociocultural, or economic—is different in its implications for females than for males.

(de Mota et al., 1990; Grantham-McGregor et al., 1991; Lucas et al., 1990; Osuntokun 1972a; Pollitt and Thompson, 1977; Rush, 1984; Smart, 1986; Stocks et al., 1982).

Onset of nutritional and toxic diseases of the nervous system, which include the tropical myeloneuropathies (Roman et al., 1987), are known to be precipitated by pregnancy and lactation. Wernicke's encephalopathy, caused by thiamine deficiency, is a known complication of severe morning sickness during pregnancy (hyperemesis gravidarum) and anorexia nervosa. Females also appear highly susceptible to effects of thiaminases in seasonal foods, such as those from the worm *anaphe venata*, commonly eaten in southwestern Nigeria and postulated as an etiological factor in seasonal epidemic ataxia (Ademolekun, 1993; Osuntokun, 1972b).

Folate and iron deficiencies, often associated with pregnancy and lactation, may be important determinants of fetal morbidity and mortality in the Sub-Saharan region. During pregnancy there is a greater requirement for folate because of the increased rate of folate metabolism (McParklin et al., 1993). Folate deficiency is widespread in African women and can contribute to a variety of neuropsychiatric syndromes, including peripheral neuropathy, dementia, and depression. The incidence of neural tube defects caused by folic acid deficiency could be as high as 7 per 1,000 deliveries (Airede, 1992), and may well be increasing in areas where maternal malnutrition has increased and folate deficits are significant. It is now well established that periconceptional folate supplementation could prevent first occurrence of neural tube defects (Czeizel and Dudas, 1992; MRC Vitamin Study Research Group, 1991). There is also greater need for folate in subjects with chronic hemolytic disease, such as hemoglobin sickle-cell disease, which afflicts about 1 percent of the West African population, and malaria.

Iron deficiency is particularly common in Sub-Saharan Africa, and more common in females than in males. A major cause of iron deficiency is hookworm infection, which afflicts millions of black Africans, especially in rural areas. Hookworm anemia is often unrecognized as an underlying cause of high maternal morbidity and mortality, apathy and poor health in children, and easy fatigability and impaired working capacity in adults (Pawlowski et al., 1991). Menorrhagia and pregnancy states predispose to iron deficiency anemia. Other risk factors for iron deficiency are the growth spurt of adolescence, with the accompanying burden of providing iron for an increased red cell mass and increased hemoglobin concentration; childhood, especially between the ages of 4 months and 3

TABLE 5-2 Disorders of the Nervous System in the African Female Across Her Life Span

Time of Life	Disorders
Intrauterine	Congenital malformations from maternal malnutrition and infections Cretinism from maternal iodine deficiency and goitrogenic diet, including cassava diet Low birthweight from maternal malnutrition may cause poor neurodevelopment, increased occurrence or risk in later life of high blood pressure; and mortality from cardiovascular disease, including stroke (Barker et al., 1989a,b; Edwards et al., 1993; Law et al., 1993, 1991; Seldman et al., 1991; Whincup et al., 1989)
Infancy (0–1 year)	Congenital malformations Impaired neurodevelopment from malnutrition Febrile convulsions Meningitides, encephalitides (including parainfectious encephalomyelitis), poliomyelitis Cerebral malaria Epilepsies
Childhood (1–9 years)	Cerebral malaria Meningitides and encephalitides (including parainfectious encephalomyelitis), poliomyelitis Epilepsies Migraine Cerebrovascular disease Lymphomas (especially Burkitt's) of nervous system
Adolescence (10–19 years)	Migraine Epilepsies Meningitides and encephalitides, cerebral abscess
Adulthood (20–45 years)	Epilepsies Migraine Meningitides, encephalitides, trypanosomiasis, cerebral malaria Head injuries Nutritional and toxic myeloneuropathies and peripheral nerve disorders Nervous system involvement from choriocarcinoma Polymyositis, myasthenia gravis Demyelinating diseases (often monophasic, as Devic's disease) Neurological complications of snake bites
Menopause/late adulthood (46–65 years)	Cerebrovascular disease Migraine Nutritional and toxic myeloneuropathies and peripheral nerve disorders Epilepsies Spinal cord and spinal nerve root disorders secondary to osteodegenerative disease of vertebral column Brain and spinal cord neoplasms (primary and secondary) Head injuries Polymyalgia rheumatica, temporal arteritis
Elderly (> 65 years)	Cerebrovascular disease Spinal cord and spinal nerve root disorders secondary to osteodegenerative disease of the vertebral column (spine) Brain and spinal cord neoplasms Head injuries Parkinson's disease Cognitive impairment/dementia

years, with the rapid rate of growth and increase in red cell mass; and diets consisting primarily of whole grain cereal and legumes with a rich iron content that is not readily absorbable. With the vital role of iron in the fundamental metabolism of the cells (including the neurons), it is not surprising that increasing evidence indicates that impaired psychomotor development and intellectual performance and changes in behavior result from even mild iron deficiency, particularly in infants between 6 months and 2 years of age (Lozoff, 1988). Such infants showed significant decreases in responsiveness and activity, increased body tension, fearfulness, and tendency to fatigue (Lozoff et al., 1982a,b; Oski et al., 1983; Walter et al., 1983), and there is some evidence that these abnormalities may persist after correction of iron deficiency.

The deficiency of riboflavin common in African women has been associated with endogenous and neurotic depression, and pyridoxine deficiency has been linked to peripheral neuropathy and affective illness (Carney, 1990). Use of oral contraceptives also contributes to pyridoxine deficiency and may increase existing nutrition-related deficits (Stamp, 1993).

In some parts of Africa, endemic cretinism is widespread and is the result of iodine deficiency, further conditioned by a cassava diet. A neurodegenerative syndrome linked to a cassava diet is also endemic in some countries (Monekosso and Wilson, 1966; Osuntokun, 1968, 1981b) and occurs in epidemics, especially at times of drought, as reported from Mozambique, Tanzania, and Zaire (Carton et al., 1986; Cliff et al., 1986; Essers et al., 1992; Howlett et al., 1990, 1992; Mozambique, Ministry of Health, 1984; Rosling, 1986; Rosling et al., 1988; Tylleskar et al., 1992). Evidence that indicates a disproportionate occurrence of these disorders in females is lacking.

Poor nutritional status may also enhance the neurotoxicity of the cyanogenic glycosides, found in cassava, manihot, millet, and other dietary items commonly consumed in some parts of Sub-Saharan Africa (Osuntokun, 1968, 1981b); the organophosphates commonly used as pesticides; and some frequently used drugs, including isoniazid, ethambutol, nitrous oxide, chloramphenicol, metronidazole, phenytoin, dapsone, chloroquine, vincristine, and nitrofurantoin (Osuntokun, 1986). Again, there are no data indicating an unusual burden of these disorders in females.

HEADACHE SYNDROMES

The prevalence of headache syndromes exceeds 50 percent, and the incidence of migraine is 6 percent or higher even in rural communities (Joubert, 1992; Levy, 1983; Lisk, 1987; Longe and Osuntokun, 1988; Osuntokun and Osuntokun, 1972; Osuntokun et al., 1982b,c, 1987b, 1992b). In some parts of Africa, migraine and tension headache are the most common modes of presentation of headache, in the community as well as in the hospital (Osuntokun, 1971b).

Migraine

Both common and classical migraine are predominantly diseases of women, with female-to-male ratios ranging from 5:2 in hospital case series, to 2:1 in two rural communities, and 6:5 in urban community studies in Nigeria. In one Nigerian study, in a sample of 19,000 people, the female predominance was high in patients under the age of 30 years, but the age-specific incidence rates in males and females over age 30 were comparable (Osuntokun et al., 1992b; see Table 5-3 below).

A community-based study among the Zulus in Natal, South Africa, found a prevalence of migraine of 8.8 percent, with a female-to-male ratio of 10:1 (Joubert, 1992). Evidence suggests that migraine, particularly common migraine as defined by the International Headache Society (IHS, 1988), is influenced by hormonal changes associated with menarche, ovulation, and menstruation, which may account for the increased susceptibility of females to migrainous headaches. Contraceptive pills may also precipitate migraine, which may then continue despite stopping the pills. The relationship of migraine to hormonal levels is complex: some individuals experience reduction in migraine during pregnancy; in others, the headaches are worse; and in a third group, the headaches reappear soon after childbirth. Unlike Caucasian patients, who suffer from cluster headaches with a male-to-female ratio of 5:1 or higher, Nigerian females outnumber males among patients with cluster headaches

TABLE 5-3 Migrainous Headaches in Nigerian Africans—Age-Specific Prevalence Ratios

Age Group (years)	Cases per 100 Persons	
	Male	Female
0–9	10.2	10.6
10–19	1.8	4.0
20–29	1.3	3.4
30–39	3.1	3.3
40–49	3.8	3.8
50–59	3.9	2.2
60–69	5.4	4.0
> 70	2.9	4.7
Age unknown	2.1	5.0
Total	5.03	5.64

(Osuntokun, 1971b; Osuntokun et al., 1982a). Nigerian migraine sufferers with hemoglobin AS genotype (usually symptomless, apart from being susceptible to painless hematuria from ischemic renal papillitis) are significantly liable to suffer from complicated migraine (Osuntokun and Osuntokun, 1972). HB AS has a frequency of 25 percent in West Africans. Among Nigerian migraine sufferers, the relative risk of epilepsy ranged from 2 to 3.2 (Osuntokun, 1971a; Osuntokun et al., 1982b). Among Caucasians, epilepsy is said to be two to six times more common in people who suffer migraines compared with people who do not (Basser, 1969; Hannington, 1974).

Tension Headache

As in Caucasians, there is an excess of females among Africans who suffer from tension headaches as defined by the IHS. In the Zulu study, all 19 patients who suffered from tension headache were females (Joubert, 1992). Among Nigerians, tension headache is twice as frequent as migraine (Osuntokun, 1971a,b), in contrast to subjects in the Zulu study, who experienced migraine with nearly four times the frequency of tension headache (Joubert, 1988; 1992).

CEREBROVASCULAR DISEASES AND USE OF ORAL CONTRACEPTIVES

Cerebrovascular disease, such as stroke (subarachnoid hemorrhage, cerebral hemorrhage, cerebral infarction, hypertensive encephalopathy), is now as common in most communities in Africa as in the developed countries (Abraham and Abdulkadir, 1981; Bahemuka, 1989; Danesi et al., 1983; Lester, 1982; Matenga et al., 1986; Putterpill et al., 1984). In a community-based study in Nigeria, the age-specific incidence rates of stroke or cerebrovascular accident were comparable to rates in the Caucasian populations in Europe and among the Japanese (Osuntokun et al., 1979). Some analysis has suggested that the age-adjusted mortality rate for stroke in a Nigerian community may surpass that of the United States (Osuntokun, et al., 1987b). In Ethiopia, Ghana, Kenya, Nigeria, Senegal, and Uganda, stroke constitutes between 4 and 10 percent of all causes of death (Osuntokun, 1980).

Since the mid-1960s, a vast amount of epidemiologic, clinical, and laboratory evidence in developed countries has linked the current use of combined oral contraceptives with certain types of cardiovascular disease (CVD), especially venous thromboembolism, thrombotic stroke, myocardial infarction, subarachnoid hemorrhage, and hypertension (Irey et al., 1978; *Lancet*, 1979; Stadel, 1981; Thorgood et al., 1981; Vessey, 1982). Whether these findings from the developed countries can be extrapolated to black African countries is debatable. To date, no valid epidemiologic data link the use of the oral contraceptives by black Africans to increased CVD risk, although it is unlikely that the metabolic changes (Fotherby, 1989) that occur in women using oral contraceptives and described in the communities of the developed countries would be different from those in African women. It is also true that the smaller-dose oral contraceptives that are now the norm are associated with a lower CVD risk than the formulations common in the 1970s and 1980s.

OTHER NEUROLOGICAL DISORDERS

Epilepsies

The prevalence ratios of epilepsy per 1,000 range from 5 to 42 in Sub-Saharan Africa, compared with 5 to 8 in developed countries (Feksi et al., 1991a,b; Gerritts, 1983; Goudsmit et al., 1983; Jilek and Aall-jilek, 1970; Osuntokun, 1992; Osuntokun et al., 1987a; Tekle-Haimanot, 1990). Data suggest that epilepsy has a higher prevalence in poor, deprived communities in Sub-Saharan Africa than in communities with improved socioeconomic status and adequate access to health care facilities (Osuntokun, 1992; Sorvon and Farmer, 1988). The high prevalence of epilepsy in Sub-Saharan Africa and other developing countries may stem from a high frequency of birth trauma and other forms of head trauma; infective, including parasitic, diseases (such as cysticercosis and cerebral malaria) of the central nervous system; febrile convulsions; and encephalopathies complicating the childhood exanthematas. Immunization against the childhood infections appeared to protect against epilepsy (Ogunniyi et al., 1988).

In some cultures it is believed that epilepsy is incurable because it is a manifestation of some divine intervention; hence many African epileptics do not seek modern treatment. Fortunately, drug treatment has proven as effective here as in the developed countries, regardless of whether anticonvulsant therapy was started early or late (Feksi et al., 1991b; Ogunniyi and Osuntokun, 1991). In Africa as elsewhere, about 70 percent of epileptics properly treated in the first year of the occurrence of seizures can go on to be seizure-free. Low compliance with a drug regimen remains a significant problem, however, and appropriate drugs are often unavailable or are too costly to be affordable for the vast majority of patients. Community surveys indicate that many epileptics are not under any form of treatment because of widespread inadequacy of the health care system. In most African countries, epilepsy continues to incur considerable social disadvantage and to cause major disruption in the sufferers' lives.

With respect to epilepsy and gender, there is a male preponderance of black African epileptics seen in hospitals, with the exception of two reports from Uganda and South Africa that documented female preponderance in a small series of 83 (38 males and 45 females) and 50 (21 males and 29 females) patients, respectively. Evidence from three Nigerian community-based studies indicating an excess of female over male epileptics, however, support the possibility that the disorder may occur more frequently in females than males in the region (Longe and Osuntokun, 1989; Osuntokun et al., 1982b, 1987b).

Demyelinating Diseases

In Africans, as in Caucasians, disseminated myelitis with optic neuritis (neuromyelitis optica, Devic's disease) affects both sexes equally (Osuntokun, 1971a; Spillane, 1973). Of the few anecdotal cases of multiple sclerosis reported in Africans, females are in slight excess (Collomb et al., 1970; Kanyerezi et al., 1980; Lisk, 1991; Tekle-Haimanot, 1985). Among Caucasians in most published series, males have been affected more often than females by multiple sclerosis, but the disease often begins earlier and runs a more rapid course in females (Acheson, 1972).

Neurologic Complications of Collagen Diseases

Collagen diseases appear to be relatively uncommon in black Africans, among whom the prevalence of autoimmune disorders is lower than in Caucasians; polymyositis/dermatomyositis, whether idiopathic or secondary to an underlying neoplasm (which may be occult), is the third most common disease of muscles after pyomyositis and the muscular dystrophies in black Africans. As in Caucasians, females predominate among

African patients with polymyositis/dermatomyositis, with a female-to-male ratio of 2:1 (Osuntokun, 1971a; Spillane, 1973). The neurological manifestations of systemic lupus erythematosus (SLE) are protean. SLE, like neurosarcoidosis, is several times more common in black Americans whose ancestral home is West Africa than in white Americans, but is relatively uncommon in black Africans. SLE is predominantly a disease of females, with female-to-male ratios ranging from 5:1 to 9:1. The female-to-male ratio in polymyalgia rheumatica is 2:1. There is a slight excess of females among patients with polyarteritis nodosa and giant cell arteritis (temporal arteritis); the latter often coexists with polymyalgia rheumatica.

Dementia

The most common cause of dementia in the elderly, Alzheimer's disease, is an age-related disorder for which age is the prime risk factor. Because females live longer than males in almost every society, there are more females than males overall who suffer from Alzheimer's disease (Jorm, 1990), but analysis of dementia prevalence studies showed no overall gender difference (Jorm et al., 1987). Nevertheless, when studies of specific dementing diseases were analyzed, both prevalence ratio and incidence rates for Alzheimer's disease tended to be higher among females than males, whereas for vascular dementia they tended to be higher for males.

The longevity revolution, or greying of the population, that has contributed to increasing rates of age-related dementias in developed countries is also occurring in the developing countries, where 52 percent of the world's population of 400 million individuals older than 65 years now live. It is estimated that this proportion will increase to 75 percent by 2020. Of the worldwide monthly increase of 1 million elderly (65 years or older), 80 percent are in the developing countries, including Africa (WHO, 1984). The elderly already exceed 5 percent or more of the population of some African countries, so it is increasingly important to determine and monitor patterns of epidemiological transition that have particular meaning for the elderly cohorts. Sub-Saharan countries would benefit if ongoing transcultural research (Evans, 1992; Osuntokun et al., 1992a) were to identify some preventable causes of the dementias of the elderly, particularly Alzheimer's disease, before the "epidemic" raging in the developed world hits Africa.

CONCLUSIONS

Evidence concerning the contribution of nervous system disorders to the overall burden of disease and disability in females in Sub-Saharan Africa is fragmentary, but disturbing. Data from the few well-conducted neuroepidemiologic studies in the region emphasize the great disability and mortality from disorders of the nervous system that will be experienced by African females during their lifetime, and these, in combination with the other evidence presented in this chapter, suggest that the burden of neuropsychiatric disorders is probably heavier in African communities than in other parts of the world.

Table 5-4 presents the times in the life span when the major nervous system disorders discussed in this chapter occur in Sub-Saharan African females. Toxic and nutritional disorders occur more frequently early in life, but are evident throughout the life span; this suggests that they may contribute in an important manner to the overall burden of neurologic disease in the region. Similarly, while the epilepsies appear to predominate in females under the age of 30 years, their chronicity and effect may lead to substantial disability in later life. The headache syndromes occur most commonly in adolescence and adulthood; their sequelae, in contrast, appear to be limited. The onset of cerebrovascular diseases, predominantly stroke, is most common in adulthood. If not fatal, however, the initial disease episode can be expected to result in substantial subsequent disability in many cases. The demyelinating and collagen diseases and dementias are, for the most part, disorders of older adulthood, and their adverse impact on mobility and health status in general can be expected to parallel those of older women in the developed world.

RESEARCH NEEDS

- The nature, extent, and sequelae of nervous system disorders in Sub-Saharan African females (and males)

TABLE 5-4   Ages of Occurrence of Nervous System Disorders and Their Sequelae in Sub-Saharan African Females

In Utero	Early Childhood (birth through age 4)	Infancy/ Childhood (ages 5–14)	Adolescence (ages 15–19)	Adulthood (ages 20–44)	Postmenopause (age 45+)
	Toxic and nutritional disorders	Toxic and nutritional disorders	Toxic and nutritional disorders	Toxic and nutritional disorders	Toxic and nutritional disorders
			Headache syndromes	Headache syndromes	
				Oral contraceptive-related cerebrovascular diseases	Oral contraceptive-related cerebro-vascular diseases
	Epilepsies	Epilepsies	Epilepsies		
					Demyelinating diseases
					Neurologic complications of collagen diseases
					Dementias

require elucidation. Research attention should be directed toward identification of major risk factors for the more important nervous system disorders in females and development of cost-effective strategies for disease prevention.

• The prevalence of epilepsies is much higher in Sub-Saharan countries than in developed countries, and there is preliminary evidence that suggests the disorder may be more common in females. There is a need to identify risk factors for epilepsy in Africans and ways to reduce subsequent morbidity and mortality (for example, from falls, household burns, and the like).

• Evidence suggests that the frequency and mortality from stroke are increasing in Sub-Saharan countries (unlike developed countries, where they are decreasing). Research is needed to identify major risk factors for stroke in women and to determine the feasibility and effectiveness of different preventive intervention measures—for example, control of high blood pressure, the most common risk factor for stroke, and to assure that all available oral contraceptives are of mini-dosage.

• There is a need to better characterize the extent and severity of nutrition-related toxic syndromes of the nervous system in Sub-Saharan African populations. Nutrition research and intervention activities should be directed, in part, toward reducing the incidence of and morbidity from these disorders.

• Research is also needed to determine how best to incorporate the management (identification, treatment, and prevention) of the common neurologic diseases of females (and males) into primary health care. Means for training and supervision of nonphysician personnel in this capacity should be developed and assessed.

REFERENCES

Abraham, G., and J. Abdulkadir. 1981. Cerebrovascular accidents in Ethiopians: a review of 48 cases. E. Afr. Med. J. 58:431-436.

Acheson, E. D. 1972. The epidemiology of multiple sclerosis. In Multiple Sclerosis: A Reappraisal. D. McAlpine, C. E. Lumsden and E. D. Acheson, eds. Edinburgh: Churchill-Livingstone.

Ademolekun, B. 1993. Anaphe venata entamophagy and seasonal ataxic syndrome in Southwest Nigeria. Lancet 141:629.

Airede, K. I. 1992. Neural tube defects in the middle belt of Nigeria. J. Trop. Paediat. 38: 27-30.

Akinkugbe, O. O. 1987. World epidemiology of hypertension in blacks. J. Clin. Hypertension 3 (Suppl. 3): 15-25.

Alonso, P. L., S. W. Lindsay, J. R. M. Armstrong, et al. 1991. The effect of insecticide treated bed nets on mortality of Gambian children. Lancet 337:1499-1502.

Assael, M. I., J. M. Namboze, G. A. German, and F. J. Bennetet. 1972. Psychiatric disturbances during pregnancy in a rural group of African women. Soc. Sci. Med. 6: 387–395.

Babaniyi, O. A., and B. D. Parakoyi. 1989. Mortality rate from neonatal tetanus in Ilorin: results of a community survey. J. Trop. Paediat. 35:137-138.

Bademosi, O., and B. O. Osuntokun. 1976. The clinical spectrum of pyogenic meningitis in Southern Nigerians, 1963-1974. E. Afr. Med. J. 53: 185-192.

Bademosi, O., B. O. Osuntokun, M. L. van de Werd, and O. A. Ojo. 1980. Obstetric neurodraxia: a study of 34 patients at Ibadan, Nigeria. Intl. J. Gynaecol. Obstet. 23:611-614.

Bahemuka, M. 1989. Cerebrovascular accidents (strokes) in young normotensive Africans: a preliminary report of a prospective study. E. Afr. Med. J. 56:661-664.

Barker, D. J. P., G. Osmond, G. P. D. Winder, et al. 1989a. Weight in infancy and death from ischaemic heart disease. Lancet 11:577-580.

Barker, D. J. P., C. Osmond, J. Golding, et al. 1989b. Growth in utero, blood pressure in childhood and adult life, and mortality from cardiovascular disease. R. Med. J. 298:564-567.

Barnaby, O. 1878. The Guardian (United Kingdom) May 19, p. 4.

Basser, L. 1969. The relation of migraine and epilepsy. Brain 92:285-300.

Bolan, G., C. V. Broomel, and R. R. Fackiam. 1986. Pneumococcal vaccine efficacy in selected populations in the United States. Ann. Intern. Med. 104:1-6.

Bradley-Moore, A. M., B. M. Greenwood, and A. K. Bradley. 1985. Malaria chemoprophylaxis in young Nigerian children, 2. Its effects on the immune response. Ann. Trop. Med. Parasitol. 75:563-572.

Carney, M. W. P. 1990. Vitamin deficiency and mental symptoms. Br. J. Psychiat. 156:878-882.

Carton, H., K. Kazadil, O. D. Kabeyal, A. Billiaul, and K. Maertans. 1986. Epidemic spastic paraparesis in Bandundu (Zaire). J. Neurol. Neurosurg. Psychiat. 49:620-627.

Chandra, R. K. 1986. Nutrition. Immunity and infection: present knowledge and future directions. Lancet 1:688-691.

Chartier-Harlin, M. C., M. Mullan, et al. 1991. A missense mutation in the amyloid precursor protein gene segregates with familial Alzheimer's disease caused by mutations at codon 717 of the betramyloid precursor protein gene. Nature 353:844-846.

Cliff, J., P. Lundquist, J. Martensson, H. Rosling, and B. Sorbo. 1985. Association of high cyanide and low sulphur intake in cassava induced spastic paraparesis. Lancet 11:1211-1213.

Cliff, J., S. Essers, and H. Rosling. 1986. Ankle clonus correlating with cyanide intake from cassava in rural children from Mozambique. J. Trop. Paediat. 32:186-189.

Collomb, H., M. Dumas, G. Lemercler, and P. L. Girard. 1970. Sclérose au Senegal. Afr. J. Med. Sci. 1:253-254.

Czeizel, A. E., and I. Dudas. 1992. Prevention of first occurrence of neural tube defects by periconceptional vitamin supplementation. N. Engl. J. Med. 327: 1832-1835.

Dallman, P. 1990. Iron. Pp. 241–250 in Present Knowledge in Nutrition, M. Brown, ed. Washington, D.C.: International Life Sciences Institute.

Danesi, M. A., V. A. Oyebola, and A. C. Onitiri. 1983. Risk factors associated with cerebrovascular accidents in Nigeria: a case control study. E. Afr. Med. J. 60:190-195.

de Mota, H. C., A. M. Anthonio, G. Lettuo, and M. Porto. 1990. Late effects of early malnutrition. Lancet 335:1158.

Donnelly, J. J. 1990. Immunogenicity of a haemophilus influenzaneisseria meningitides outer membrane protein complex conjugate vaccine. J. Immunol. 145: 3071-3079.

Edwards, C. R., W. Benediktson, R. S., Lindsay, and J. R. Seckl. 1993. Dysfunction of placental glucocorticoid barrier: link between foetal environment and adult hypertension. Lancet 341: 355-357.

Einhorn, M. S., G. S. Winberg, and E. L. Anderson. 1986. Immunogenicity in infants of Haemophilus influenza type B. Polysaccharide in conjugate vaccine with Neisseria meningitidis outer membrane protein. Lancet 2:299-303.

Eskola, J., H. Kayhty, and L. Gordon. 1988. Simultaneous administration of Haemophilus influenza type B capsular polysaccharide diphtheria toxoid conjugate vaccine with routine diphtheria-tetanuspertussis and inactivated poliovirus vaccinations of children. Pediatr. Infect. Dis. J. 7: 480-484.

Essers A. I. A., P. Alsen, and H. Gosling. 1992. Insufficient processing of cassava induced acute intoxications and the paralytic disease konzo in a rural area of Mozambique. Ecol. Food Nutr. 27:17-27.

Evans, D. A. 1992. Alzheimer's disease—where will we find the etiologic clues? Challenges and opportunities in cross-cultural studies. Ethnic. Dis. 2:321-325.

Fedson, D. S. 1988. Pheumococcal vaccine. Pp. 271–299 in Vaccines, S. A. Plotkin and E. A. Mortimer, eds. Philadelphia: W. B. Saunders.

Feksi, M. A. T., J. Kaamugishae, S. Gatiti, J. W. A. S. Saunders, and S. D. Sorvon. 1991a. A comprehensive community epilepsy programme. The Nakuro projecet. Epilepsy Res. 8:252.

Feksi, M. A. T., J. Kaamugisha, J. W. A. S. Saunders, S. Gatiti, and S. D. Sorvon. 1991b. Comprehensive primary health care anti-epileptic drug treatment programme in rural and semi-urban Kenya. Lancet 337:406-409.

Fotherby, K. 1989. Oral contraceptives and lipids. Br. Med. J. 298:1049-1050.

Galler, J. R. 1983. The influence of early malnutrition on subsequent behavioral development. J. Am. Acad. Psychiat. 22:16-22.

Gebre-Ab, T., Z. Wolde Gabriel, M. Malfi, Z. Ahmed, T. Ayele, and H. Fantal. 1978. Neurolathyrism: a review and a report of an epidemic. Ethiop. Med. J. 16:1-11.

Gerritts, C. A. 1983. West African epilepsy focus. Lancet 1:358.

Goate, A. M., M. Chartler-Harlin, C. Mullanel, et al. 1991. A missense mutation in the amyloid precursor protein gene segregates with familial Alzheimer's disease. Nature 349:704-706.

Goudsmit, J., F. W. van der Waals, and D. C. Gajdusek. 1983. Epilepsy in the Gbawein and Wroughbarh clan of Grand Bassa County, Liberia: the endemic occurrence of See-ee in the native population. Neuroepidemiol. 2:24-34.

Gout, O., A. Gessaiu, F. Bolgert, et al. 1986. Chronic myelopathies associated with human T-Lymphocytic virus type 1. A clinical, serological and immunological study of ten patients in France. Arch. Neurol. 46:255-260.

Grantham-McGregor, S. 1987. Field studies in early nutrition and later achievement Pp. 128–174 in Early Nutrition and Later Achievement, J. Dabbing, ed. London: Academic.

Grantham-McGregor, S. M., S. A. Powell, S. P. Walker, and J. I. H. Hines. 1991. Nutritional supplementation, psychosocial stimulation and mental development of stunted children. The Jamaican Study. Lancet 338:1-5.

Greenwood, B. M., and S. Wah. 1980. Control of meningococcal meningitis in the African meningitis belt by selective vaccination. Lancet 1:729-732.

Gur, R. C., P. D. Mozley, S. M. Resnick, et al. 1991. Gender differences in age effect on brain atrophy measured by magnetic resonance imaging. Proc. Natl. Acad. Sci. U.S.A. 88:2845-2849.

Hachinskil, V. 1992. Preventable senility: a call for action against the vascular dementia. Lancet 340:641-648.

Hannington, K. 1974. Migraine. London: Priority.

Howlett, W. P., G. R. Brubaker, N. Milingl, and H. Rosling. 1990. Konzo: an epidemic upper motor neuron disease studied in Tanzania. Brain 113: 223-235.

Howlett, W. P., C. Brubaker, N. Milingi, and H. Rosling. 1992. A geographical cluster of Konzo in Tanzania. Trop. Geogr. Neurol. 2:102-108.

Humphries, S. V. 1937. A study of hypertension in the Bahamas. S. Afr. Med. J. 31: 1031-1033.

Hypertension Prevention Collaborative Research Group. 1992. The effects of nonpharmacologic interventions on blood pressure of persons with high normal levels. J. Am. Med. Assoc. 267:1213-1218.

Iloeje S. O. 1991. Febrile convulsions in a rural and an urban population. E. Afr. Med. J. 68:43-51.

IHS (International Headache Society). Headache Classification Committee. 1988. Classification and diagnostic criteria for headache disorders, cranial neuralgins and factal pain. Headache 3 (Suppl. 7).

Irey, N. S., H. A. McAllister, and J. M. Henry. 1978. Oral contraceptives and stroke in young women: a clinicopathologic correlation. Neurology 28:1216-1219.

Jilek, W. C., and I. M. Aall-jilek. 1970. The problem of epilepsy in a rural Tanzanian tribe. Afr. J. Med. Sci. 1:305-307.

Jorm, A. F. 1990. The Epidemiology of Alzheimer's Disease and Related Disorders. London: Chapman and Hill.

Jorm, A. F., Korten, A. B., and A. E. Henderson. 1987. The prevalence of dementia: a quantitative integration of the literature. Acta Psychiat. Scand. 76:465-479.

Joubert, J. 1988. Cluster headaches in black patients. A report of 7 cases. S. Afr. Med. J. 73:552-554.

Joubert, J. 1992. Migraine. S. Afr. Med. J. 81:587-589.

Kanyerezi R. R., C. F. Kilre, and A. Obaceal. 1980. Multiple sclerosis in Mulago Hospital, Uganda. E. Afr. Med. J. 57:262-270.

Kwasa, T. O. O. 1992. The pattern of neurological disease at Kenyatta National Hospital. E. Afr. Med. J. 69:326-339.

Ladipo, G. O. A., and Y. F. Fakunle. 1977. Tropical myositis in the Nigerian Savannah. Trop. Geogr. Med. 29:220-228.

Lamborey, J. L., and A. E. Elmendorf. 1992. Combating AIDS and other Sexually Transmitted Diseases in Africa. I. Washington D.C.: World Bank.

Lancet. 1979. Editorial. Cardiovascular risks and oral contraceptives. Lancet 1: 1063.

Lancet. 1988. Annotation. HTLV–1 comes of age. Lancet 1: 127-129.

Lancet. 1989. Editorial. Meningococcal meningitis. Lancet 1:647-648.

Law, C. M., D. J. P. Barker, A. R. Bull, et al. 1991. Maternal and fetal influences on blood pressure. Arch. Dis. Child. 66:1291-1295.

Law, C. M., A. de Swiet, S. Osmond, et al. 1993. Initiation of hypertension in utero and its implication throughout life. Br. Med. J. 306:24-27.

Lester, F. T. 1982. Medical diseases in the elderly Ethiopian. Ethiop. Med. J. 20:55-61.

Levy, L. M. 1983. An epidemiological study of headaches in an urban population in Zimbabwe. Headache 23:1-9.

Lewis, B., J. I. Mann, and M. Mancini. 1986. Reducing the risks of coronary heart disease in individuals in the population. Lancet 1: 956-959.

Li, G., Y. C. Shen, C. T. Chen, et al. 1988. An epidemiological survey of age-related dementia in an urban area of Beliang. Acta Pschiat. Scand. 78:257-264.

Lisk, D. R. 1991. Multiple sclerosis in a West African. Afr. J. Neurol. Sci. 10:10-11.

Lisk, D. R. 1987. Severe headaches in the African. Report of 250 cases from Sierra Leone, West Africa. Headache 27:447-483.

Lloyd-Still, J. D. 1976. Clinical studies on the effects of malnutrition during infancy and subsequent physical and intellectual development. Pp. 103–140 in Malnutrition and Intellectual Development, J. D. Lloyd-Still, ed. Lancaster: MTP.

Longe, A. C., and B. O. Osuntokun. 1988. Prevalence of migraine in Udo, a rural community in Bendel State. E. Afr. Med. J. 65:621-625.

Longe, A. C., and B. O. Osuntokun. 1989. Prevalence of neurological disorders in Udo, a rural community in Bendel State. Trop. Geogr. Med. 41:36-40.

Lozoff, B. 1988. Behavioral alterations in iron deficiency. Adv. Pediatr. 35:331-359.

Lozoff, B., G. M. Brittenham, F. E. Viteri, A. W. Wolf, and J. J. Urrutial. 1982a. The effects of short–term oral iron therapy on developmental deficits in iron deficient anemic infants. J. Pediatr. 100: 351-357.

Lozoff, B., G. M. Brittenham, F. E. Viteri, A. W. Wolf, and J. J. Verrutia. 1982b. Developmental deficits in iron-deficient infants: effects of age and severity of iron lack. J. Pediatr. 101:948-952.

Lucas, A. O. 1964. Pneumococcal meningitis in pregnancy and the puerperium. Br. Med. J. 5375: 92-95.

Lucas, A., R. Morley, T. J. Cole, et al. 1990. Early diet in preterm babies and developmental status at 18 months. Lancet 335:1477-1481.

Mant, D., L. Villaed-Mackintosh, M. P. Vessey, and D. Yeates. 1987. Myocardial infarction and angina pectoris in young women. J. Epidemiol. Commun. Hlth. 41:215-219.

Matenga, J., I. Kital, and L. Levy. 1986. Strokes among black people in Harare, Zimbabwe: results of computed tomography and associated risk factors. Br. Med. J. 292:1649-1651.

McCormick, J., and P. Skrabanek. 1988. Coronary heart disease is not preventable by population intervention. Lancet 2:839-841.

McParklin, J., A. Halligan, I. M. Scott, M. Darling, and D. G. Weir. 1993. Accelerated folate breakdown in pregnancy. Lancet 341:148-149.

Melnick, J. L. 1992. Poliomyelitis: eradication in site. Epidemiol. Infect. 108:1-18.

Milord, F., J. Pepin, L. Loko, L. Ethier, and B. Mpia. 1992. Efficacy and toxicity of eflorinithine for treatment of trypanosomia brucel namblense sleeping sickness. Lancet 340:632-635.

Mirza, N. B., and I. A. Wamola. 1980. Trends in meningococcal meningitis over the past thirteen years at Kenyatta National Hospital, 1967-1979. E. Afr. Med. J. 57:883-889.

Mishell, D. R. 1989. Contraception. N. Engl. J. Med. 320:777-787.

Mohammed, I., and K. Zaruba. 1981. Control of epidemic meningococcal meningitis by mass vaccination. Lancet 2:80-82.

Mohammed, E. C., G. C. Onyemelukwe, E. N. Oluneche, N. Gupta, and G. O. Oyeyinka. 1984. Control of epidemic meningococcal meningitis by mass vaccination. J. Infect. 9:197-202.

Monekosso, G. L., and J. Wilson. 1966. Plasma thiocyanate and vitamin B12 in Nigerian patients with degenerative neurological diseases. Lancet 1:1062-1064.

Mozambique, Ministry of Health. 1984. Mantakassa—an epidemic of spastic paraparesis associated with chronic cyanide intoxication in a cassava staple area in Mozambique. Bull. WHO 62:477-92.

MRC Vitamin Study Research Group. 1991. Prevention of neural tube defects: results of the Medical Research Council Vitamin Study. Lancet 338:131-137.

Murell, J., M. Farlow, B. Ghettil, and M. D. Benson. 1991. A mutation in the amyloid precursor protein associated with hereditary Alzheimer's disease. Science 254:97-99.

Nissinen, A., J. Toumilehto, T. T. Lottke, and P. Puska. 1986. Cost-effectiveness of the North Karella Hypertension Program, 1972–1977, Med. Care 24:767-780.

Odeku, E. L. 1973. Congenital malformations of the neural axis in the Africans. P. 179 in Proceedings of the 10th International Congress of Neurology, A. Subirana and J. M. Burrows, eds. Amsterdam: Excerpta Medica.

Odio, M., I. Faingezicht, M. Paris, M. Nassar, A. Baltodano, J. Rogers, J. Suez-Liorens, K. D. Olsen, and N. H. McCracken. 1991. The beneficial affects of early dexamethasone administration in infants and children with bacterial meningitis. N. Engl. J. Med. 324:1525-1531.

Odugbemi, T., O. Ademidun, A. Agbabiaka, and E. Panjo. 1991. Nasopharyngeal carrier of Neisseria meningitides among school children at Ijede, Lagos State, Nigeria. Ethiop. Med. J. 10:33-36.

Ogunniyi, A. O. 1984. Prevalence of headache among Nigerian University students. Headache 4: 127-130.

Ogunniyi, A. O., and B. O. Osuntokun. 1991. Effectiveness of anticonvulsant therapy in the epilepsies in Nigerian Africans. E. Afr. Med. J. 68:707-713.

Ogunniyi, A., B. O. Osuntokun, O. Bademosi, et al. 1988. Risk factors for epilepsy: case-controlled study in Nigerians. Epilepsia 28:280-285.

Ogunniyi, A., U. G. Lekwauwa, and B. O. Osuntokun. 1991. The influence of education on aspects of cognitive functions in non-demented elderly Nigerians. Neuroepidemiol. 10:246-250.

Ogunniyi, A. O., B. O. Osuntokun, U. G. Lekwauwa, and Z. F. Falope. 1992. Rarity of dementia (by DSM-lll) in an urban community in Nigeria. E. Afr. Med. J. 69:10-14.

Ohaegbulam, S. C. 1981. Congenital malformation of the central nervous system. Post-graduate Doctor (Africa) 3:280-284.

Ohaeri, J. U., and O. A. Odejide. In press. Admissions for drugs and alcohol-related problems in Nigerian psychiatric care facilities in one year. Drug and Alcohol Dependence.

Oliver, M. 1984. Coronary risk factors: Should we not forget about mass control? World Hlth. Forum 5:5-11.

Onadeko, M. O., and J. B. Familusi. 1990. Observations on the age and spatial distribution of paralytic poliomyelitis in Ibadan, Nigeria. Ann. Trop. Paediat. 10:133-138.

Oski, F. A., A. S. Honig, B. Helu, and P. Howanitz. 1983. Effect of iron therapy on behavior performance in non-anemia-iron-deficient infants. Pediatrics 71:877-880.

Osuntokun, B. O. 1968. An ataxic neuropathy in Nigeria: a clinical biochemical and electrophysiological study. Brain 91:215-248.

Osuntokun, B. O. 1970. Primary disease of muscles in Nigerians: experience at Ibadan in Actualités de pathologie neuromusculaire. Pp. 289–290 in Actualites de pathologie neuromusculaire. Marseilles.

Osuntokun, B. O. 1971a. Pattern of neurologic illness in Tropical Africa. J. Neurol. Sci. 12:417-422.

Osuntokun, B. O. 1971b. Headache as a presenting symptom in Nigerians. A five-year study, 1966-1971. J. Nigeria Med. Assoc. 1:14-17.

Osuntokun, B. O. 1972a. The effects of malnutrition on the development of cognitive functions of the nervous system in childhood. Trop. Geogr. Med. 24:295-310.

Osuntokun, B. O. 1972b. Epidemic ataxia in Western Nigeria. Br. Med. J. 2:589.

Osuntokun, B. O. 1980. Neuroepidemiology in Africa. Pp. 57–86 in Clinical Neuroepidemiology, F. C. Rose, ed. London: Pitman Medical.

Osuntokun, B. O. 1981a. Neurological syndrome, management, and prognosis in sickle-cell disease. Trop. Doctor 11:1-9.

Osuntokun, B. O. 1981b. Cassava diet, chronic cyanide intoxication, and neuropathy in the Nigerian Africans. Wld. Rev. Nutr. Diet 36:141-173.

Osuntokun, B. O. 1986. Epidemiology of peripheral neuropathies. Pp. 257–273 in Neurology, K. Poeck, H. Freund, and H. Canshirt, eds. Hamburg: Springer-Verlag.

Osuntokun, B. O. 1992. Clinical and social implication of the epidemiology of epilepsy in African populations. Pp. 43–54 in Clinical Relevance in the Epidemiology of Epilepsies, P. Jallon, ed. Paris: Sanofi Pharma.

Osuntokun, B. O., and O. Osuntokun. 1972. Complicated migraine and haemoglobin AS. Br. Med. J. 2:621-622.

Osuntokun, B. O., O. Bademosi, A. B. O. O. Oyediran, et al. 1979. Incidence of stroke in an African city. Stroke 10:205-208.

Osuntokun, B. O., O. Bademosi, and O. Osuntokun. 1982a. Migraine in Nigeria. Pp. 25-38 in Advances in Migraine Research, F. C. Rose, ed. New York: Raven.

Osuntokun, B. O., B. S. Schoenberg, V. Nottidge, et al. 1982b. Research protocol for measuring the prevalence of neurologic disorders in developing countries: results of a pilot study in Nigeria. Neuroepidemiol. 1:143-153.

Osuntokun, B. O., B. S. Schoenberg, V. Nottidge, et al. 1982c. Headache in a rural community in Nigeria: results of a pilot study. Epidemiol. 1:31-39.

Osuntokun, B. O., A. O. G. Adeujal, V. A. Nottidge, et al. 1987a. Prevalence of the epilepsies in Nigerian Africans: a community-based study. Epilepsis 28:272-279.

Osuntokun, B. O., A. O. G. Adeuja, B. S. Schoenberg, et al. 1987b. Neurological disorders in Nigerians: a community-based study. Acta Neurol. Sci. 6:18-22.

Osuntokun, B. O., A. O. Ogunniyi, U. G. Lekwauwal, and A. B. O. O. Oyediran. 1991. Epidemiology of age-related dementias in the third world and etiological clues of Alzheimer's disease. J. Trop. Geogr. Med. 43:345-351.

Osuntokun, B. O., H. C. Hendrie, K. Hall, A. Ogunniyi, et al. 1992a. Cross-cultural studies in Alzheimer's disease. Ethnic. Dis. 2:352-357.

Osuntokun, B. O., A. O. G. Adeuja, V. A. Nottidge, et al. 1992b. Prevalence of headache and migrainous headache in Nigerian Africans: a community-based study. E. Afr. Med. J. 69:31-34.

Otten, M. W., M. S. Derming, E. O. Jaiteh, et al. 1992. Epidemic poliomyelitis in The Gambia following the control of poliomyelitis as an endemic disease. Am. J. Epidemiol. 135:381-392.

Oyediran, A. B. O. O., B. O. Osuntokun, O. O. Akinkugbel, R. Carlisle, O. Bademosil, and I. A. Olatunde. 1975. Community control of hypertension: results in Epe of blood pressure and urinary survey and preliminary response to control measures. Nigerian Med. J. 6:448-453.

Oyefeso, A. O., and A. R. Adegoke. 1992. Psychological adjustment of Yoruba adolescents as influenced by family type: A research note. J. Child Psychol. Psychiat. Allied Disc. 33(4): 785-788.

Parakoyi, B., and O. A. Babaniyi. 1990. Prevalence of paralytic poliomyelitis in children of Kwara State, Nigeria. Report of a house to house survey. E. Afr. Med. J. 67:545-549.

Patriarca, P. A., P. F. Wright, and J. T. John. 1991. Factors affecting the immunogenicity of oral poliovirus vaccine in developing countries—a review. Rev. Infect. Dis. 13:926-938.

Pawlowski Z. S., G. A. Schad, and M. Scott, eds. 1991. Hookworm Infection and Anaemia: Approaches to Prevention and Control. Geneva: WHO.

Pearson, T. A. 1989. Influences on the CHD incidence and case fatality: medical management of risk factors. Intl. J. Epidemiol. 18 (Suppl.):S2l7-S222.

Pearson, T. A., D. T. Jamison, and J. Treiz-Gutlerrez. 1990. Health sector priorities review: Cardiovascular disease. Population, Health and Nutrition Division, The World Bank, Washington, D.C.

Piot, P., B. M. Kapita, E. N. Nnugi, J. M. Mann, R. Colebunders, and R. Wabitsch. 1992. AIDS in Africa. A Manual for Physicians, Geneva: WHO.

Pollitt, E., and C. Thompson. 1977. Protein-calorie, malnutrition and behavior—a view from psychology. Pp. 281–306 in Nutrition and the Brain, R. J. Wurtman and J. J. Wurtman, eds. New York: Raven.

Putterpill, J. S., P. B. Disler, E. Dacka, M. D. Hoffman, A. R. Sayed, and G. S. Watermeyer. 1984. Coping with chronic illness. Part II, Cerebrovascular accidents. S. Afr. Med. J. 65:891-895.

Quagliarello, V., and W. M. Scheld. 1992. Bacterial meningitis: pathogenesis, pathophysiology and progress. N. Engl. J. Med. 327:864-872.

Ramsay, W. 1993. HIV, AIDS and Africa. Lancet 341:366-367.

Robertson, S. E., H. P. Gaverso, J. A. Brucker, et al. 1988. Clinical efficacy of a new enhanced potency inactivated polio virus. Lancet 1:897-902.

Roman, G., P. S. Spencer, and B. S. Schoenberg. 1985. Tropical myeloneuropathies. The hidden endemias. Neurology 35:1158-1170.

Roman, G. C., P. S. Spencer, B. S. Schoenberg, J. Hogan, A. Ludolph, P. Rodgers-Johnson, B. O. Osuntokun, and C. F. Shamlaye. 1987. Tropical spastic paraparesis in the Seychelles Islands. A clinical and case-control epidemiological study. Neurology 37:1323-1328.

Rosen, M. E. 1988. When to act: the appropriateness of cardiovascular disease intervention. Hlth. Pol. Plan. 3:261-270.

Rosling, H. 1986. Cassava, cyanide and epidemic spastic paraparesis. A study in Mozambique on dietary cyanide exposure. Acta Univers. Upsall.: 7-42.

Rosling, H., A. Gessain, G. de The, et al. 1988. Tropical and epidemic spastic paraparesis are different. Lancet 1:1222-1223.

Rush, D. 1984. The behavioral consequences of protein-energy deprivation and supplementation early in life: an epidemiological perspective. Pp. 119–154 in Human Nutrition: A Comprehensive Treatise, J. D. Guller, ed. New York: Plenum.

Schoenberg, B. S. 1987. Recent studies of the epidemiology of epilepsy in developing countries: a coordinated programme for prevention and control. Epilepsia 28:721-722.

Seldman, D. S., A. Laor, R. Gale, et al. 1991. Birthweight, current body weight, and blood pressure in late adolescence. Br. Med. J. 302:1235-1237.

Shann, F. 1990. Modern vaccines: Pneumococcus and influenza. Lancet 335:1219-1220.

Shapiro, E. D., A. T. Berg, and R. Austrian. 1991. The protective efficacy of polyvalent pneumococcal polysaccharide vaccine. N. Engl. J. Med. 325:1453-1460.

Smart, J. L. 1986. Undernutrition, learning and memory, review of experimental studies. Pp. 74–78 in Proceedings of XIII International Congress of Nutrition, T. C. Taylor and N. Jenkins, eds. London: Joan Libbey.

Sorvon, S. D., and P. J. Farmer. 1988. Epilepsy in developing countries: a review of epidemiological, sociocultural and treatment aspects. Epilepsia 29 (Suppl. 1):536-554.

Spillane, J. D., ed. 1973. Tropical Neurology. London: Oxford University Press.

Stadel, B. V. 1981. Oral contraceptives and cardiovascular disease. New Engl. J. Med. 305:612-618; 672-677.

Stamp, T. J. 1993. Who really cares for Africa? World Hlth. Forum 14:34-36.

St. George-Hyslop, P. H., H. Haines, L. A. Farrer, et al. 1990. Genetic linkage studies suggest that Alzheimer's disease is not a single homogeneous disorder. Nature 347:194-197.

Stocks, M. B., P. M. Smythe, A. O. Moodie, and D. Bradshaw. 1982. Psychosocial outcome and CT finding after gross undernutrition during infancy: a 20-year developmental study. Develop. Med. Chil. Neurol. 24:419-436.

Stuart, J. M., K. A. V. Cartwright, P. M. Robinson, and N. D. Noah. 1989. Effect of smoking on meningococcal carriage. Lancet 2:723-725.

Tahzib, F. 1990. Nigeria: Talking about food. Lancet 336:1371.

Tekle-Haimanot, R. 1985. Multiple sclerosis. A case report on an Ethiopian. Ethiopia Med. J. 23:27-29.

Tekle-Haimanot, R. 1990. Neurological disorders in Ethiopia: a community-based study in pattern and prevalence. Umen University Medical Dissertations n.s. 291.

Tekle-Haimanot, R., I. Forgren, M. Abebel, A. Gabre-Mariam, J. Heiabel, G. Homgren, and J. Ekstedet. 1990. Clinical and electroencephalographic characteristics of epilepsy in rural Ethiopia: a community-based study. Epilepsy Res. 7:230-239.

Thorgood, M., S. A. Adam, and J. Nlann. 1981. Fatal subarachnoid haemorrhage in young women: role of oral contraceptives. Br. Med. J. 283:762.

Tylleskar, T., M. Banea, N. Bikangi, L. Fresco, L. A. Persson, and H. Rosling. 1991. Epidemiological evidence from Zaire for a dietary aetiology of Konzo: an upper motor neurone disease. Bull. WHO 69:581-590.

Tylleskar, T., M. Baneal, M. Rikangil, R. Cooke, and N. Poolter. 1992. Cassava cyanogens and Konzo: an upper motor neurone disease found in Zaire. Lancet 339:208-211.

Vessey, M. P. 1982. Oral contraceptive and cardiovascular disease Br. Med. J. 284:615-616.

Walsh, J. A. 1988. Establishing Health Priorities in the Developing World. New York: United Nations Development Programme.

Walter, T., J. Kovalaskys, and A. Stekel. 1983. Effects of mild iron deficiency on infant mental developmenent scores. J. Pediatr. 104:710-713.

Whincup, P. H., D. G. Cook, and A. G. Shaper. 1989. Early influences on blood pressure: a study of children aged 5-7 years. Br. Med. J. 299:587-591.

WHO (World Health Organization). 1984. The Uses of Epidemiology in the Study of the Elderly. WHO Technical Report Services, 9. Geneva.

Williams, A. O. 1992. AIDS. African perspective. Boca Raton, Fla.:CRC.

6

Mental Health Problems

For many years mental illnesses were thought to be rare in Africa, or at least less severe or of milder consequence compared with other countries, particularly in the more industrialized parts of the world. This belief has gradually been replaced by growing evidence, supported by epidemiologic studies, that such illnesses are at least as frequent in Africa as in the developed world, if not more so. In addition, a number of studies have shown that, as in other societies, there are indeed gender differences in the rate and the course of many mental disorders in African societies.

The aim of this chapter is to provide a review of the current state of knowledge about women and psychiatric disorders in African countries, underlining the similarities and differences between the two sexes in the rate, phenomenology, course, and outcome of these disorders. With respect to the rates of occurrence, it is their similarity in the two sexes that is remarkable: as Table 6-1 indicates, the only psychiatric disorders that appear to impose a disproportionate and, in this instance, unique burden on Sub-Saharan females are those associated with pregnancy and the puerperium. The similarities and differences will also be compared with the picture in non-African societies, particularly the societies where most epidemiological investigations have been carried out.

MENTAL HEALTH AND MENTAL ILLNESS IN AFRICA: GENERAL ISSUES

The belief that mental disorders were generally less common and less severe in Africa than in other regions arose primarily from the expectation that a rural traditional life, lived in harmony with nature, could only lead to mental health, without psychological stress and suffering. This belief was also supported by some superficial observations regarding the mentally ill in these settings. For instance, in most African countries, few people with mental illness find their way into the European-inspired health system. The majority of people with psychological problems customarily remain with their families and are eventually treated by traditional healers. Those who do come to health clinics and hospitals tend to be brought by law enforcement agencies and have been violent and destructive; there is a greater chance that they will be male. Since many observations concerning the rate of occurrence of mental disorders are based on institutional statistics, it has been easy to sustain the assumption that the smaller number of females admitted to specialized psychiatric hospitals and clinics reflect a true difference in prevalence rates between the sexes, with females at lower risk.

It was also thought that women were essentially dependent, and thus by definition more likely to be kept in the community. The very process of getting an excited person to the hospital is also resource-intensive and expensive,

TABLE 6-1 Mental Health Problems in Sub-Saharan Africa: Gender-Related Burden

Problem	Exclusive to Females	Greater for Females than for Males	Burdens for Females and Males Comparable, but of Particular Significance for Females
Psychological disorders associated with pregnancy and the puerperium	X		

NOTE: Significance is defined here as having impact on health that, for any reason—biological, reproductive, sociocultural, or economic—is different in its implications for females than for males.

so that such effort is more likely to be made for men, who generally have a higher socioeconomic status. For all these reasons it was—and still is—true that more men than women are admitted to mental hospitals in Africa, as demonstrated by a number of epidemiological investigations providing data about the percentage of male and female users of psychiatric in- and outpatient services (Ihezue, 1982; Khandelwal and Workneh, 1988; Levin et al., 1981; Orley, 1972).

The preponderance of excited patients admitted to mental hospitals for social control purposes was also a factor that led to the erroneous conclusion that the depressive disorders were rare in Africa. Misdiagnosis of weakness and multiple somatic complaints as only somatic, rather than in any way psychological, was another factor, especially in the tumultuous context of busy outpatient departments that allow just a few minutes for each patient and only a limited number of treatment responses.

With better understanding of the nature of many mental disorders, and with the growing number of epidemiologic studies in community samples or among general health clinic clients, it became clear that most mental disorders are, in reality, frequent in Africa. A better understanding of changing rural lifestyles further helped to dispel the notion that African populations are free of stress and that their culture somehow protects them from the pressures that normally affect others.

Despite this wider awareness, until recently many European and American observers held on to the notion that stressful situations have different, generally milder, consequences among African women than among women elsewhere. Some have believed that African mothers are relatively immune to the grief that comes with the death of a child; apparent helplessness in the face of such events has been mistaken for coolness, rather than anguish.

It is clear that the stresses on Sub-Saharan women as they go through life are intense, even in the most traditional societies. In the many parts of the region where disruption, famine, war, and forced migration prevail, the pressures are all the greater (Toole and Waldman, 1990). The customs and expectations of women's roles, although variable among African societies, can also lead to stress on women, even where there is no disaster or disruption of family and social ties. In some societies, a young woman will move to her husband's home after her marriage and break many of the ties with her natal family. A "bride price" is often paid to her family, which can mean that if she wishes to return, even for a good reason such as maltreatment, her family will be reluctant to take her back because they would be obliged to return the wealth they had been paid for her. If she bears no children, this too is reason to withhold installments on the price that may have been held back pending proof of fecundity; this puts her at a disadvantage with both her husband's family and her natal family.

The great value placed on a woman as a bearer of children should mean that the menopause might be a time of great stress. Yet this can also become a time of caring for grandchildren, although this may depend, at least in the virilocal marriage situation that is normative in much of Africa, on her having borne sons. Even for women who have not borne children, their childless state can be somewhat attenuated by living in a polygamous household and having access to other wives' grandchildren or to a husband's brother's grandchildren. At the same time, living in a polygamous household may be still another source of strain: the frequent jealousy of co-wives can lead them to deliberately harm one other. Although not conducted in Africa, a recent, well-designed epidemiologic study carried out in a sample of women in Dubai, one of the seven Arab Emirates, confirmed that polygamous marriages are psychologically stressful (Ghubash et al., 1992). In this study, the overall prevalence of any psychiatric disorder, assessed on the basis of the PSE Index of Definition/CATEGO system (a computerized method for determining "caseness"), was about 23 percent; women who were living in polygamous marriages were more than twice as likely to be psychiatric cases as women in monogamous marriages.

Another recent study, carried out in a sample of 116 Yoruba adolescents in Nigeria (69 males and 47 females) with a mean age of 17.8, investigated the psychological adjustment of the two groups in relation to their type of birth family (Oyefeso and Adegoke, 1992). Male adolescents from monogamous families seemed to be better adjusted psychologically than those from polygamous families, while no such difference seemed to exist in the levels of psychological adjustment of female adolescents. These findings suggest that: (1) sex-role prescription can influence psychological adjustment of adolescents in Yoruba societies, and (2) female children may enjoy a more protective upbringing in polygamous families than their male counterparts experience.

Added to these stresses on women is the nature and size of their workload. The various household duties of cleaning, cooking, and washing must be performed along with the agricultural work, which men traditionally leave to women, except perhaps for occasional heavy digging and clearing. When men go off to the cities to find work, women are left to carry the whole burden of family life. Their burden may be lightened a little by presents or occasional cash brought back from the city by the emigrés, but this would not seem to be the norm.

It is not surprising, therefore, to see that mental illness is frequent in Africa, and may not be less so among women. Many of the precursors are there—in the frequent severe life events and difficulties they face—even in contexts where social support may be available. In a study of young women living in an urban environment in Zimbabwe, added stresses were reported, including marital disharmony associated with violence and the threat of AIDS. In such situations the women found themselves powerless, removed as they were from their traditional support systems (Broadhead and Abas, 1993).

GENDER DIFFERENCES IN THE RATE, COURSE, AND OUTCOMES OF MENTAL DISORDERS: GLOBAL ISSUES

The gender difference in the rate, course, and outcomes of various mental disorders across the world has attracted the attention of researchers and clinicians. It is appropriate to briefly discuss this global issue before examining the African situation in more detail. Several well-conducted epidemiologic studies from outside Africa have indeed shown that there are remarkable differences in the rates of occurrence of various mental disorders between the two sexes, with females generally showing higher incidence and prevalence rates compared with males. This result has been confirmed in a number of reviews (Dohrenwend and Dohrenwend, 1969, 1974; Goldman and Ravid, 1980; Gove and Tudor, 1973; Weissman and Klerman, 1977). In the most recent review of 11 major epidemiologic studies based on direct assessment by standardized research interviews and generally carried out through a two-stage procedure, Goldberg and Huxley (1992) found an overall one-month prevalence rate in random samples of the general population for any psychiatric disorder (excluding cognitive impairment, substance use, and antisocial personality) of 12.1 percent among males, compared with 20.2 percent among females. In the only study conducted in Africa among the 11 considered, however, the prevalence rate was approximately the same among males and females.

Despite the consistency of this finding of gender differences in most parts of the world, with that single African "exception," Jenkins (1985) has demonstrated that if samples of males and females are chosen in order to be completely comparable in social adjustment, the sex difference disappears, or is greatly reduced. In addition, some major surveys have not supported the general finding of a sex difference in prevalence rates. For instance, in the Epidemiologic Catchment Area (ECA) Program study for the United States, a large survey carried out in five American sites in an overall sample of over 18,000 people, more men than women reported some kind of psychiatric disorder over their lifetime (36 percent versus 30 percent). Nevertheless, men and women did not differ in the proportions of those with an active disorder in the year immediately prior to the survey, when there was a 20 percent prevalence rate in both sexes (Robins and Regier, 1991). According to the authors, one of the more noteworthy results of the ECA is that it brought into question the overall excess of mental disorder among women compared with men that had been reported in many earlier surveys.

This discordance is resolved by disaggregating interactions of gender according to disorder, as noted over two decades ago by Dohrenwend and Dohrenwend (1969). There is generally an excess of alcohol and substance abuse and antisocial personality among males, while there is an excess of depressive and neurotic disorders among females. From a variety of clinical and epidemiological studies, gender emerges strongly and consistently as a major risk factor for depression, with women outnumbering men, on average, by a 2:1 ratio (Goodwin and Blehar, 1993). A major review by Nolen-Hoeksema (1987) found a mean female-to-male ratio across all clinic-based studies of treated cases of depression of 1.95:1 in the United States and 2.39:1 outside the United States; these gender differences were statistically significant. Moreover, considering data from 12 studies that provided only summary data on all affective disorders, used idiosyncratic criteria for diagnoses, or were based on small samples, the mean female-to-male ratio was 1.5:1 (p < .01). Three of these studies were carried out in African countries (Kenya, Nigeria, and Zimbabwe).

On the whole, from epidemiologic studies carried out in a variety of countries and sociocultural settings throughout the world, it appears that there are significant gender differences in the rate of selected mental disorders when these are sorted by type, with an excess of males for some disorders and an excess of females for others. In addition, several clinical and follow-up studies have also shown gender differences in age of onset, course, and outcomes of various mental disorders. To take two major examples, it has been shown repeatedly that, on average, schizophrenia starts five years earlier in men than in women (Warner and de Girolamo, 1995), and that it has a milder course and a better outcome among females. In contrast, depression seems to have a more severe course in females than in men, and females appear to be at higher risk of relapse (Brown, 1991).

THE EPIDEMIOLOGIC EVIDENCE IN AFRICA

Data concerning psychological symptoms and psychiatric disorders in Africa are not abundant. Epidemiologic studies are few, and most have been carried out on people presenting at health clinics, so that they suffer from all the usual problems associated with biases leading to clinic attendance. Although many studies do segregate data from males and females, they do not customarily provide data broken down by age. Very few studies look beyond simple "head-counting" for a selected number of diagnoses.

A number of mental health problems are mentioned in this chapter in passing, because although they represent a significant cause of morbidity and burden, they do not differentially affect women; indeed, in some cases women may be relatively spared. Problems such as depression, anxiety, schizophrenia, and puerperal illness, which do affect women differentially, are addressed in more detail. When samples for studies are drawn in some relatively unselected way from within a total community, these will be referred to as "community-based," and the results should be understood to reflect the rates of disorder expected within the population as a whole. Where studies have been done on individuals attending a clinic (even a general outpatient clinic), they are referred to as "clinic-based," and their results should not be viewed as generalizable to community samples because a variety of factors differentially affect help-seeking behavior in males and females.

Two comprehensive reviews that focus on the extent of mental health problems in Africa today are important—German (1987) and Odejide and colleagues (1989). The first author emphasizes that while early estimates of the prevalence of psychiatric disorder in black Africa were universally low, primarily because they were mainly hospital-based, more recent studies that have sampled diverse populations suggest a burden of psychiatric morbidity in black Africa not dissimilar to that found in more developed countries. Some of the studies reviewed suggest that rates in Africa may be even higher than in developed countries. Similar conclusions were reached by the authors of the second review. Unfortunately, neither of these reviews discussed the gender issue in any detail. Nevertheless, they provide a crucial starting point by underlining the magnitude of mental health problems among Africans and pointing to the need for a closer examination of this important topic.

GENDER DIFFERENCES IN AFRICA FOR ALL PSYCHOLOGICAL DISORDERS

The study carried out in Nigeria by Leighton and coworkers (1963a) was the seminal psychiatric investigation for the African continent, as well as for cross-cultural psychiatry. This extensive investigation was carried out in the late 1950s and early 1960s, and it was aimed at estimating the prevalence of psychiatric disorders among the

Yoruba people in the western region of Nigeria. The sampling methods were sound, with scientifically acceptable applicability or generalization of the observations. Findings from the Stirling County study, a major community-based epidemiologic investigation carried out in rural Canada (Leighton et al., 1963b), provided the main comparative data. In general, the Yoruba group seemed to have more symptoms but fewer cases of clearly evident psychiatric disorder. While in the Stirling County study the prevalence of psychiatric disorder, especially psychoneurotic symptoms, was considerably greater among women than men (65 percent versus 47 percent), in the Yoruba sample this pattern was reversed, although the sex difference was small (42 percent among males and 39 percent among females). The Yoruba group also showed a higher prevalence of psychiatric symptoms based primarily on organic disorder than the Stirling County population, a finding that was compatible with the greater amount of severe endemic disease and malnutrition in the Nigerian population.

Another seminal community survey was carried out by Orley in the early 1970s (Orley and Wing, 1979) in two Ugandan villages, and its results were compared with those obtained in a survey conducted with the same methodology in a working-class area in southeast London (Camberwell) among 237 women. The brief form of the ninth edition of the Present State Examination was used, translated into the Luganda language, and all the interviews in the Ugandan villages were conducted in that language. The data were analyzed using the PSE Index of Definition/CATEGO system. The three major psychiatric illnesses detected were depression, hypomania, and anxiety states, and higher rates were found for all three diagnoses in the Ugandan villages. The highest rates were for depression—the Ugandan rates were twice as high as those in Camberwell, both at threshold and for more definite cases. There was no significant difference in the overall rate of disorders between the two sexes in the Ugandan sample; combining all cases at threshold level and above, according to the Index of Definition, 27 percent of the women and 24 percent of the men had psychiatric disorders. For comparison, 11 percent of the women surveyed in the London sample were cases at threshold level and above. The PSE mean total scores were not significantly different between the two sexes in the Ugandan sample (male, 5.22; female, 5.71).

A number of other community surveys of various sample sizes and employing methodologies with different degrees of sophistication have been carried out in other African countries, including Sudan (Baasher, 1961; Rahim and Cederblad, 1989) and Senegal (Beiser et al., 1972; Diop et al., 1982). The Senegal studies did not break down psychiatric morbidity rates by gender, and thus will not be discussed further. In Sudan, Baasher (1961) surveyed the inhabitants of a village with 1,860 residents. A team including a psychiatrist visited all households and interviewed family members in order to pick up any cases of mental disorders. (The short report on the study does not specify how many people were actually interviewed.) The author found an overall prevalence rate for most common psychiatric disorders of 6.3 percent; females outnumbered males almost 4:1. The author points out that this result was the opposite of that found in a Khartoum clinic studied, where the ratio of males to females was 3:1. Two explanations were advanced to account for the excess of females in rates of psychiatric disorders within the general population: (1) the absence of husbands for 38 percent of married women; and (2) a high infant mortality rate (up to 116/1,000), which was expected to have a significant psychological impact on females' mental status.

In the later study in Sudan, Rahim and Cederblad (1989) randomly selected 204 subjects between the ages of 22 and 35 from a newly urbanized part of Khartoum. Subjects were assessed using the Self-Reporting Questionnaire, the Eysenck Personality Inventory, and a Sudanese rating scale of anxiety and depression. A psychiatric interview and a medical examination were also administered. It was found that 40.3 percent of the subjects had at least one psychiatric symptom; 16.6 percent received clinical diagnoses according to DSM-III. The most common diagnoses were neurotic and endogenous depressive illness (8.4 percent) and generalized anxiety (3.4 percent). Alcohol abuse was very rare (0.4 percent). No gender differences in the rates of the disorders assessed were encountered.

AFFECTIVE AND NEUROTIC DISORDERS

Despite the contention of some researchers in the past that depression, and particularly guilt, were uncommon in African populations (Carothers, 1953), subsequent investigations contradict such conclusions and reveal a remarkable rate of depressive disorders and symptoms in the samples surveyed. In the 1963 studies by Leighton and colleagues (1963a,b) cited above, depressive symptoms were four times more common in their Nigerian series than among the population of Stirling County, Canada. In the Orley and Wing (1979) study, also cited above, there were approximately twice as many cases of depression in their Ugandan series as in the female sample from a London inner-suburb. In a later review of this topic, Jegede (1979) also noted a considerable frequency of depression among Africans and stressed the common somatic presentation of this disorder.

It has already been noted that most epidemiologic investigations carried out in community samples in various sites, predominantly in industrialized countries, have found a remarkable difference in rates of depressive disorders between males and females. Bebbington (1988, p. 8) has stated, "Perhaps, the most consistent finding in psychiatric epidemiology is that women suffer from depression more frequently than men."

The situation in Africa appears to be more complicated. For instance, the Nigeria study referred to above (Leighton et al., 1963a) found no significant difference between the reports by men and women of depressive symptoms, although formal clinical diagnoses were not made. While one analysis of the Ugandan data showed a significant excess of women with depressive disorders, however, this was largely accounted for by the exclusion from that analysis of subjects over 65 years of age: four of the eight men over age 65 in the group had a depressive disorder, but none of the seven women did. Adding the four men to the "depressed" sample served to narrow the gender gap, although the predominance of depressive symptoms among women persisted. Beyond the results obtained in these two studies, we lack population-based data, which might help clarify the issue, although there is an accumulation of data gathered through clinic-based investigations. Unfortunately, the clinic-based results cannot be generalized to total populations because of the potential biases inherent in presenting samples, which can be extreme between the two sexes in any clinical setting. For instance, a study was conducted in Ghana among all patients showing depressive symptoms who contacted a psychiatric inpatient or outpatient service over a period of several weeks. These patients were then evaluated using the WHO Schedule for the Assessment of Depressive Disorders (SADD) (Majodina and Johnson, 1983), and two-thirds of the study population showing depressive symptoms were females. Yet in a similar study conducted at the outpatient psychiatric clinic of a hospital in Addis Ababa over a period of three years, a slight excess of males over females (27 versus 25) was encountered (Keegstra, 1986).

Another—and crucial—issue is the relationship between life events and depression. An investigation carried out in Kenya using methodology comparable to that used in studies in Britain (Brown and Harris, 1978) found that the group identified as depressed had experienced more life events in the 12 months preceding the onset of depression than the controls in that same period (Ndetei and Vadher, 1984; Vadher and Ndetei, 1981). These results are similar to those obtained by researchers in Western settings and underscore the centrality of this issue to any future study that purports to unravel the determinants of depression in African settings.

As for manic disorder, one relatively large study looked at all patients presenting over a two-year period at the two psychiatric units of a teaching hospital in Nigeria who met the Research Diagnostic Criteria for manic disorder (Makanjuola, 1985). Out of a total of 104 patients diagnosed, 61 were males and 43 were females. Although there was an excess of females in the group diagnosed with bipolar disorder compared with the groups with recurrent unipolar manic disorder or with a single manic episode, the difference was not statistically significant.

Conversion hysteria and anxiety and panic disorders have also been studied in African settings, providing institutional statistics about the differential sex prevalence among psychiatric patients treated for these disorders and the various aspects of their phenomenology, determinants, and course (Awaritefe, 1988; Benjamin et al., 1975). Because these studies suffer from the service bias noted earlier, they are not discussed in detail here. And, despite the great problems that many African countries face as a result of natural and man-made disasters, there have been no studies that systematically set out to assess the extent, course, and outcome of post-traumatic stress and related disorders among African populations.

In sum, there is ample scope for community-based epidemiologic investigations of different African populations—conducted with comparable designs and methodologies, with samples of sufficient size and rigor of selection—to provide a better understanding of the full spectrum of disorders addressed above.

SCHIZOPHRENIA

Incidence

The only study carried out in Africa focusing on the incidence of schizophrenia was part of the WHO Study on the Determinants of Outcome of Severe Mental Disorders (the "Outcome Study"; see Jablensky et al., 1992), which included a site at Ibadan, Nigeria. Unfortunately, the Ibadan portion, in common with 4 other sites out of the total of 13 participating in the Outcome Study, was unable to achieve adequate coverage of the "helping agencies" that were likely to serve as the first contact for psychotic patients. This aspect of the study methodology had been considered essential to grasping the "true" incidence rates of all new schizophrenia cases, independent of any possible service bias. Because of this incomplete coverage in the five sites that included Ibadan, incidence rates were expected to be, and indeed proved, lower than rates in the sites with complete coverage. In any event, the final report of the WHO study does not mention the specific rates for those five sites, and it is therefore impossible to discuss gender differences in the incidence of this disorder in the African population in even a tentative way. Although the study has provided a wealth of additional data about many aspects of premorbid adaptation, antecedents, and initial symptomatology of subjects with a diagnosis of schizophrenia, these data are disaggregated by gender in only a very limited fashion, and therefore preclude even speculation about these aspects of the disorder as they might apply differently to males and females in the Nigerian site.

Nevertheless, an interesting result was obtained from the site that is worth mentioning. In studying the subgroup of patients worldwide ($n = 386$) with acute-onset schizophrenia, the investigators found that stressful life events had preceded onset of the disorder in a substantial proportion of cases, about 65 percent of the total (Day et al., 1987). While in six of nine sites, event rates per person were similar both to each other and to rates recorded in London by Brown and Harris (1978), rates were lower in the Nigerian and Indian centers, and the rate was the lowest of all in the African site. Despite the possibility advanced by the authors that the rate was artificially low because of methodological limitations of the study, it is still the case that the Nigerian site reported more very acute onsets of schizophrenia than sites in developed countries, and many of these did not appear to have been related to stressful life events. This distinctive pattern remains to be investigated.

Prevalence

In a recent review on the epidemiology of schizophrenia (Warner and de Girolamo, 1995), three African prevalence studies were retrieved that had been carried out in Botswana, Ghana, and Sudan. In the first study, the authors ascertained an age-corrected, one-year prevalence rate among individuals aged 15 years or older living in 6 villages in a remote area of Botswana (Ben-Tovim and Cushnie, 1986); all cases were diagnosed by two experienced psychiatrists according to ICD-9 criteria. The age-adjusted prevalence rate found was 5.3 per 1,000 population. Unfortunately, the two authors did not provide any information about the gender distribution of the cases identified.

In the Ghana study in a relatively urbanized suburb of Accra, the authors found an age-adjusted point prevalence rate of 1.1 per 1,000 population (Sikanerty and Eaton, 1984). In this study, as well as in two other previous investigations mentioned by these authors, a male-to-female ratio greater than 1.5:1 was encountered. As noted in the original report of the study, the male-to-female ratio for other disorders (for example, depression and neurosis) showed an excess of females, but the magnitude of this excess is not specified. Nonetheless, there again appear to be variations in gender ratios that depend on the nature of the disorder under study.

In the third study, carried out in Sudan and mentioned earlier in this chapter, Baasher (1961) found a point prevalence rate (without age correction) of 6.9 per 1,000 population in a sample of 1,860 inhabitants of a Sudanese village. Again, no data on gender ratios were provided.

Course and Outcome

Insofar as the course and outcome of schizophrenia are concerned, it has been consistently demonstrated, especially in the two major WHO multicentric studies (WHO, 1979; Jablensky et al., 1992), that schizophrenia has a significantly better course and outcome among patients living in developing countries than in those living in developed countries.[1] The International Pilot Study of Schizophrenia (IPSS) (WHO, 1979), in which the African site of Ibadan (Nigeria) took part, included two follow-ups of the patients enrolled in the study at intervals of two and five years. A major finding was that the onset, symptomatology, and help-seeking behavior of people diagnosed with schizophrenia differed in significant ways across settings. Onset of schizophrenia was much more likely to be acute than insidious in developing countries; catatonia was more common in the two sites of Ibadan and Agra (India) than elsewhere; and, to repeat, the course and outcome of schizophrenia were significantly better in the developing than in the developed countries studied. Among all nine sites in the study, patients in Ibadan had the best prognosis of all.

In the Outcome Study mentioned at the beginning of this section, there were surprisingly few gender-related differences in course and outcome when data from centers in developed and developing countries were aggregated. When centers in developed and developing countries were taken separately, however, some suggestion of gender differences appeared. As shown in Table 6-2, females in the Ibadan site outnumbered males in the group with the best course (that is, single psychotic episode followed by complete remission; 60.5 percent versus 43.6 percent), while there was a relative predominance of males with poor course (two or more psychotic episodes with incomplete remissions between most of them; 16.4 percent versus 2.3 percent). This was consistent with the result found for all developing countries considered together. Although the authors provided a distribution of selected course variables by gender (including percentage of time spent in psychotic episodes, in complete remission, on antipsychotic medication, in hospital treatment, and percentage of time of unimpaired social functioning), the results of this in-depth analysis are not available for individual study sites, so it is impossible to take a closer look at the gender differences in the African center alone. Still, in the overall study, female subjects tended to have more favorable outcomes than male subjects, and the data from the Nigerian center do not appear to contradict this general trend.

TABLE 6-2   Pattern of Course of Schizophrenia by Gender in the Ibadan Center, Outcome Study (percentage distribution)

Pattern of Course	Males (n = 55)	Females (n = 43)
Single psychotic episode followed by complete remission	43.6	60.5
Single psychotic episode followed by incomplete remission	5.5	2.3
Single psychotic episode followed by one or more nonpsychotic episodes, with complete remissions between all or most of the episodes	5.5	4.7
Single psychotic episode followed by one or more nonpsychotic episodes, with incomplete remissions between all or most of the episodes	—	2.3
Two or more psychotic episodes with complete remissions between all or most of the episodes	25.5	25.6
Two or more psychotic episodes with incomplete remissions between all or most of the episodes	16.4	2.3
Continuous psychotic illness (no remission); psychotic symptoms present most of the time		
Continuous nonpsychotic illness (no remission); psychotic symptoms may be present for some time, but nonpsychotic symptoms predominant throughout	—	—
Information inadequate for rating the pattern of course	1.8	—

SOURCE: Data taken from Jablensky et al., 1992.

PSYCHOLOGICAL DISORDERS IN GENERAL MEDICAL SETTINGS

As stated above, most epidemiologic studies in Africa have been conducted in primary care or general medical settings, generally surveying consecutive patients attending the clinic(s) participating in the study. While such approaches are more feasible than community-based surveys, which often require large investments of research staff and funds, they have substantial limitations, as noted earlier.

Table 6-3 lists the principal studies carried out in general medical settings in African countries, with a breakdown of their characteristics and the rates of disorders found among males and females. Three studies (Abiodun et al., 1993; Binitie, 1981; Jegede et al., 1990) that did not provide separate rates of disorders for males and females have been included nonetheless, because they provide some textual comments on differential rates of disorders in the two sexes.

It can be seen that in three of the studies listed in Table 6-3, females showed higher rates of psychiatric disorders than males. The study by Abiodun (1993) also found a statistically significant excess of psychiatric morbidity among females compared with males, although it did not provide the actual numbers. In one study, the rate was exactly the same for the two sexes; in another three studies—in the police force hospital, mentioned in the paper by Giel and Van Luijk (1969); in the study by Binitie (1981); and in the WHO multisite study (Sartorius et al., 1993)—males outnumbered females. Jegede and colleagues (1990) did not provide differential rates by sex, but reported approximately similar PSE scores for males (9.73, SD ± 62.7) and females (11.34, SD ± 8.44), without any significant difference. While the results reported by Giel and Van Luijk (1969) and by Binitie may be explained by the settings where the studies were carried out (in the former case, a clinic attached to a special hospital for police personnel and their families; in the latter, an overall sample with males greatly outnumbering females), the findings of the WHO multisite study are of particular interest and deserve a more in-depth discussion.

The WHO multisite study was designed to investigate the form, frequency, course, and outcome of psychological problems seen in primary health care settings in 15 sites around the world (Sartorius et al., 1993). The research employed a two-stage sampling design in which the 12-item General Health Questionnaire (GHQ-12) was administered to 26,422 persons aged 18 to 65 years who were consulting health care services. Of these, 5,604 were selected for detailed examination using standardized instruments and were followed up at three months and one year to provide information on course and outcome; here we will only refer to the results of the initial examination. The study included an African site, again located in Ibadan (Nigeria). In this site, the study was conducted in the general outpatient department (GOPD) of the University College Hospital (UCH), a tertiary hospital with specialist clinics in many areas of medicine. These specialized clinics serve no defined catchment area and receive referrals not only from Ibadan, but also from hospitals throughout the southwestern area of Nigeria. Unlike the specialist clinics of hospitals, which usually require physician referral, the GOPD is a walk-in clinic, and many patients come on a self-referral basis. Thus, the GOPD tends to draw its patients from the entire city of Ibadan. Of 1,433 patients approached for screening, 1,431 (99.9 percent) took part, with only two refusals. Of the 524 patients eligible for the second-stage interview, 435 (83 percent) completed it. Consistent with patterns in epidemiologic studies in so many primary care settings, more women than men were screened and interviewed; the same pattern appeared in most of the other centers in the overall study. The mean age of the sample was about 33 years. More than a quarter of the participants were in their late teens and early twenties, about another quarter were aged 45 or more, with the remainder between 25 and 44 years. This pattern of age distribution closely approximated those in Bangalore and Ankara, two other developing-country centers, and was generally different from centers in Europe and North America, where subjects tended to be older. Only 34.7 percent of the subjects were judged by clinic doctors to have any mild to severe physical disorders, and 11.8 percent were rated by the clinic doctors as having mild or moderate psychological problems. None was thought to have severe psychological problems.

Table 6-4 shows the diagnostic breakdown by gender of the patients actually interviewed; the percentage of the various diagnoses of the total sample; and the estimated prevalences, adequately weighted to reflect the percentage of individuals with a given disorder among consecutive presenters at the health center. On the whole, well-defined ICD-10 disorders had a weighted prevalence of 10.4 percent in this population. Major depression had the highest prevalence (4.2 percent). Alcohol dependence and neurasthenia were present in 0.4 percent and 1.1

TABLE 6-3 Prevalence of Psychiatric Disorders among Subjects Attending General Health Care Clinics, Selected African Countries

Author and Year	Country	Sample (N) F	M	(M + F)	Assessment Method	Diagnostic System	Overall Prevalence Rate	Males with any Disorder (%)	Females with any Disorder (%)
Abiodun et. al. (1993)	Nigeria			(272)	PSE	ICD-9	21	—	—
Binitie (1981)	Nigeria			(1,654)	Clinical assessment	?	05	—	—
Giel and Van Luijk (1969)	Ethiopia (general hospital)	100	90		Clinical assessment	?	—	16	21
Giel and Van Luijk (1969)	Ethiopia (provincial hospital)	576	246		Clinical assessment	?	—	07	07
Giel and Van Luijk (1969)	Ethiopia (health center)	234	146		Clinical assessment	?	—	15	27
Giel and Van Luijk (1969)	Ethiopia (police force hospital)	287	209		Clinical assessment	?	—	18	14
Jegede et al. (1990)	Nigeria	41	62		PSE	ICD-9	40	—	—
Ndetei and Muhangi (1979)	Kenya			(103)	Clinical assessment	?	—	19	22
Ustün and Sartorius (1995)	Nigeria	97	172		CIDI	ICD-10	—	19	07

TABLE 6-4 Prevalence of Current ICD-10 Psychological Disorders by Gender, Ibadan Site, WHO Multicentre Collaborative Study

Category	Number of Male Patients Interviewed	Estimated Prevalence in Males (%)	Number of Female Patients Interviewed	Estimated Prevalence in Females (%)
Alcohol dependence	2	1.5	0	0.0
Harmful use of alcohol	3	3.0	0	0.0
Current depression	8	5.3	15	3.8
Dysthymia	4	1.8	4	1.1
Agoraphobia	0	0.0	1	0.2
Panic disorder	2	1.5	2	0.3
Generalized anxiety disorder	7	4.9	8	2.2
Somatization disorder	1	0.5	2	0.3
Neurasthenia	5	3.4	1	0.2
One mental disorder (from the above)	17	13.3	21	5.6
Two or more mental disorders (from the above)	9	5.8	7	1.6
All patients	97	100.0	172	100.0

NOTE: Information is weighted to reflect baseline prevalence rates among consecutive attenders.

SOURCE: Üstün and Sartorius, 1995.

percent of the health clinic population, respectively. Generalized anxiety was present in 2.9 percent of the sample, and panic disorder and agoraphobia had a weighted prevalence of 0.7 percent and 0.1 percent respectively.

The weighted prevalence rate for all psychiatric disorders mentioned above is much lower than the weighted rate of 27.8 percent reported from an earlier study conducted in a primary care clinic in Ibadan, and in which identical instruments for case detection were used (Gureje et al., 1992). A number of factors may be responsible for this discrepancy. First, in the earlier study, the reported rate had included the diagnostic category of "undifferentiated somatoform disorder," with a prevalence of 10.8 percent. Second, the subjects of the earlier study were older and had received considerably less formal education than those in the later study; 6.7 percent of the later sample had four years or less of education, compared with up to 38 percent of the sample of the earlier study with no formal education. Disorders that were considerably more common in the earlier sample, such as generalized anxiety disorder, were associated with increasing age and with less education. A third factor that may explain the different rates between the two studies is the idiosyncracies of the two settings themselves. The earlier study was conducted in a setting where the patient population on any given day included a substantial number of patients being followed up for ongoing treatment of an existing condition. The later study was conducted in a setting where the population of patients was always dominated by those seeking care for acute disorders; follow-ups were few because most patients in need of further care had been referred to other clinics in the hospital, so that only a few patients would have been ill for a sufficiently long period at the time of the study to meet the criterion of duration of illness. Thus, for example, only a few patients would meet the criterion of six months of illness that would make them eligible for an ICD-10 diagnosis of generalized anxiety disorder (WHO, 1993).

The gender differences in rates of disorders found in the later study are of particular interest, for they show an unusual preponderance of males over females: 13.3 percent of males had one mental disorder compared with 5.6 percent of the females, a statistically significant difference ($X^2 = 4.41$; $P < .03$). An additional 5.8 percent of males had two or more mental disorders compared with 1.6 percent of females, a difference in rates that was not statistically significant. Except for agoraphobia, for which the number of cases was so small that it precluded any meaningful conclusion, there was no disorder among those investigated with a higher rate for females than for males. Alcohol dependence and harmful use of alcohol were exclusively male disorders in this setting.

Beyond these studies of the rates of disorders among users of health clinics, other investigations carried out in similar settings have focused on other indicators of ill health. For instance, the prevalence and pattern of psychotropic drug use were investigated in an urban walk-in clinic in Nigeria during the course of a two-stage epidemiological survey (Gureje and Obikoya, 1991). A total of 14.9 percent of the patients were using psychotropic drugs, with almost all the users taking anxiolytics. At odds with the results of many studies carried out in developed countries, which consistently show an excess of females taking psychotropic drugs, there was no significant gender difference in the prevalence of drug use. Almost half of the users had been on the drug in question for over 12 months. Increasing age was associated with psychotropic drug use in females, while being married had a similar association in males. Although an increasing score on the GHQ-12 was associated with drug use, over two-thirds of patients with DSM-IIIR disorders identified during the second-stage interview were not taking any psychotropic drug.

PSYCHOLOGICAL DISORDERS IN PREGNANCY AND THE PUERPERIUM

A number of studies have looked at the frequency, form, and determinants of psychological disorders found among African women during pregnancy and the puerperium. The great importance that reproductive life plays for African women living in traditional societies has already been noted, and the fulfillment of female roles linked to reproduction is regarded as an essential step in any woman's life. For these reasons, it is reasonable to predict a substantial rate of psychological problems associated with this central component of female life. In addition, the mortality rate associated with pregnancy in Africa, the highest in the world according to WHO data, makes pregnancy a particularly stressful event for the many African women living in traditional settings, which are not always well-equipped with maternal health facilities.

Cox (1979) conducted one of the most extensive investigations around this topic. He surveyed 263 pregnant women in Uganda and compared them with 89 nonpregnant, nonpuerperal women through administration of a semistructured psychiatric questionnaire. Pregnant women showed increased frequency of psychiatric morbidity compared with the control group, and separated women were at particular risk. The author found no association between antenatal psychiatric morbidity and age, number of children, number of co-wives, or duration of pregnancy. This study supported findings previously reported by Assael and colleagues (1972), who had found an association between psychiatric morbidity and marital separation; in their sample, 24 percent of pregnant Baganda women showed conspicuous psychiatric morbidity.

In another careful investigation, 240 pregnant women consecutively attending an antenatal clinic in Nigeria over a period of eight weeks were assessed by a two-stage procedure, using the 30-item General Health Questionnaire (GHQ-30) and the Present State Examination schedule (PSE) (Abiodun, 1993). Overall prevalence of psychiatric disorder was 12.5 percent, with anxiety states and neurotic depression the most common diagnoses. Prevalence of psychiatric morbidity was found to be significantly associated with younger age (under 24 years), being primigravid, having been married for less than one year, having an unsupportive husband, and a previous history of induced abortion.

Other investigations have confirmed a substantial rate of psychological disturbances among pregnant African women (Cheetham et al., 1981; Jinadu and Daramola, 1990), at least equalling the prevalence range encountered among women in developed countries (Cox, 1983). In many of the mothers surveyed, psychiatric symptoms (particularly anxiety) present during pregnancy tended to remit after childbirth, suggesting at least some concerns about the birth event itself. Nevertheless, a substantial proportion of mothers continue to exhibit depressive symptoms during the puerperium (Cox, 1983). The question of whether this interferes with the quality of childcare has simply not been addressed.

Apart from these studies related to pregnancy, which of necessity must have women as their subjects, there is one further study of an urban community sample of 200 young women (average age, 32 years) from Zimbabwe. Both life events and difficulties and mental state (in those who passed a screening interview) were assessed for the previous 12 months. Thirty percent had suffered a major depression (average duration, 5 months) in the period, often related to severe life events. One-fifth of these had attempted suicide or had previously considered it. Many had been markedly disabled by their condition, leading to reduced family income and child neglect (Broadhead and Abas, 1993). These prevalence rates are comparable to those obtained in developed countries for socially disadvantaged women, and they indicate that African women are not spared from high rates of depression, given poor social conditions.

CONCLUSIONS

Table 6-5 presents a picture of the ages at which mental health problems occur in Sub-Saharan African females; the picture must be considered approximate because of the almost total lack of data for most disorders concerning age at onset. The table suggests that adolescence and early adulthood are life span stages of risk for depression, schizophrenia, and psychological morbidity associated with pregnancy and the puerperium, a finding consistent with those for females in the developed world. Considerations of age aside, the limited data available seem to point to two conclusions: (1) the magnitude of psychiatric morbidity in Africa is substantial and comparable to that found in developed countries; and (2) African women, despite their substantial burdens in various settings, do not seem to show the excess in rates of defined psychological disorders compared with males that have been recorded for women in developed countries. As Table 6-1 indicates, the only psychiatric disorders that appear to impose a disproportionate and, in this instance, unique burden on Sub-Saharan females are those associated with pregnancy and the puerperium. Even in the case of depression, for which there is the greatest evidence of an excess among females in most studies throughout the rest of the world, the African picture seems to be quite different, with males showing a comparable, or even a higher, rate of depressive disorders compared with females. It should be stressed that this conclusion is supported mainly by community-based studies. It is also true that the large majority of studies assessing the actual number of people in treatment at psychiatric facilities in Africa consistently shows an excess of males to females; this excess is certainly caused by differences in help-seeking behavior between the two sexes.

It is difficult to explain this finding, bearing in mind that African women have to face substantial problems, adversities, and burdens. A clarification of this issue is surely a research priority for researchers and clinicians active in African countries. It may also provide valuable clues to a better understanding of the complex interplay of risk factors, protective factors, coping styles, and interpersonal relationships that is at the origin of many psychological disorders and strongly affects the course and the outcome of many others.

It has been postulated that the low figures reported for certain disorders (including mental disorders) among women in Africa are the result of the underutilization of health services by women. While data for the mental health field do indicate that women are less inclined to be referred and admitted to inpatient facilities, the data obtained for general medical outpatients in the very thorough WHO study cited above (Üstün and Sartorius, 1995) indicate higher utilization by women than by men. Nor were these women attending primarily because they were bringing their children to the clinic. It thus seems likely that the data from the WHO study indicating higher rates of psychiatric disorder in men than women attending the clinic are not an artifact.

TABLE 6-5   Ages of Occurrence of Mental Health Problems in Sub-Saharan African Females

In Utero	Infancy/ Early Childhood (birth through age 4)	Childhood (ages 5–14)	Adolescence (ages 15–19)	Adulthood (ages 20–44)	Postmenopause (age 45+)
			Depression	Depression	
			Schizophrenia	Schizophrenia	
			Psychological morbidity associated with pregnancy and the puerperium	Psychological morbidity associated with pregnancy and the puerperium	

Insofar as the course and outcome of psychological disorders are concerned, in the case of schizophrenia the most important data come from the WHO Outcome Study and point to a better course and outcome for females than for males with a diagnosis of schizophrenia in Africa (and in developing countries in general). These data are also consistent with those obtained in follow-up studies in developed countries. Important additional data on the course and outcome of less severe disorders will be provided by the follow-up of the patients enrolled in the WHO study on psychological disorders in general medical settings (Üstün and Sartorius, 1995).

With regard to reproductive life, some studies seem to show that the Rousseauesque belief that African women have a stress-free, "natural" pregnancy is not substantiated. For a variety of reasons—including the high risk of physical morbidity and mortality associated with pregnancy in African countries, the anxiety associated with it, and the extremely high value assigned to the fulfillment of a mother's role—pregnancy seems to be a particularly high-risk situation for psychological morbidity, and therefore deserves special efforts in scientific investigations and the refinement of effective preventive and treatment methods.

RESEARCH NEEDS

The following general recommendations for future studies and research to be carried out in the African continent are proposed.

- There is a need to further investigate why women in Africa have the same, or perhaps fewer, psychiatric disorders, including depression, than men in Africa. It is still unclear whether this is the result of African men suffering from an excess of the disorder when compared with men in the developed world, or whether African women are somehow protected from mental disorders more than their counterparts in developed countries. The existing studies seem to indicate that both men and women, and particularly men, suffer from more psychiatric disorder in Africa than in the more developed world. Nevertheless, there are few studies, and more should be done to explore this important issue. These studies should employ reliable methodologies that enable comparisons to be made with findings obtained in other countries. The experience of several researchers has shown that it is indeed possible to carry out careful investigations in African countries using the same methodology employed in developed nations, adapted for local situations and the specificities of African cultures. For this purpose, collaborative, cooperative, or coordinated studies offer a valuable tool, as demonstrated by several WHO multicenter studies, which have included at least one African center as well as other centers from developing countries (for example, IPSS, Outcome Study, the study on psychological problems in general health care settings, and the study of the neuropsychiatric manifestations of AIDS).

- It is well known that life events and expressed emotion are important in the genesis and maintenance of depression, as well as schizophrenia. Because depression is known to be a significant cause of disability worldwide and occurs frequently in African women, it is necessary to better clarify how depression interacts with these factors in African populations, and to what extent these variables are responsible for sex differences in the rate, course, and outcome of psychiatric disorders.

- Another area that merits special efforts is related to post-traumatic stress disorders and related disorders. Natural disasters, social disruption, famine, war, and forced migration are not uncommon in many African countries, and it would be important to assess the magnitude of stress-related psychiatric disorders among the affected communities and to investigate the determinants and the variables affecting the onset, the course, and the outcome of these disorders. This is also an area that warrants special efforts in order to define effective methods of prevention and treatment, to be disseminated among various levels of health workers.

- Finally, the possible effects of puerperal depression on the health of the babies born to these mothers deserve investigation. In situations where infant mortality rates are already high, any added factors may tip the balance of an infant's health adversely, and thus may have an important effect on the mortality rates and the genesis of sporadic cases of infant malnutrition.

NOTE

1. Within the WHO studies on schizophrenia quoted in this chapter, the "developing countries" were Colombia, India, and Nigeria. This follows the classification used within the United Nations and by WHO.

REFERENCES

Abiodun, O. A. 1993. A study of mental morbidity among primary care patients in Nigeria. Comp. Psychiat. 34(1):10–13.

Abiodun, O. A., O. O. Adetoro, and O. O. Ogunbode. 1993. Psychiatric morbidity in a pregnant population in Nigeria. Gen. Hosp. Psychiat. 15:125–128.

Assael, M. I., J. M. Namboze, G. A. German, and F. J. Bennett. 1972. Psychiatric disturbances during pregnancy in a rural group of African women. Soc. Sci. Med. 6:387–395.

Awaritefe, A. 1988. Clinical anxiety in Nigeria. Acta Psychiat. Scand. 77(6):729–735.

Baasher, T. 1961. Survey of mental illness in Wadi Halfa. Paper presented at the Sixth International Congress on Mental Health, September. (Cited in J. Racy, 1970; Psychiatry in the Arab East, Acta Psychiat. Scand. Suppl. 211: 1–171: pp. 92–93).

Bebbington, P. E. 1988. The social epidemiology of clinical depression. In Handbook of Social Psychiatry, G. H. Burroughs and A. S. Henderson, eds. Amsterdam: Elsevier.

Beiser, M., J. L. Ravel, H. Collomb, and C. Egelhoff. 1972. Assessing psychiatric disorder among the Serer of Senegal. J. Nerv. Mental Dis. 154(2):141–151.

Benjamin, O., O. Osuntokun, and A. Boroffka. 1975. Hysteria in Nigerians. Nigerian Med. J. 5(1):6–13.

Ben-Tovim, D. I., and J. M. Cushnie. 1986. The prevalence of schizophrenia in a remote area of Botswana. Br. J. Psychiat. 148:576–580.

Binitie, A. 1981. Psychiatric disorders in a rural practice in the Bendel State of Nigeria. Acta Psychiat. Scand. 64:273–280.

Broadhead, J., and M. Abas. 1993. The Presentation and Management of Mental Illness at the Primary Care Level in Developing Countries. Working Paper 5, Series on International Mental and Behavioral Health. Cambridge, Mass.: Program in Medical Anthropology, Harvard University.

Brown, G. W. 1991. Some public health aspects of depression. Pp. 59–72 in The Public Health Impact of Mental Disorders, D. Goldberg and D. Tantam, eds. Bern: Hogrefe and Huber.

Brown, G. W., and T. Harris. 1978. Social Origins of Depression: A Study of Psychiatric Disorder in Women. Cambridge: University Printing House.

Carothers, J. J. 1953. The African Mind in Health and Disease. World Health Organization Monograph Series. No. 17. Geneva: WHO.

Cheetham, R. W. S., A. Rzadkowolski, and S. Raaemane. 1981. Psychiatric disorders of the puerperium in South African women of Nguni origin. S. Afr. Med. J. September:502–506.

Cox, J. L. 1979. Psychiatric morbidity and pregnancy: A controlled study of 263 semi-rural Ugandan women. Br. J. Psychiat. 134:401–405.

Cox, J. L. 1983. Post-natal depression: A comparison of African and Scottish women. Soc. Psychiat. 18:25–28.

Day, R., A. Nielsen, A. Korten, G. Ernberg, K. C. Dube, J. Gebhart, A. Jablensky, C. Leon, A. Marsella, M. Olatawura, N. Sartorius, E. Stromgren, R. Takahashi, N. Wig, and L. C. Wynne. 1987. Stressful life events preceding the acute onset of schizophrenia: a cross-national study from the World Health Organization. Cult. Med. Psychiat. 11:123–205.

Diop, B., R. Collingnon, M. Guèye, and T. W. Harding. 1982. Diagnosis and symptoms of mental disorder in a rural area of Senegal. Afr. J. Med. Med. Sci. 11:95–103.

Dohrenwend, B. P., and B. S. Dohrenwend. 1969. Social Status and Psychological Disorder: A Causal Inquiry. New York: John Wiley and Sons.

Dohrenwend, B. P., and B. S. Dohrenwend. 1974. Social and cultural influences on psychopathology. Ann. Rev. Psychol. 25:417–452.

German, G. A. 1987. Mental health in Africa. I. The extent of mental health problems in Africa today. An update of epidemiological knowledge. Br. J. of Psychiat. 151:435–439.

Ghubash R., E. Hamdi, and P. Bebbington. 1992. The Dubai community psychiatric survey. I. Prevalence and socio-demographic correlates. Soc. Psychiat. 27:53–61.

Giel, R., and J. N. Van Luijk. 1969. Psychiatric morbidity in a small Ethiopian town. Br. J. Psychiat. 115:149–162.

Goldberg, D., and P. Huxley. 1992. Common Mental Disorders. A Bio-social Model. London: Routledge/Tavistock.

Goldman, N., and R. Ravid. 1980. Community surveys: Sex differences in mental illness. In The Mental Health of Women, M. Guttentag, S. Salasin, and D. Belle, eds. New York: Academic Press.

Goodwin, F. K., and M. C. Blehar. 1993. Special edition: Toward a new psychobiology of depression in women. J. Aff. Dis. 29:75–76.

Gove, W. R., and J. Tudor. 1973. Adult sex roles and mental illness. Am. J. Sociol. 78:812–835.

Grantham-McGregor, S. 1987. Field studies in early nutrition and later achievement. Pp. 128–174 in Early Nutrition and Later Achievement, J. Dabbing, ed. London: Academic Press.

Gureje, O., and B. Obikoya. 1991. Psychotropic drug use in an urban primary care clinic. Soc. Psychiat. Psychia. Epidemiol. 26(3):143–146.

Gureje, O., B. Obikoya, and B. A. Ikuesan. 1992. Prevalence of specific disorders in an urban primary care clinic. E. Afr. Med. J. 69:282–287.

Ihezue, U. H. 1982. Some observations and comments on the psychosocial profile of first-ever referrals to the psychiatric hospital, Enugu, Nigeria. Acta Psychiat. Scand. 65(5):355-364.

Jablensky, A., N. Sartorius, G. Ernberg, M. Anker, A. Korten, J. Cooper, R. Day, and A. Bertelsen. 1992. Schizophrenia: manifestations, incidence and course in different cultures. Psychological Medicine Monograph Supplementum 21. Cambridge, U.K.: Cambridge University Press.

Jegede, R. O. 1979. Depression in Africans revisited: A critical review of the literature. Afr. J. Med. Med. Sci. 8:125–132.

Jegede, R. O., J. U. Ohaeri, E. A. Bamgboye, and A. O. Okunade. 1990. Psychiatric morbidity in a Nigerian general out-patient clinic. W. Afr. J. Med. 9:177–186.

Jenkins, R. 1985. Sex differences in minor psychiatric morbidity. Psychological Medicine Monograph Supplementum 7. Cambridge, U.K.: Cambridge University Press.

Jinadu, M. K., and S. M. Daramola. 1990. Emotional changes in pregnancy and early puerperium among the Yoruba women of Nigeria. Intl. J. Soc. Psychiat. 36(2):93–98.

Keegstra, H. J. 1986. Depressive disorders in Ethiopia. A standardized assessment using the SADD schedule. Acta Psychiat. Scand. 73:658–664.

Khandelwal, S. K., and F. Workneh. 1988. Psychiatric outpatients in a general hospital of Ethiopia: Diagnostic and sociodemographic characteristics. Intl. J. Soc. Psychiat. 34(3):230–235.

Leighton, A. H., T. A. Lambo, C. C. Hughes, D. C. Leighton, J. M. Murphy, and D. B. Macklin. 1963a. Psychiatric Disorder among the Yoruba. Ithaca, N.Y.: Cornell University Press.

Leighton, D. C., J. S. Harding, D. B. Macklin, A. M. Macmillan, and A. H. Leighton. 1963b. The Character of Danger. The Stirling County Study. New York: Basic Books.

Levin, A., L. Schlebusch, L. Willgoose, and N. K. Naidoo. 1981. Admissions to a South African general hospital psychiatric unit. Gen. Hosp. Psychiat. 3(2):165-170.

Majodina, M. Z., and F. Y. Attah Johnson. 1983. Standardized assessment of depressive disorders (SADD) in Ghana. Br. J. Psychiat. 143:442–446.

Makanjuola, R. O. A. 1985. Recurrent unipolar manic disorder in the Yoruba Nigerian: Further evidence. Br. J. Psychiat. 147:434–437.

Ndetei, D. M., and J. Muhangi. 1979. The prevalence and clinical presentation of psychiatric illness in a rural setting in Kenya. Br. J. Psychiat. 135:269–272.

Ndetei, D. M., and A. Vadher. 1984. Life events occurring before and after onset of depression in a Kenyian setting—any significance? Acta Psychiat. Scand. 69:327–332.

Nolen-Hoeksema, S. 1987. Sex differences in unipolar depression: evidence and theory. Psychol. Bull. 101:259–282.

Odejide, A. O., L. K. Oyewunmi, and J. U. Ohaeri. 1989. Psychiatry in Africa: An overview. Am. J. Psychiat. 146(6):708–716.

Orley, J. 1972. A prospective study of 372 consecutive admissions to Butabika Hospital, Kampala. E. Afr. Med. J. 49:16–26.

Orley, J., and J. K. Wing. 1979. Psychiatric disorders in two African villages. Arch. Gen. Psychiat. 36: 513–520.

Osuntokun, B. O., and A. Boroffka. 1975. Hysteria in Nigerians. Nigerian Med. J. 5(1):6–13.

Oyefeso, A. O., and A. R. Adegoke. 1992. Psychological adjustment of Yoruba adolescents as influenced by family type: A research note. J. Child Psychol. Psychiat. Allied Disc. 33(4): 785–788.

Rahim, S. I. A., and M. Cederblad. 1989. Epidemiology of mental disorders in young adults of a newly urbanized area in Khartoum, Sudan. Br. J. Psychiat. 155:44–47.

Robins, L. N., and D. A. Regier. 1991. Psychiatric Disorders in America. New York: The Free Press.

Sartorius N., T. B. Ustün, J. A. Costa e Silva, D. Goldberg, Y. Lecrubier, H. Ormel, M. Von Korff, and U. Wittchen. 1993. An international study of psychological problems in primary care. Preliminary report from the WHO collaborative project on "Psychological Problems in General Health Care." Arch. Gen. Psychiat. 50:819–824.

Sikanerty, T., and W. W. Eaton. 1984. Prevalence of schizophrenia in the Labadi district of Ghana. Br. J. Psychiat. 69:156–161.

Toole, M. J., and R. J. Waldman. 1990. Prevention of excess mortality in refugee and displaced populations in developing countries. J. Am. Med. Assoc. 263:3296–3302.

Ustün, T. B., and N. Sartorius, eds. 1995. Mental Illness in General Health Care: An International Study. Chichester, U.K.: John Wiley and Sons.

Vadher, A., and D. M. Ndetei. 1981. Life events and depression in a Kenyan setting. Br. J. Psychiat. 139:134–137.

Warner, R., and G. de Girolamo. 1995. Epidemiology of Mental Disorders and Psychosocial Problems—Schizophrenia. Geneva: WHO.

Weissman, M. M., and G. L. Klerman. 1977. Sex differences in the epidemiology of depression. Arch. Gen. Psychiat. 34:98–111.

WHO (World Health Organization). 1979. Schizophrenia: The International Follow-up Study of Schizophrenia. Chichester, U.K.: Wiley.

WHO (World Health Organization). 1993. The ICD-10 Classification of Mental and Behavioural Disorders—Diagnostic Criteria for Research. Geneva: WHO.

7

Cardiovascular Diseases, Cancers, and Chronic Obstructive Pulmonary Diseases

An increasing number of studies suggest that noncommunicable diseases will soon be the most important cause of morbidity and mortality in developing countries (Commission on Health Research for Development, 1990; Dodu, 1988; Feachem et al., 1992; Ghali, 1991; Manton, 1988; World Bank, 1993). The reasons for this are several, and include the changing demographic profile of Sub-Saharan Africa (see the Appendix to this volume), as well as changes in environmental, economic, and other sociocultural variables (Commission on Health Research for Development, 1990; Feachem and Jamison, 1991; Ghali, 1991; Manton, 1988). Issues such as increased access to health care, population aging patterns, and modifications in lifestyle patterns—especially in connection with established risk factors such as smoking—are also equally pertinent considerations in any discussions of these disease transitions.

The historic dominance of the communicable diseases and the emphasis to date on their treatment and control partially explain the lack of information and reliable data on the noncommunicable diseases. Lack of interest and appropriately trained medical personnel, especially in epidemiology, and the absence of coherent policies concerning data collection, information management, and research in general, however, are more critical in explaining the present dearth of understanding concerning the large and important category of noncommunicable and chronic diseases (Commission on Health Research for Development, 1990; Feachem and Jamison, 1991).

This chapter begins with a discussion of cardiovascular diseases (CVD), which as a group are rapidly becoming a major cause of mortality and morbidity in Sub-Saharan Africans. The discussion is structured in two parts: (1) emerging problems, including coronary artery disease and stroke and their risk factors, such as smoking, hypertension, dyslipidemias, obesity, and diabetes; and (2) continuing problems, including rheumatic heart disease and the cardiomyopathies. An overview of selected cancers in women follows, and this section is also divided into two parts: (1) emerging problems, including breast cancer; cancers of the uterus, ovary, and choriocarcinoma; colorectal and lung cancers; and liver cancer; and (2) continuing problems, including cancer of the cervix; the leukemias and lymphomas; skin cancers; and cancer of the bladder. The evidence on chronic obstructive pulmonary diseases is then reviewed, and the chapter ends with a presentation of conclusions and a summary of research needs. Where specific information and data are not available for Sub-Saharan populations, the chapter offers analogies (or extrapolations) from current trends in other populations and their implications.

Table 7-1 identifies the chronic diseases reviewed in this chapter that appear to show a disproportionately high burden in African females compared with males. Of the eight listed, four—including rheumatic heart disease and cancers of the breast, skin, and possibly bladder associated with *Schistosoma haematobium* infection—occur both

TABLE 7-1 Noncommunicable Diseases in Sub-Saharan Africa: Gender-Related Burden

Disorder	Exclusive to Females	Greater for Females than for Males	Burdens for Females and Males Comparable, but of Particular Significance for Females
Cancer			
Breast		X	
Uterus, ovary, choriocarcinoma	X		
Cervix	X		
Skin		X	
Bladder		X?	
Cardiomyopathies associated with pregnancy	X		
Gestational diabetes mellitus	X		
Rheumatic heart disease		X	

NOTE: Significance is defined here as having an impact on health that, for any reason—biological, reproductive, sociocultural, or economic—is different in its implications for females than for males.

in males and females, but show a disproportionate burden in females. The other four disorders—including gestational diabetes mellitus; the cardiomyopathies associated with pregnancy; and cancers of the uterus, ovary, and cervix and choriocarcinoma—are unique to females. The other major chronic diseases covered in this chapter currently show no differences in occurrence or outcome by gender; this may reflect inadequacies in the evidentiary base, as well as a possible true lack of gender-specific burden.

CARDIOVASCULAR DISEASES

Emerging Problems

Coronary Artery Disease

The frequency of coronary artery disease (CAD) and related complications in the Sub-Saharan region is much lower than that in developed countries, and CAD is only infrequently the reason an individual is hospitalized for cardiovascular problems (Bertrand et al., 1991; Hutt, 1991; Ticolat et al., 1991) (see Tables 7-2 and 7-3). Nevertheless, recent trends in urbanization, lifestyle changes, and acquisition of appropriate technology are thought to be responsible for what seems to be an increasing number of reports and hospitalizations for this condition (Hutt, 1991; Ticolat et al., 1991). Approximately 6 percent of all admissions into a cardiovascular unit in Côte d'Ivoire between 1988 and 1990 were for CAD; the frequency about a decade ago was less than 3 percent in that same unit (Bertrand, 1991; Bertrand et al., 1991).

In all the studies cited above, myocardial infarction, and CAD in general, are more common in men than in women. Although a direct extrapolation to Sub-Saharan African women cannot be made, it has been shown in some populations that while survival rates with CAD are similar in black men and women, the prognosis is considerably worse in black women for reasons that are not well understood (Liao et al., 1992; Tofler, et al., 1987; Willerson et al., 1987). Because Sub-Saharan women tend to live longer than men (see Appendix), studies will be needed to determine if this added longevity produces a selective effect.

TABLE 7-2 Hospitalizations in a Cardiovascular Unit: Five Most Common Cardiovascular Disorders

Disorder	Number of Admissions	Percentage
Hypertension	574	39.3
Rheumatic heart	212	14.5
Congenital heart	182	12.5
Cerebrovascular	159	10.9
Cardiomyopathies	135	9.1

NOTE: Based on 1,458 admissions over a two-year period.

SOURCE: Bertrand et al., 1991.

TABLE 7-3 Common Disorders in a Population of Hospitalized Patients of a General Internal Medicine Service

Disorders	Number of Admissions			Percentage		
	Men	Women	Total	Men	Women	Total
Hypertension	634	366	1,000	9.8	5.6	15.4
Diabetes	523	262	785	8.0	4.0	12.0
Nonhypertensive cardiac disorders	402	305	707	6.2	4.7	10.9
Hepatitis	326	74	400	5.0	1.1	6.1
Renal	296	85	381	4.5	1.3	5.8
Respiratory	178	151	329	2.7	2.3	5.0

NOTE: Based on 6,515 admissions over a three-year period.

SOURCE: Data supplied by the National Epidemiology Board of Cameroon, 1993.

Stroke

As shown in Table 7-2, cerebrovascular disease—or stroke—is the fourth leading cause of hospitalization in a large reference cardiovascular unit of this region (Bertrand, 1991; Bertrand et al., 1991). As in the case of cardiovascular disease, the incidence of stroke increases with age, and this may again place older Sub-Saharan women at increased risk (Bam and Yako, 1984).

Factors Influencing Coronary Artery Disease and Stroke Risk

Smoking

In addition to its implications in CVD, smoking is a pivotal risk factor in a large number of chronic disorders, with significant impact on burdens of morbidity and mortality. While the frequency of tobacco use and the absolute number of smokers are generally on the decrease in many developed countries, the reverse is true in much

TABLE 7-4 Cardiovascular Risk Factors: Frequency of Hypertension[a] and Smoking[b] in Selected Age Groups in Cameroon

Age Range	Hypertension (%[c])			Smokers (%[c])		
	Total	Females	Males	Total	Females	Males
0–1	3.6	2.0	1.0	—	—	—
3–15	7.3	3.4	7.8	4.5	1.5	3.0
10–20	5.5	6.0	5.1	14.6	3.3	11.3
18–30	5.0	5.9	4.5	15.5	2.0	13.5
25–64[d]	12.3	7.7	13.5	16.5	3.5	13.0

[a]For the 0–1-year age group, systolic blood pressure only was used, and values greater than the mean plus 2 standard deviations were considered to be in the hypertensive range. For the age groups younger than 15 years, both systolic and diastolic readings were used, with the values higher than the mean plus two standard deviations considered to be in the hypertensive range. For the age groups older than 15 years, WHO criteria were used to define hypertension.

[b]Have smoked cigarettes daily or weekly for at least six months.

[c]All percentages shown are pooled averages from one or more studies, using the same or a similar protocol on the same or similar population groups.

[d]This age group concerns studies involving the general population. All other age groups shown are from studies involving institutions such as hospitals, schools, and universities in urban or semiurban areas. Total number of subjects involved in the studies from which the data above were generated = 11,200. (See text for further discussion.)

of Sub-Saharan Africa (WHO, 1992). The present estimate is that the prevalence of smoking increases at a rate of about 3.4 percent a year in developing countries overall, while a reduction of about 0.2 percent a year is recorded for the developed countries (WHO, 1992).

As for the behavior of specific subpopulations, a group of great size and particular risk—and, obviously, a primary matter of concern for this report—is the world's population of girls and women. About 10 percent of African women report that they smoke cigarettes daily (WHO, 1992). Although earlier data from Cameroon suggested a figure of less than 3.5 percent across all age groups (see Table 7-4), it is unlikely that this figure will hold. Recent, unpublished results from that country suggest that a significant number of girls under age 12 may already have established smoking habits. A study involving female university students in Nigeria showed an increase in smoking prevalence from 3 to 24 percent between 1973 and 1982 (Elegboleye and Femi-Perse, 1976; WHO, 1992), with an even more alarming increase among student teachers, among whom a prevalence of 50 percent was encountered. Similar trends have been noted in Ghana (Report from Ghana, 1984). The major culprits identified in these changes, in Africa and elsewhere in the developing world, are rapid urbanization and acculturation, associated changes in lifestyle, and the dumping of tobacco products into these countries (WHO, 1992).

Our current understanding of the effects of environmental smoke (and passive smoking in general) also suggests that young people who live around adult smokers run significant smoking-related health risks. Consequently, all children may be exposed to the ill-effects of environmental tobacco smoke at practically all ages (Taylor et al., 1992).

Hypertension

Hypertension is commonly defined as sustained elevated arterial blood pressure, measured indirectly by an inflatable cuff and pressure manometer. Hypertension is the most common cardiovascular disorder in Sub-Saharan Africa. It results in more hospital admissions than any other disorder in almost all cardiovascular hospital units (see Table 7-2) and in general internal medicine units (see Table 7-3). Hypertension has been shown to increase the risk of developing stroke, coronary heart disease, congestive heart failure, peripheral vascular disease, and nephrosclerosis (NRC, 1989; Philips and Whisnant, 1992). It can also directly affect many organ systems, including the heart, endocrine organs, kidneys, and central and autonomic nervous systems (NRC, 1989). Thus, hypertension can be considered both a risk factor for CVD and a cardiovascular disorder in its own right. The classification of hypertension most commonly used for adults in the studies cited below is that of the World Health Organization Expert Committee published in 1978 (WHO, 1978): systolic blood pressure   160 mmHg, or diastolic blood pressure   95 mmHg.

Risk factors for hypertension include a positive family history of the disorder, increased body mass, obesity, and elevated salt intake (Dyer et al., 1994; NRC, 1989; Stamler et al., 1991). Race has also been shown to be an important risk factor; many studies demonstrate that blood pressure is higher and hypertension more prevalent among blacks of African origin than in Caucasians living in similar environments (DHHS, 1986; Stamler et al., 1975).

Now that acceptable blood pressure levels for different age groups have been defined, we are also able to recognize hypertension in childhood. Table 7-4 summarizes the results of several cross-sectional studies from Cameroon that included screening for hypertension across various age groups. These studies show prevalence rates of hypertension of less than 8 percent among subjects between 0 and 30 years of age, and of less than 14 percent among subjects aged 25–64. A greater percentage of females aged 0–30 years were labeled hypertensive than males of the same age. Beyond the 18-to-30-year-old group, males predominate, but it is unclear when this transition occurs. While most hospital-based and screening studies in the adult general population suggest that hypertension rates are much higher in men (see Table 7-3), some studies suggest that the prevalence of hypertension is much higher in women than in men, with higher rates among Sub-Saharan Africans in general (Bam and Yako, 1984; M'Buyamba-Kabangu et al., 1987; Seedat and Seedat, 1982). These seemingly contradictory observations again highlight the problems of differential access and utilization of health care and reporting bias in the attempt to achieve a clear picture of regional mortality and morbidity by gender.

Additional data from Cameroon and other Sub-Saharan countries may raise more questions than they answer. Table 7-5 presents population-based rates of hypertension derived from several comparable studies in six countries of the region. Hypertension rates in the rural populations of those countries vary between about 5 percent and 15 percent, while rates for urban population groups vary between 7 and 24 percent. Rates for women are generally one-third to one-half the rates for men; rarely are both rates the same. Table 7-5 also shows higher rates of hypertension in the urban than the rural population of Ghana and the South African Zulu population, but higher rates in rural than in urban areas of Cameroon and the Congo (M'Buyamba-Kabangu et al., 1987; Seedat and Seedat, 1982). Age may play a role in those differences, because migration of large numbers of young people into urban areas will affect distributions, although other factors may be involved (M'Buyamba-Kabangu et al., 1987; Seedat and Seedat, 1982).

The relevance of hypertension to the health of Sub-Saharan Africa's female population is far from trivial.

TABLE 7-5 Rates of Hypertension[a] in Selected Countries of Sub-Saharan Africa

Country	Population	
	Rural Rates (%)	Urban Rates (%)
Ghana	5.9	11.3
Nigeria	10.2	—
South Africa (Zulu)	5–6.6	23.8
Côte d'Ivoire	—	13.8
Cameroon	14.8	10.2
Congo, The	12.4	6.8

[a]WHO criteria used for definition. Composite data derived from published reports (see text for further details).

Women are especially vulnerable from hypertension associated with pregnancy; among its consequences are elevated risk for eclampsia and preeclampsia, with potentially fatal implications (Dulay, 1990; Merz et al., 1992; Schoon et al., 1990). Hypertension may also produce excess morbidity and mortality in black African women in older age groups because of a documented contribution to increased frequency of stroke (Bertrand, 1991; Hutt, 1991; Seedat and Seedat, 1982; Bam and Yako, 1984; Philips and Whisnant, 1992), although reporting bias and other issues related to access to care will need to be taken into account in future studies of this association.

Dyslipidemias

There are relatively few reports on lipid levels in Sub-Saharan populations (Bensadoun et al., 1984; Hutt, 1991; Ngongang and Titanji, 1985; Raisonnier et al., 1988; Shaper, 1974). Both women and men in these populations have relatively higher HDL cholesterol levels than their counterparts in other developing countries, which may explain the "relative protection" of black Africans against CVD. Obese women may, however, have atherogenic levels—that is, lipid levels that initiate, increase, or accelerate the process leading to atherosclerosis (Ngongang et al., 1988). Studies have shown that some East African tribes appear to have cholesterol and lipid levels indistinguishable from those found in a number of Western societies (Barnicot et al., 1972; Shaper et al., 1969). Studies involving other important lipid fractions that also control for potential confounding variables will be required, however, before firm conclusions can be drawn about similarities and differences between such populations and those in the West.

Obesity

Obesity (see also Chapter 3, Nutritional Status) is an important risk factor for a number of disorders: cardio-vascular disorders, a variety of conditions related to women's reproductive health, and a number of cancers. There is a strong association between obesity and other cardiovascular risk factors, including hypertension and metabolic disorders such as diabetes (Bonham and Brock, 1985; Gillum and Grant, 1982; Joint National Committee on Detection, Evaluation, and Treatment of High Blood Pressure, 1986; Sims and Berchtold, 1982).

Although relatively few studies have involved Sub-Saharan population groups (Alade and Ezeokeke, 1990), most studies conclude that obesity—generally defined in these studies as a body mass index (BMI) greater than $27km/m^2$—is more common in women than in men, and there is presently no reason to think that Sub-Saharan Africa diverges from this pattern (Johnson, 1970; Kumanyika and Adams-Campbell, 1991; Njitoyap et al., 1991; Sloan, 1960). Obesity rates of 8.3 percent for men and 35.7 percent for women have been reported in Nigeria, and rates in the neighborhood of 50 percent have been recorded for the Bantus of South Africa (Johnson, 1970; Sloan, 1960). Akintewe and Adetuyibi (1986) report a significant association between obesity and hypertension in diabetics in the Sub-Saharan region, particularly in females. All in all, the prevalence of obesity in Sub-Saharan female populations would seem to constitute a real health problem for those populations. A determination of which of these populations, where, and under what circumstances obesity reaches problematic levels is a matter of future study, as are the varying cultural perceptions of the condition—that is, its acceptability, and even desirability.

Diabetes Mellitus

While the frequencies of degenerative and metabolic diseases in Sub-Saharan populations remain unknown, increasing clinical awareness of disorders such as diabetes mellitus (DM) suggests that they are either more common than initially thought, or that their prevalence is increasing (King and Rewers, 1991) (see Table 7-3). Like hypertension, diabetes mellitus is considered both a disease and an independent risk factor for CVD. There is also a suggestion that diabetes mellitus is associated with poorer CVD prognosis in women.

Reported prevalence rates for diabetes (See Table 7-6) are generally under 5 percent for Sub-Saharan populations (King and Rewers, 1991), and there seems to be a general impression among clinicians in the region that the DM subclass, insulin-dependent diabetes mellitus (IDDM), may be less common in Sub-Saharan African popula-

TABLE 7-6 Percentage Prevalence Rates for Diabetes and Impaired Glucose Tolerance for Selected Populations of Sub-Saharan Africa

Country and Population Group	Diabetes Mellitus General Population	Men	Women	Impaired Glucose Tolerance Men	Women
Tanzania		3	1	9	16
Kenya (Wachaga/Masai)		1	1	8	10
Ghana (civil servants)		0.5	0.6		
Nigeria (urban)	1.7				
Cameroon	0.5–3				
Mali	1				

SOURCE: King and Rewers, 1991.

tions than in populations of developed countries, but the basis for this impression is probably compromised by biases in access, utilization, and reporting and issues of cost.

The prevalence of impaired glucose tolerance, however, considered a stage in the progression to diabetes in some individuals, may be almost double the 5 percent figure in some Sub-Saharan populations, and it is invariably higher among women (King and Rewers, 1991). In Tanzania, which has the highest prevalence rates of six countries studied, prevalence of impaired glucose tolerance was 9 percent in men and 16 percent in women (see Table 7-6). At the same time, a study of three years of hospital admissions in a general internal medicine service in Cameroon found that, of over 500 admissions for diabetes during that period, 8 percent were males and 4 percent were females (information from the National Epidemiology Board of Cameroon, 1991). Since male admissions overall ran at almost 2:1 compared with female admissions for six common disorders, it would be unwise to draw a conclusion from these figures, which may only reflect differential utilization of tertiary facilities by gender.

Diabetes is especially compromising for females. For already diabetic women, the complex metabolic alterations that accompany pregnancy may complicate disease control and place both mother and fetus in jeopardy, with particularly grave risks for the fetus. Gestational diabetes mellitus (GDM), a special category for pregnant women, is defined as carbohydrate intolerance of variable severity, with onset or first recognition during the present pregnancy. There is considerable demographic and phenotypic heterogeneity in the prevalence of gestational diabetes mellitus (Dooley et al., 1991), and optimum case management includes screening for GDM in any pregnant woman, because the consequences of unrecognized or untreated GDM include increased fetal and neonatal loss and higher neonatal and maternal morbidity.

Oral Contraceptive Use

The use of contraceptive pills has increased substantially among Sub-Saharan African females, especially in the middle and upper socioeconomic groups who can afford their cost. Since the mid-1960s a considerable amount of epidemiological clinical and laboratory evidence has linked current use of combined oral contraceptives with certain types of CVD, especially venous thromboembolism, thrombotic stroke, myocardial infarction, subarachnoid hemorrhage, and hypertension (Irey et al., 1978; *Lancet*, 1979; Stadel, 1981; Thorgood et al., 1981). The risk of CVD from oral contraceptive use is independent of smoking, although, except for venous thromboembolism, that risk is increased by smoking. There may also be some residual excess risk of myocardial infarction in women aged 40 or over with 5 or more years of pill use in the past (Mishell, 1989). Still, there is also evidence that current users of low-dose estrogen oral contraceptives showed no increase in risk (relative risk of 0.87) of myocardial infarction (Mant et al., 1987), and that use of oral contraceptive formulations containing less than 50 micrograms of estrogen by healthy, nonsmoking women up to age 45 is not associated with increased risk of serious CVD (Mishell, 1989). Whether these findings from developed countries can be extrapolated to Africa is debatable. So far, there are no valid epidemiologic data to link the use of oral contraceptives by black Africans with an increased risk factor of CVD.

The risk factors discussed above do not constitute an exhaustive listing of all the factors implicated in the general picture of all risks for cardiovascular disorders. They were addressed because of current estimates and projections of their relative prevalence in Sub-Saharan populations. It is unfortunate that there is still a considerable void in our understanding of the magnitude and implications of these factors in the region, a void that has negative implications for regional capability for prevention and control, for containing the elevated costs of managing most cardiovascular disorders in the situation of limited resources faced by the countries of Sub-Saharan Africa, and for long-term health care planning in general.

Continuing Problems

Rheumatic Heart Disease

Rheumatic heart disease (RHD) is second only to hypertension and its complications among cardiovascular disorders resulting in hospital admissions in Sub-Saharan Africa (Bertrand, 1991; Ekra and Bertrand, 1992; Hutt, 1991) (see Table 7-2). Screening studies among schoolchildren suggest a prevalence for RHD that may range from less than 1 per 1,000 to over 15 per 1,000 (WHO, 1988). A history of rheumatic fever, generally considered a prelude to the subsequent development of RHD, is present in less than 50 percent of the cases (Hutt, 1991). RHD accounts for over 14 percent of hospital admissions for cardiovascular disease (see Table 7-2) (Bertrand, 1991; Hutt, 1991; Serme, 1992), and it appears to be more common and associated with higher rates of morbidity and mortality in Sub-Saharan African women than in men (Cole, 1980; Sankale and Koate, 1970; Serme, 1992). The prevalence of RHD is highest among the young, and consequently morbidity and mortality are particularly high in this age group.

Cardiomyopathies

The cardiomyopathies comprise a group of heart muscle disorders of obscure etiology and, in some cases, pathophysiology as well. Cardiomyopathies invariably lead to intractable heart failure and are the fifth leading cause of hospitalization in cardiovascular or related units in the Sub-Saharan region (Bertrand et al., 1991) (see Table 7-2). Although some infectious and parasitic agents are known to attack the heart muscle directly—or indirectly, through immunological mechanisms—the Sub-Saharan African region is endemic for idiopathic cardiomyopathies characterized by cardiac dilatation, with or without muscle hypertrophy (Hutt, 1991; WHO, 1984). There is no evidence that women are particularly prone to heart failure, with the exception of some forms of cardiomyopathy—for example, peripartum and postpartum cardiomyopathy—that are intimately related to pregnancy and childbirth, and consequently exclusive to women (Bertrand et al., 1985; Talabi et al., 1985). Although excessive salt consumption and undiagnosed hypertension have been suggested as possible mechanisms operative in the cardiomyopathies observed during pregnancy and childbirth, or shortly afterward, their etiology remains obscure. They are suspected to have a nonnegligible impact on maternal morbidity and mortality, but the frequency and the amplitude of this impact requires carefully designed, controlled studies.

CANCERS

Neoplastic disorders are another increasingly prominent cause of morbidity and mortality in Sub-Saharan African countries (Bassett et al., 1992; Hutt, 1991; Mbakop et al., 1992; Parkin et al., 1988; Sobo, 1982; Tuyns and

Ravisse, 1970). This increase, similar to that observed for cardiovascular disorders, is probably the result of a combination of factors, including decreasing childhood mortality and increasing longevity, availability of trained manpower, improved health care and related diagnostic technology, changes in lifestyle and diet, and other environmental factors (WHO, 1990). In a seminal study in 1981, Doll and Peto estimated that approximately 35 percent (range, 10 to 70 percent) of all cancer *mortality* in the United States was related to diet. In 1977, Wynder and Gori estimated that 40 percent of cancer *incidence* among men and nearly 60 percent among women was related to diet. In 1989, the National Research Council commented that, because few of the relationships between specific dietary components and cancer risk are well established, the contribution of diet to individual cancers, and thus to total cancer rates, cannot be quantified precisely (NRC, 1989). Nevertheless, these now fundamental estimates emphasize the importance of diet in the etiology and prevention of cancer in the United States and, by extension, its importance worldwide.

Dietary influence aside, females are at risks of cancer that differ from male risk profiles simply because of differences in their basic physiologies. Neoplasms affecting the breast, cervix, and uterus belong exclusively to the female domain, with the exception of rare cases of breast cancer in males. According to studies to date, the most common neoplasms in African women are cancers of the cervix, followed by breast cancer, with cancer of the lymphatic system in third position (see Bassett et al., 1992, Zimbabwe; Mbakop et al., 1992, Cameroon; Parkin et al., 1988, worldwide frequencies of 16 major cancers; Sobo, 1982, Liberia; Stanley et al., 1987, worldwide statistics; Tuyns and Ravisse, 1970, the Congo). Estimated annual incidence rates for these neoplasms are 37, 27, and 12 per 100,000, respectively.

Emerging Problems

Cancer of the Breast

There are no reliable studies on the true frequency of breast cancer in Sub-Saharan Africa, because routine breast examinations, either by individuals or health professionals, are not commonly practiced. Clinical experience suggests, however, as indicated above, that breast cancers may be the second most common neoplasm in women of this region (Bassett et al., 1992; Mbakop et al., 1992; Parkin et al., 1988; Sobo, 1982; Stanley et al., 1987).

As for etiology, it is possible that changes in hormonal profiles brought about by greater longevity, as well as shifts in patterns of childbearing in response to such socioeconomic factors as urbanization, will affect the frequency of cases of breast cancer, if they have not done so already. Dietary factors have been implicated as a possible contributor to breast cancer, and socioeconomic factors may also be producing dietary modifications that could be meaningful (Howe et al., 1990; Lubin et al., 1986; WHO, 1990) It may also be, as conditions improve and screening programs are developed, that the combination of all these changes with improvements in case-finding will generate higher frequencies, so that breast cancer may be found to be more common than cervical cancer (Miller, 1992). As with the other forms of gynecologic cancer in Sub-Saharan Africa, diagnosis in most cases of breast cancer is made relatively late in the course of the disease, significantly reducing survival. Thus, unlike so many other cancers, a thorough clinical examination and patient education in self-examination can have a crucial impact on early identification of breast cancer; its diagnosis; and, ultimately, enhanced survival (Koroltchouk, 1990).

Cancers of the Uterus and Ovary and Choriocarcinoma

The exact frequency of these three cancers in the Sub-Saharan region is a subject of considerable debate, despite the low rates currently reported—generally less than 5 per 100,000 (Bassett, et al., 1992; Doll and Peto, 1981; Hutt, 1991; Mbakop et al., 1992; Mmiro, 1987; Omigbodun, and Akanmu, 1991; Parkin et al., 1988; Sobo, 1982; Stanley et al., 1987). Some risk factors for endometrial and ovarian cancer—such as early menarche, late menopause, and obesity (for cancer of the uterus)—are characteristic of many female populations in this region. And, as in the case of the etiology of breast cancer, dietary factors have been implicated (Howe et al., 1990; Lubin et al., 1986; WHO, 1990). The debate results largely from ignorance of the facts, which are obscured by the lack of clinical and laboratory skills necessary for accurate diagnosis, as well as by cultural resistance to autopsy. In countries that have acquired the appropriate diagnostic technology and trained manpower, reports of cases of these cancers are becoming more common, so there is reason to suspect that this will occur more generally in the Sub-Saharan region as diagnostic capabilities improve.

Colorectal and Lung Cancers

Colorectal cancer appears to be relatively uncommon in the Sub-Saharan region. As in the case of breast cancer and some gynecologic cancers, changes in diet and life-style have been implicated as etiologic factors (Bassett et al., 1992; Hutt, 1991; Mbakop et al., 1992; Parkin et al., 1988; Sobo, 1982; WHO, 1990). The risk levels of the various populations and whether women are at any special risk are unknown (Soubeyrand et al., 1984).

Similarly, while lung cancers rarely have been found in women in Sub-Saharan Africa, this profile may change with time, given the increased smoking at earlier ages observed among women in the region. In addition, improvements in diagnostic capabilities can be expected in themselves to increase cases of lung cancer in women.

Continuing Problems

Cancer of the Cervix

Cancer of the cervix is the most common form of malignancy in Sub-Saharan African women, and it may be the most common of all malignancies in the population as a whole (Doll and Peto, 1981; Hutt, 1991; Mbakop et al., 1992; Mmiro, 1987; Omigbodun and Akanmu, 1991; Sobo, 1982; Stanley et al., 1987; Tuyns and Ravisse, 1970; WHO, 1990). In some Sub-Saharan regions, cervical cancer may constitute as much 35 percent of all malignancies in women, and reported incidence rates range between 20 and 28 per 100,000.

Cervical cancer is generally considered a sexually transmitted disease that is intimately linked to the presence of human papillomavirus (HPV; see also Chapter 11). The disease may remain undetected until a relatively advanced stage. Sadly, the critical diagnostic techniques that would catch the disease at an earlier stage, when it is curable—ideally, in its premalignant phase—are not readily available in most countries of the region.

Leukemias and Lymphomas

Leukemias and some lymphomas (e.g., Burkitt's) are also relatively common in some Sub-Saharan countries and have been reported to be the third most common cancer in African women (Bassett et al., 1992; Feldmeier and Kranz, 1992; Stanley et al., 1987). Further studies will be required to determine with more accuracy how these frequencies compare with those in males in the region (Hutt, 1991).

Skin Cancers

Cancers of the skin are of special concern in Sub-Saharan African women (Bassett et al., 1992; Doll and Peto, 1981; Hutt, 1991; Mbakop et al., 1992; Mmiro, 1987; Omigbodun and Akanmu, 1991; Parkin et al., 1988; Sobo, 1982; Stanley et al., 1987). They have been reported as the fourth leading cancer among women in Zimbabwe (Bassett et al., 1992), and it has been suggested that certain skin and other systemic disorders may be related to use of skin-lightening creams and ointments containing steroids and known toxic chemicals (Gwet-Bell, 1990). In addition, chronic tropical ulcers have a tendency to degenerate into malignant skin-based lesions (Hutt, 1991). By virtue of their daily agricultural and other domestic duties, Sub-Saharan African women can be expected to be prone to such ulcers, and they are consequently at risk for this particular lesion. Whether they differ from males in this respect is unknown.

Liver Cancer

Cancer of the liver has been described in some populations of Sub-Saharan women (Bassett et al., 1992; Doll and Peto, 1981; Hutt, 1991; Mbakop et al., 1992; Mmiro, 1987; Omigbodun and Akanmu, 1991; Parkin et al., 1988; Sobo, 1982; Stanley et al., 1987), although the extent and magnitude of the disease remain unknown. Environmental factors associated with increased risk of liver cancer include infection with Hepatitis B virus, exposure to aflatoxin, and alcohol consumption (Barnum and Greenberg, 1993). That these factors are common to many Sub-Saharan African populations would suggest that liver cancer has been, and continues to be, an important malignancy in the region. The degree to which the disease affects African females disproportionately compared with males remains unknown.

Bladder Cancer

Bladder cancers are also relatively common in the Sub-Saharan region and have been intimately linked to chronic infection by *Schistosoma haematobium*. Where the nature of women's agricultural work enhances their chances of infection, in contrast to the chances of males, or where gender-linked limitations on access to appropriate health care are at issue, females may be at higher risk not only for infection and reinfection, but also for receiving inadequate therapy. Whether this differential is real remains to be resolved (Bassett et al., 1992; Feldmeier and Kranz, 1992; Parkin et al., 1988).

CHRONIC OBSTRUCTIVE PULMONARY DISEASES

Chronic obstructive pulmonary (lung) disease (COPD) refers to several disease entities, including asthma, emphysema, chronic bronchitis, peripheral airways disease, right-sided heart disease, and cor pulmonale (heart disease with an underlying pulmonary deficiency). These conditions are ill-defined and rarely characterized separately in descriptive epidemiologic studies of COPD. Risk factors for COPD include cigarette smoking, childhood respiratory tract infections, occupational dust exposure, and both indoor and outdoor air pollution (Bumgarner and Speizer, 1993; Elo and Preston, 1992; Hutt, 1991; Malik et al., 1983).

Data on COPD mortality and morbidity are scarce in Sub-Saharan Africa and elsewhere in the developing world. This scarcity reflects both a relative lack of attention and a lack of consistency in classification and reporting of COPD internationally. Evidence from industrialized countries indicates an inverse association of COPD rates with socioeconomic status, a factor that may act as a surrogate for other influences, such as cigarette smoking, poor nutrition, and higher levels of ambient pollution, including indoor air pollution. Data also demonstrate consistently higher mortality rates in males than females, most probably because of the longer and heavier smoking experience among men. It is believed, however, that COPD is a more important cause of mortality and morbidity in the developing than in the developed world, and that the burden of COPD may be growing disproportionately in Sub-Saharan African females, particularly the poor, for reasons noted below (Bumgarner and Speizer, 1993).

Cigarette Smoking

The relative increase in smoking prevalence in Sub-Saharan African females described earlier heralds increasing COPD incidence in this group. Prospective studies in other regions of the world have demonstrated higher COPD mortality and earlier disease onset in cigarette smokers (Peters and Ferris, 1967), and there is no reason to believe that African females will be immune to these effects.

Indoor Air Pollution

Outdoor air pollution has long been recognized to exacerbate COPD. While many studies in industrialized countries have failed to establish a conclusive link between COPD risk and air pollution levels, smoking behavior alone has not been sufficient to explain geographic variations in the prevalence of symptoms. Similarly, in studies in developing countries outside of the Sub-Saharan region, prevalence rates of cigarette smoking cannot explain all the variation seen in COPD rates, because mortality and prevalence rates often appear to be higher than in industrialized countries, and the sex ratios more equal (Bumgarner and Speizer, 1993; Chen et al., 1990; Saha and Jain, 1970). This last point is significant, because the relative increase in COPD rates in females in these studies may be indicative of other gender-specific exposures, such as indoor air pollution.

In one study in the Kenyan highlands, Clifford (1972) estimated the exposure to (mainly indoor) airborn total suspended particles at 25,000 milligrams annually. In another study in India, women in kitchens were found to be inhaling levels of benzopyrene, a known carcinogen present in cigarette smoke, at levels equivalent to smoking 20 cigarettes a day (Smith et al., 1983). Although benzopyrene exposure has not been linked to COPD risk, its presence clearly indicates that the microenvironment in the kitchens studied contained significant amounts of smoke. Although the materials used for cooking can be expected to vary in Sub-Saharan African households, there are no reasons to suggest that kitchens and indoor spaces in the region are necessarily better-ventilated or "cleaner" than those in the Indian study. These findings suggest that COPD may have a greater effect on females, particularly poor women and girls, in Sub-Saharan Africa than might otherwise be expected.

In summary, the etiology of most COPD remains obscure, although environmental factors, including cigarette smoking, appear to play a major role in causation, as well as in disease management and prognosis. Current trends in cigarette smoking indicate that COPD rates can be expected to rise disproportionately in Sub-Saharan females in the coming years. Prolonged exposure to smoke and its various component substances in poorly ventilated kitchens, homes, and related structures and pollen and dust particle exposure in settings where farming and field work are principal activities for Sub-Saharan women (see Chapter 9) may place females at increased risk for this disorder.

CONCLUSIONS

Chronic disorders—especially cardiovascular and neoplastic diseases—are important emerging health issues for Sub-Saharan populations, although descriptive data on demographic trends in chronic disease incidence and mortality, especially for females, are limited. It is currently projected that these maladies will rapidly become leading causes of morbidity and mortality. In addition, current and past experience in developed countries suggest that health care resources and planning to manage chronic diseases will be a major challenge for Sub-Saharan African countries in the near future.

Table 7-7 indicates the approximate ages at which chronic diseases and their sequelae occur in Sub-Saharan African females. The following conclusions can be drawn on the basis of existing data:

• Because of their relatively early age of onset and persistence across the life span, the cardiovascular disorders—hypertension, rheumatic heart disease, and cardiomyopathies associated with pregnancy—appear to be among the chronic disorders that may most adversely affect female health status in the region.

• Metabolic disorders such as diabetes mellitus constitute a major source of added morbidity and mortality for Sub-Saharan African women. This entity presents specific problems for women during pregnancy, for the fetus, and for both mother and child during delivery.

• Among the neoplastic disorders, clinical experience suggests that breast and cervical cancers are increasingly important causes of morbidity and mortality. While the screening and diagnosis of cervical cancer will continue to represent a major technological challenge for Sub-Saharan countries in general, opportunities for early screening for breast cancer do exist, but their potential is far from being realized. Leukemias and lymphomas and cancers of the skin and bladder may also represent important causes of female mortality and morbidity in the region.

• Gender-related environmental or occupational exposures—for example, cooking fires in enclosed spaces—may place Sub-Saharan African women at particular risk for COPD.

TABLE 7-7 Ages of Occurrence of Noncommunicable Diseases and their Sequelae in Sub-Saharan African Females

In Utero	Infancy Early Childhood (birth through age 4)	Childhood (ages 5–14)	Adolescence (ages 15–19)	Adulthood (ages 20–44)	Postmenopause (age 45+)
			Hypertension	Hypertension	Hypertension
			Rheumatic heart disease	Rheumatic heart disease	Rheumatic heart disease
			Cardiomyopathies associated with pregnancy	Cardiomyopathies associated with pregnancy	
			Gestational diabetes mellitus	Gestational diabetes mellitus	
				Breast cancer	Breast cancer
				Cancer of the cervix	Cancer of the cervix
		Leukemias and lymphomas	Leukemias and lymphomas	Leukemias and lymphomas	Leukemias and lymphomas
				Skin cancer	Skin cancer
				Bladder cancer	Bladder cancer
					Chronic obstructive pulmonary diseases

RESEARCH NEEDS

• There is an urgent need to create or support existing units concerned with data collection, evaluation, and surveillance of the major chronic disorders in Sub-Saharan Africa. Gender disaggregation in the collection and analysis of such data will be required in order to discover and understand specific issues related to women's health. The chronic disorders that should be surveyed include, in particular, rheumatic heart disease; hypertension and stroke; cardiomyopathies; coronary artery disease; leukemias and lymphomas and cancers of the cervix, breast, uterus, ovary, skin, and bladder and choriocarcinoma; diabetes mellitus; and COPD. In collecting and interpreting these data, special attention must be given to reporting bias and other issues related to access of care.

• Because strokes may be an increasingly important cause of morbidity and mortality in Sub-Saharan African women, future controlled studies should be conducted to determine to what extent factors such as obesity, smoking, alcohol use, and age contribute to stroke-related morbidity and mortality in women. The results of such studies could have useful implications for treatment and, especially, prevention.

• Comparative surveys to determine the distribution of, and trends in, major risk factors for the other chronic diseases described in this chapter are also needed. These surveys should build on the methods and data of current comparative studies in other regions of the world such as the MONICA study, which provides for efficient assessment of disease severity across different countries and identification of putative risk factors. Special attention should be paid to the strengths and limitations of past longitudinal studies of specific populations in the region—for example, the six African studies described in Feachem and Jamison (1991; pp. 245–247). (For additional description of these studies, see the Appendix to this volume). Specific risk factors that should be assessed in these comparative studies include hypertension, serum cholesterol and lipid fractions, obesity, and nutritional status. Better knowledge of the prevalence of these risk factors—and identification of other risk factors for chronic diseases in women—are crucial to prevention and control, as well as to long-term health care planning, given the elevated costs for managing most chronic diseases that are the norm in much of the Western world.

• Because of evidence of growing rates of cigarette smoking in Sub-Saharan females and the role of smoking as a risk factor for multiple chronic diseases, research in this area is urgent and essential. There are currently no reliable studies surveying the prevalence of, and trends in, smoking in Sub-Saharan females. Experience in Cameroon suggests that a significant number of girls already have established smoking habits at age 12. Special attention should be directed to identification of risk factors for smoking initiation in adolescent females and to the development of intervention programs appropriate to the target audience.

• The higher prevalence and mortality rates for rheumatic heart disease in Sub-Saharan African females observed in hospital case series is striking and needs to be confirmed. The presence of a history of rheumatic fever, generally considered a prelude to the subsequent development of RHD, in less than 50 percent of those cases requires investigation.

• Women of African descent with coronary artery disease have been shown in some studies to have a poorer prognosis than males. The reasons for this gender disparity and their implications for Sub-Saharan African women need to be clarified.

• Skin cancer has been reported to be the fourth leading cause of cancer in some groups of women of the region. The relation of daily agricultural and other female household duties to risk of chronic tropical ulcers and associated malignant skin-based lesions needs to be investigated. The suggestion of a greater frequency of skin and other systemic disorders related to use of skin-lightening creams and ointments containing steroids and other toxic chemicals requires evaluation.

• The higher rates of glucose intolerance in Sub-Saharan women compared with men that has been observed in a few studies should be confirmed, particularly given the relation of diabetes to complications during pregnancy and childbirth.

• Attention should be given to identification of environmental and occupational risk factors for cancers and COPD that are particular to the domestic and work environments of Sub-Saharan African females.

REFERENCES

Akintewe, T. A., and A. Adetuyibi. 1986. Obesity and hypertension in diabetic Nigerians. Trop. Geogr. Med. 38:146–149.

Alade, I., and J. N. Ezeokeke 1990. Combattre l'obesité par l'education (lettre). Forum Mond. Santé 11:466–467.

Bam, W. J., and P. M. Yako. 1984. Correlation between hypertension and cerebrovascular accidents in black patients. S. Afr. Med. J. 65:638–641.

Barnicot, N. A., F. J. Bennett, J. C. Woodburn, T. R. E. Pilkington, and A. Antonis. 1972. Blood pressure and serum cholesterol in the Hadza of Tanzania. Hum. Biol. 44:87.

Barnum, H., and E. R. Greenberg. 1993. Cancers. In Disease Control Priorities in Developing Countries, D. T. Jamison, W. H. Mosley, A. R. Measham, and J. L. Bobadilla, eds. New York: Oxford University Press for the World Bank.

Bassett, M. T., L. M. Levy, C. Chetsanga, and E. Chokunonga. 1992. Zimbabwe National Cancer Registry: Summary data 1986–1989. Centr. Afr. J. Med. 38:91–94.

Bensadoun, G., L. Ravinet, F. Luccioni, and E. D. Bertrand. 1984. Intérêt du bilan lipidique dans l'évaluation du risque coronarien de la population générale ivoirienne; étude effectuée sur 1368 personnes. Cardiol. Trop. 10:117–124.

Bertrand, E. D. 1991. Maladies cardiovasculaires en Afrique noire. Cardiol. Trop. 17 (Special 1):81–82.

Bertrand, E. D., A. Ekra, M. Odi Assamoi, G. Clerc, M. Hanna, D. Levy, J. Renambot, A. Adoh, and M. Ravinet. 1985. L'insuffisance myocardique latente du post-partum normal. Cardiol. Trop. 11:57–67.

Bertrand, E. D., A. O. Coulibaly, and R. Ticolat. 1991. Annual incidence of the main nosological groups of cardiovascular diseases among African in-patients at the Abidjan Institute of Cardiology. Cardiol. Trop. 17:151–155.

Bonham, G. S., and D. B. Brock. 1985. The relationship of diabetes with race, sex, and obesity. Am. J. Clin. Nutr. 41:776–783.

Bonita, R. 1992. Epidemiology of stroke. Lancet 339:342–347.

Bumgarner, J. R., and F. E. Speizer. 1993. Chronic obstructive pulmonary disease. In Disease Control Priorities in Developing Countries, D. T. Jamison, W. H. Mosley, A. R. Measham, and J. L. Bobadilla, eds. New York: Oxford University Press for the World Bank.

Chen, B. H., C. J. Hong, M. R. Pandey, and K. R. Smith. 1990. Indoor air pollution in developing countries. Wld. Hlth. Stat. 43:127–137.

Clifford, P. 1972. Carcinogen in the nose and throat: nasopharyngeal carcinoma in Kenya. Proc. R. Soc. Med. 65:682–686.

Cole, T. O. 1980. Pattern of rheumatic heart disease in Nigerians. Trop. Cardiol. 6:69–76.

Commission on Health Research for Development. 1990. Health Research: Essential Link to Equity in Development. New York: Oxford University Press.

DHHS (U.S. Department of Health and Human Services). 1986. Blood Pressure Levels in Persons 18–74 Years of Age in 1976–80, and Trends in Blood Pressure from 1960 to 1980 in the United States. Data from the National Health Survey, Ser. 11, No. 234. DHHS Publ. No. (PHS) 86–1684. Hyattsville, Md.: National Center for Health Statistics, Public Health Service, U.S. Department of Health and Human Services.

Dodu, S. R. A. 1988. Emergence of cardiovascular disease in developing countries. Cardiol. 75:56–64.

Doll, R., and R. Peto. 1981. The Causes of Cancer. Oxford, U.K.: Oxford University Press.

Dooley, S. L., B. E. Metzger, N. Cho, and K. Liu. 1991. The influence of demographic and phenotypic heterogeneity on the prevalence of gestational diabetes mellitus. Intl. J. Gynecol. Obstet. 35:13–18.

Dulay, L. 1990. Maternal mortality associated with hypertensive disorders of pregnancy in Africa, Asia, Latin America and the Caribbean. Br. J. Obstet. Gynaecol. 99:547–553.

Dyer, A. R., P. Elliott, M. Shipley, R. Stamler, and J. Stamler. 1994. Body mass index and associations of sodium and potassium with blood pressure in INTERSALT. Hypertension 23:729–736.

Ekra, A., and E. Bertrand. 1992. Les cardiomyopathies rhumatismales en Afrique. Forum Mond. Santé 13:360–362.

Elegboleye, O. O., and D. Femi-Perse. 1976. Incidence and variables contributing to the onset of cigarette smoking among secondary school children and medical students in Lagos, Nigeria. Br. J. Prev. Soc. Med. 30:66–70.

Elo, I. T., and S. H. Preston. 1992. Effects of early life on adult mortality: A review. Pop. Index 58:186–212.

Feachem, R. G. A., and D. T. Jamison, eds. 1991. Disease and Mortality in Sub-Saharan Africa. New York: Oxford University Press for the World Bank.

Feachem, R. G. A., T. Kjellstrom, C. J. L. Murray, M. Over, and M. A. Phillips, eds. 1992. The Health of Adults in the Developing World. New York: Oxford University Press.

Feldmeier. H., and I. Kranz. 1992. A synoptic inventory of needs for research on women and tropical parasitic diseases with an application for schistosomiasis. In Women and Tropical Disease, P. Wijeyaratne, E. M. Rathgeber, and E. St. Onge, eds. IDRC Manuscript Report MR314e. Ottawa: International Development Research Centre.

Ghali, J. K. 1991. Should cardiovascular diseases be a health priority for developing countries? A brief overview of mortality data. Ethnic. Dis. 1:295–299.

Gillum, R. F., and C. T. Grant. 1982. Coronary heart disease in Black populations, II: Risk factors. Mosby Yearb. 104:852–864.

Gwet-Bell, E. 1990. Troubles du cycle liés a l'utilisations intensives et prolongées des dermocorticoides. 2ème Conference Medicale Nationale, No. 46, 19 au 22 Mars 1990. Palais des Congrès de Yaounde.

Howe, G. R., T. Hirohata, T. G. Hilsop, et al. 1990. Dietary factors and the risk of breast cancer: Combined analysis of 12 case-control studies. J. Natl. Cancer Inst. 82:561–569.

Hutt, M. S. R. 1991. Cancer and cardiovascular diseases. In Disease and Mortality in Sub-Saharan Africa, R. G. Feachem and D. T. Jamison, eds. New York: Oxford University Press for the World Bank.

INCLEN Multicenter Collaborative Group. 1992. Risk factors for cardiovascular in the developing world: A multicenter collaborative study in the international clinical epidemiology network. J. Clin. Epidemiol. 45:841–847.

Irey, N. S., H. A. McAllister, and J. M. Henry. 1978. Oral contraceptives and stroke in young women: a clinicopathologic correlation. Neurology 28:1216–1219.

Johnson, T. O. 1970. Prevalence of overweight and obesity among adult subjects of an urban African population sample. Br. J. Prev. Soc. Med. 24:105–109.

Joint National Committee on Detection, Evaluation, and Treatment of High Blood Pressure, 1984. 1986. Non-pharmacological approaches to the control of high blood pressure: Final report of the Subcommittee on Non-pharmacological Therapy. Hypertension 8:444–467.

King, H., and M. Rewers. 1991. Diabetes in adults is now a Third World problem. Bull. WHO 69:643–648.

Koroltchouk, V. 1990. The control of breast cancer: A World Health Organization perspective. Cancer 65:2803–2810.

Kumanyika, S., and L. L. Adams-Campbell. 1991. Methodological issues in studies of obesity, psychosocial factors, and hypertension. In Cardiovascular Disease in Blacks, E. Saunders, ed. Philadelphia: F.A. Davis.

Lancet. Editorial. 1979. Cardiovascular risks and oral contraceptives. Lancet 1:1063

Liao, Y., R. S. Cooper, J. K. Ghali, and A. Szocka. 1992. Survival rates with coronary artery disease for black women compared with black men. J. Am. Med. Soc. 268:1867–1871.

Longstreth, W. T., L. M. Nelson, T. D. Koepsel, and G. van Belle. 1992. Cigarette smoking, alcohol use, and subarachnoid hemorrhage. Stroke 23:1242–1249.

Lubin, F., Y. Wax, and B. Modan. 1986. Role of fat, animal protein and dietary fiber in breast cancer etiology. A case-control study. J. Natl. Cancer Inst. 77:605–612.

Malik, S. K., D. Behera, and S. K. Jindal. 1983. Reverse smoking and chronic obstructive lung disease. Brit. J. Dis. Chest 77:199–201.

Mant, D., L. Villaed-Mackintosh, M. P. Vessey, and D. Yeates. 1987. Myocardial infarction and angina pectoris in young women. J. Epidemiol. Commun. Hlth. 41:215–219.

Manton, K. G. 1988. The global impact of noncommunicable diseases: estimates and projections. World Hlth. Q. 41:255–266.

Mbakop, A., J. L. Oyono Essame, Ngbangako C., and A. Abondo. 1992. Epidémiologic actuelle des cancers au Cameroun (Afrique Centrale). Bull. Cancer 79:1101–1104.

M'Buyamba-Kabangu, J. R., R. Fagard, J. Sraessen, P. Lijnen, and A. Amery. 1987. Correlates of blood pressure in rural and urban Zaire. J. Hyperten. 5:371–375.

Merz, R., A. Said, S. Bergstrom, A. Bugalho, and M. Samucidine. 1992. Pregnancy-associated hypertension in Maputo. A study on maternal characteristics and perinatal outcome in 1,275 consecutive cases. Intl. J. Gynecol. Obstet. 39:11–15.

Miller, A. B. 1992. Le rôle du dépistage dans la lutte contre le cancer du sein. Forum Mond. Santé 13:303–312.

Mishell, D. R. 1989. Contraception. N. Engl. J. Med. 320:777–787.

Mmiro, F. A. 1987. Gynaecology and oncology in Africa. J. Obst. Gyn. E. Centr. Afr. 6:66–68.

NRC (National Research Council). 1989. Diet and Health: Implications for Reducing Chronic Disease Risk. Washington, D.C.: National Academy Press.

Ngongang, J., and V. P. K. Titanji. 1985. The concentration of apolipoproteins and lipoprotein cholesterol in sera of normal and hypertensive African subjects from Yaounde, Cameroon. E. Afr. Med. J. 62:446–451.

Ngongang, J., A. Raisonnier, and W. J. Muna. 1988. Obésité et metabolisme lipidique chez la femme camerounaise vivant en zone urbaine. Cardiol. Trop. 14:173.

Njitoyap, E., C. Ndam, H. Kamga Gonsu, P. F. Tchokoteu, F. J. Gonsu, O. Njoya, T. A. Guemne, and W. Muna. 1991. Etude de l'obésité au Cameroun: Aspects épidemiologiques et cliniques chez 120 patients. Med. Nutr. 27:71–75.

Omigbodun, A. O., and T. I. Akanmu. 1991. Clinico-pathologic correlates of disease stage in Nigerian cervical cancer patients. J. Obstet. Gynecol. E. Centr. Afr. 9:79–81.

Parkin, D. M., E. Laara, and C. S. Muir. 1988. Estimates of the worldwide frequency of sixteen major cancers in 1980. Intl. J. Cancer 41:184–197.

Peters, J. M., and B. G. Ferris. 1967. Smoking and morbidity in a college-age group. Am. Rev. Resp. Dis. 95:783–789.

Philips, S. J., and J. P. Whisnant. 1992. Hypertension and the brain. Arch. Intern. Med. 152:938–945.

Raisonnier, A., G. P. Tagny, T. Kamso-Tchakounte, H. Sile, and W. Muna. 1988. Apolipoprotein composition of low-density lipoprotein and high-density lipoprotein in Cameroonians: a very low artherogenic risk. Ann. Univ. Sc. Sante. 5:755–763.

Report from Ghana. 1984. In smoking and health issues in selected English-speaking African countries. Report of a HQ/AFRO Regional Seminar on Smoking and Health, Lusaka, 26–28 June.

Saha, N. C., and S. K. Jain. 1970. Chronic obstructive lung disease in Delhi: a comparative study. Indian J. Chest Dis. 12:40–51.

Sankale, M., and P. Koate. 1970. Cardiopathies rheumatismales chez le noir Africain, à propos de 386 cas hospitaliers observés à Dakar. Med. Afr. Noire 17:885–896.

Schoon, M. G., W. J. Van der Walt, J. Fourie, and H. Kruger. 1990. Blood pressure profiles and perinatal outcome in pregnant black women in Pelonomi Hospital, Bloemfontein, South Africa. Intl. J. Gynecol. Obstet. 33:111–114.

Seedat, Y. K., and M. A. Seedat. 1982. An inter-racial study of the prevalence of hypertension in an urban South African population. Trans. R. Soc. Trop. Med. Hyg. 76:62–71.

Serme, D. 1992. Etude Epidemiologique, clinique et évolutive de valvulopathies rhumatismales observées à Ouagadougou. Cardiol. Trop. 18:93–99.

Shaper, A. G. 1974. Coronary heart disease. In Cardiovascular Disease in the Tropics, A. G. Shaper, M. S. R. Hutt, and G. Fejfar, eds. London: British Medical Association.

Shaper, A. G., D. H. Wright, and J. Kyobe. 1969. Blood pressure and body build in three nomadic tribes of Northern Kenya. E. Afr. Med. J. 46:273.

Sims, E. A. H., and P. Berchtold. 1982. Obesity and hypertension: Mechanisms and implications for management. J. Am. Med. Soc. 247:49–52.

Sloan, C. 1960. Weight, height and skinfold thickness of Zulu adults in Durban. S. Afr. Med. J. 34:505–509.

Smith, K. R., A. L. Aggarwal, and R. M. Dave. 1983. Air pollution and rural biomass fuels in developing countries: a pilot village study in India and implications for research and policy. Atmos. Environ. 17:2343–2362.

Sobo, A. O. 1982. Cancer in Liberia: A review of cases registered from the Liberia Cancer Registry 1973–1977. Cancer 49:1945–1951.

Soubeyrand, J., B. Y. Attia, J. M. Condat, J. P. Leleu, E. Niamkey, D. Diallo, and B. Y. Beda. 1984. Realité et originalité de la pathologie colique en Côte d'Ivoire. Med. Afr. Noire 31:437–449.

Stadel, B. V. 1981. Oral contraceptives and cardiovascular disease. N. Engl. J. Med. 305:612–618; 672–677.

Stamler, J., D. M. Berkson, A. Dyer, M. H. Lepper, H. A. Lindberg, O. Paul, H. McKean, P. Rhomberg, J. A. Schoenberger, R. B. Shekelle, and R. Stamler. 1975. Relationship of multiple variables to blood pressure—findings from four Chicago epidemiologic studies. Pp. 307–356 in Epidemiology and Control of Blood Pressure, O. Paul, ed. New York: Stratton Intercontinental Medical.

Stamler, J., G. Rose, P. Elliott, A. Dyer, M. Marmot, H. Kesteloot, and R. Stamler. 1991. Findings of the International Cooperative INTERSALT Study. Hypertension 17:I9–I15.

Stanley, K., J. Stjernsward, and V. Koroltchouk. 1987. Women and cancer. Wld. Hlth. Stat. Q. 40:267–278.

Talabi, A. I., F. E. Gaba, and B. O. George. 1985. Puerperal cardiomyopathy in Lagos. Cardiol. Trop. 11:73–79.

Taylor, A. E., D. C. Johnson, and H. Kazemi. 1992. Environmental tobacco smoke and cardiovascular disease. A position paper from the Council on Cardiopulmonary and Critical Care. American Heart Association. Circulation 86:699–702.

Thorgood, M., S. A. Adam, and J. Nlann. 1981. Fatal subarachnoid haemorrhage in young women: role of oral contraceptives. Brit. Med. J. 283:762.

Ticolat, P., E. Bertrand, P. Barabe, et al. 1991. Epidemiological findings concerning coronary disease in black Africans (103 cases). Results of a multicentric study "CORONAFRIC." Cardiol. Trop. 17:7–20.

Tofler, G. H., P. H. Stone, J. E. Muller, S. N. Willich, V. G. Davis, K. W. Poole, H. W. Strauss, and J. T. Vessey. 1987. Oral contraceptive and cardiovascular disease. Brit. Med. J. 284:615–616.

Tuyns, A. J., and P. Ravisse. 1970. Cancer in Brazzaville, the Congo. J. Natl. Cancer Inst. 44:1121–1127.

Willerson, A. S. Jaffe, T. Robertson, E. Passamani, E. Braunwald, and the MILIS Study Group. 1987. Effects of gender and race on prognosis after myocardial infarction: adverse prognosis for women, particularly black women. J. Am. Coll. Cardiol. 9:473–482.

World Bank. 1993. World Development Report, 1993: Investing in Health. New York: Oxford University Press.

WHO (World Health Organization). 1978. Arterial Hypertension. Report of a WHO Expert Committee. Technical Report Series 628. Geneva.

WHO (World Health Organization). 1984. The Cardiomyopathies. Geneva.

WHO (World Health Organization). 1988. Rheumatic Fever and Rheumatic Heart Disease. Technical Report Series 764. Geneva.

WHO (World Health Organization). 1990. Diet, nutrition, and the prevention of chronic diseases. WHO Technical Report Series No. 797. Geneva.

WHO (World Health Organization). 1992. Les Femmes et le Tabac. Geneva.

Wynder, E. L., and G. B. Gori. 1977. Contribution of the environment to cancer incidence: an epidemiologic exercise. J. Natl. Cancer Inst. 58:825–832.

8

Injury

Data on injuries in the Sub-Saharan region are limited for both females and males. There are few injury prevention programs operating within any African ministry of health and, with the exception of a handful of researchers in Nigeria and in the Republic of South Africa, there are few professionals conducting research or descriptive studies on injury in the region. Nevertheless, based on the experiences of other developing areas—the Middle East, Southeast Asia, and the Indian subcontinent—injuries are becoming an increasing public health problem that affects development, decreases the quality of life, and increases the costs of health care. There is no reason to believe that Sub-Saharan Africa is exempt in this regard.

In this chapter an attempt is made to synthesize data from other developing regions and to extrapolate these findings to the Sub-Saharan region, a task complicated by the lack of substantial evidence on injury disaggregated by gender. The study of injury viewed through the prism of female health thus presents a challenging task of inference from what is known about social, economic, political, labor, and gender relations in Sub-Saharan Africa and the health hazards typical of this region. What the data presented in this chapter suggest, and Table 8-1 demonstrates, however, is that there are three categories of injury that disproportionately affect females in the region: household burns, domestic abuse, and rape and sexual assault. The evidence for each is reviewed. While other intentional and unintentional injuries—including violence, motor vehicle and other road traffic accidents, and falls—appear to affect Sub-Saharan African males more commonly than they do women, it is expected that rates between males and females will equalize over time for reasons described later in this chapter. Thus, the evidence for these other kinds of injury is described as well.

The approach adopted here first attempts to provide a rationale for recognizing the significance of injury as a general public health problem. The chapter then briefly reviews what is known about injury patterns in the developing world. The life span perspective is employed, where possible, in the systematic evaluation of adverse health outcomes of injury across the female life span. Finally, public health research implications are drawn from a consideration of the information presented. It must be noted at the outset that substantial cross-national differences probably exist for most of what is covered in this chapter. The approach adopted will attempt to be as inclusive of such differences as possible in the hope that it will facilitate application of the variants discovered to future study of individual countries, or subpopulations within them.

TABLE 8-1   Injuries in Sub-Saharan Africa: Gender-Related Burden

Problem	Exclusive to Females	Greater for Females than for Males	Burden for Females and Males Comparable, but of Particular Significance for Females
Domestic abuse		X	
Household burns		X	
Rape and sexual assault		X	

NOTE: Significance is defined here as having an impact on health that, for any reason—biological, reproductive, sociocultural, or economic—is different in its implications for females than for males.

DEFINITIONS

An injury is physical damage to the body resulting from acute exposure to thermal, mechanical, electrical, or chemical energy or from the absence of such essentials as heat or oxygen. Often the term "injury" is used interchangeably with "trauma." Injuries are grouped into three major categories, based on their intent or the context in which they occur. Although the "intent" of an injury is not always clear, classification by intent allows the identification of possible risk factors and the development of prevention strategies. Unintentional injuries are those caused by motor vehicles and other forms of transportation, drowning, poisoning, burns, or falls. Unintentional injuries are sometimes referred to as "accidents." Intentional injuries (also called "violent injuries") are homicides, suicides, interpersonal assaults, and intergroup violence resulting from war, torture, or genocide. Certain intentional injuries, such as rape, battering, sexual abuse, and domestic violence, affect females almost exclusively. Occupational injuries are the unintentional and intentional injuries that occur at work or traveling to and from a work setting. They do not include injuries that occur in nonwage employment such as homemaking.

INJURIES WORLDWIDE

Injuries as a Public Health Issue

Injuries traditionally have been considered by many health professionals and policymakers as "accidents," uncontrollable events outside the domain of sound public health practice. This belief has been changing, and significant progress is being made in both policy and prevention strategies. For instance, during the past decade, reductions in motor vehicle fatality rates, decreases in unintentional poisonings, and lowering rates of home fire fatalities have been realized in countries with injury prevention programs. In some countries the term "accident" is no longer used to describe an injury-producing event because of its connotation as something uncontrollable or random. "Injury prevention and control" is the term now used to describe the health-directed, scientific approach to reducing the impact of injury—intentional, unintentional, or occupational—on a society.

There are a number of reasons why injury programs should be rapidly established in all countries. First, *injuries have significant impact on morbidity and mortality.* In developed countries, they account for more deaths in persons between the ages 1 and 44 than all infectious diseases combined. They also result in more premature death as measured in years of productive life lost (YPLL) than all other health conditions combined. With the decreasing rates of childhood mortality and increased longevity observed in much of the Sub-Saharan region (see the Appendix), there is reason to expect that injuries will become an ever greater contributor to morbidity and mortality in the region. The second reason to establish injury prevention programs is that *injuries impact significantly on health care and societal costs.* In the United States, injuries imposed a $180 billion burden on the economy in 1988 (Rice et al., 1989). The final reason for establishing injury prevention and control programs is that *injuries are preventable*. Although more research into risk factors and prevention and control strategies for injuries is needed, we have available today many strategies to prevent injuries (NRC, 1985).

INJURIES IN THE DEVELOPING WORLD

Trends in the epidemiology of injury in developing countries raise some troubling questions about the relationship between development and injury (Stansfield et al., 1993) and compel scrutiny.

Epidemiologic Transition

An epidemiologic transition occurs as countries move from a disease pattern dominated by infectious diseases to one characterized by noncommunicable diseases such as heart disease, cancer, and injury (Omram, 1971). Epidemiologic transition from infectious to noncommunicable diseases increases the *relative* importance of injuries compared with infectious disease. For instance, in Mexico the proportion of deaths from infectious diseases decreased from 43 percent to 17 percent during the 25-year period from 1955 to 1980. During this same time, the proportion of deaths resulting from unintentional injury increased from 4 percent to 11 percent. In Nigeria, the proportion of deaths from traffic accidents compared with the number of deaths from 16 common infectious diseases increased from 38.9 percent to 60.2 percent in 10 years (Asogawa, 1978).

In addition to a shift in the *relative* importance of injuries, demographic changes, technological changes, and social changes affect the epidemiology of injuries and influence the *absolute* importance of injury as an epidemiologic category. Changing demographics, produced by improved child survival, elevate the proportion of older persons in a population, so that injuries such as occupational injuries and falls may become more important. Countries such as Thailand, Egypt, and Indonesia are experiencing increased numbers of deaths because of occupational injuries, especially those related to manufacturing. Technological changes, such as greater use of the automobile, local manufacturing, and rural electrification can also produce increases in the absolute numbers and rate of injuries. In Nigeria the number of road traffic fatalities more than doubled in seven years, and the rate of motor vehicle fatalities per 10,000 motor vehicles increased 127 percent in only 10 years (Asogawa, 1978). Similar increases have been seen in other developing countries and are obviously related to the rapid introduction of motor vehicles (see Figure 8-1).

Finally, economic and social changes in Sub-Saharan Africa leading to greater urbanization, new family roles, and more alcohol use are likely to expand the absolute numbers of injuries simply by increasing the number of risk factors for injury. In Egypt, for example, the number of suicides among young women living in urban areas is said to be growing because of the conflicting pressures of traditional forced marriages and new kinds of socialization outside of the family (Megid, 1992).

INJURY PATTERNS IN DEVELOPING COUNTRIES

A few broad statements can be made about injuries in developing countries. First, in countries where national data are available, mortality rates for unintentional and intentional injuries, although they vary considerably among countries, are similar to those observed in developed countries (Smith and Barss, 1991). Injury deaths are usually among the top five causes of death among all age groups; when compared with other causes of death, injuries represent from 3 to 11 percent of all causes (WHO, various years). In Egypt, injuries were the fifth leading cause of death in 1987, accounting for 4.1 percent of all deaths. In Shanghai County, China, injuries are the leading cause of death for people between the ages of 1 and 44 (Gu and Chen, 1982). In most countries of the Americas, unintentional injuries, including motor vehicle injuries, are the leading cause of YPLL. Fatality rates for unintentional injuries vary considerably among countries and age groups. In the United States, peak injury rates are seen in young adult males, largely as a result of motor vehicle crashes; in developing countries, this peak is not always seen because of the relative unavailability of motor vehicles in younger age groups. Table 8-2 shows the rates of unintentional injuries, excluding motor vehicle injuries, per 100,000 population in selected countries for which WHO data were available. These rates show mounting rates of injury deaths in older age groups, with

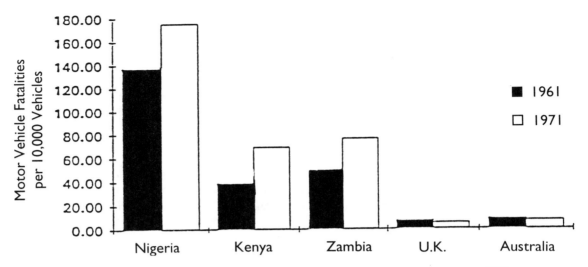

FIGURE 8-1   Motor vehicle fatalities per 10,000 vehicles: 1961 and 1971. SOURCE: Asogawa, 1978.

rates generally lower in the group aged 5–14. Rates in older age groups tend to increase for both males and females in all countries. Across all age groups, males generally have higher rates of unintentional injuries than females.

National data or systematic reports on *intentional* injuries are available for no African nation. Based on limited data from Latin American countries and anecdotal reports in Egypt, Nigeria, Zimbabwe, and Zambia, rates for homicides and suicides are probably at least as high as those in the United States, and these injuries occur primarily in young adults, ages 15–24 (PAHO, 1990). Rates of intentional injuries vary among racial groups. In a study of mortality among South African adolescents during a two-year period, assault was found to be the most common cause of death in blacks and coloreds; road traffic deaths were most common for whites (Fisher et al., 1992). In two reports describing a series of injuries treated at a Nigerian hospital, intentional injuries caused by stab or gunshot wounds comprised from 18 to 29 percent of injuries seen in each series (Roux and Fisher, 1992; Udoeyop and Iwatt, 1991). Intergroup violence in Africa is also a significant cause of injury mortality and morbidity. An estimated one million persons died in Uganda during the last two decades, and recent figures from Rwanda indicate that between 200,000 and 500,000 people died in ethnic violence between April and July 1994. In times of war, civilians seem to be most at risk of being killed or injured. In one case series in South Africa, shotgun pellets used by police during civil disturbances accounted for 5 percent of chest injuries seen in 128 children during a five-and-a-half-year period (Roux and Fisher, 1992). Between 80 and 90 percent of all war-related fatalities are among civilians (Werner, 1989). War also directly affects health status by diverting funds needed for health to defense (Ogba, 1989).

Injuries significantly affect morbidity and are a leading reason for hospital admission and clinic visit. Outpatient clinic data, although not population-based, strikingly demonstrate the impact of injuries for a country's health care system. In Zimbabwe, injuries were the among the top four reasons for outpatient clinic visits among individuals over the age of 5 years during 1987–1989, and they accounted for over 7.1 percent of all visits in this age group. For children under 5, injuries were at least the seventh leading cause for outpatient visits during this same period (Zimbabwe Ministry of Health, 1989). In one rural health unit in Egypt, injuries constituted 23.1 percent of all patient visits. Wounds, falls, and burns were the primary causes for those visits; males accounted for slightly more visits than females; and intentional injury accounted for 6 percent of the total of all injury visits (Mostafa, 1993).

TABLE 8-2 Unintentional Injury Deaths per 100,000, by Age Group and Year*a*

		<1	1–4	5–14	15–24	25–34	35–44	45–54	55–64	65–74	75+	All Ages
Egypt	Males	15	25	11	19	19	13	16	17	24	36	17
1979	Females	11	20	11	27	19	14	12	16	20	37	17
Mauritius	Males	42	13	10	20	42	37	61	65	75	170	32
1986	Females	57	16	5	24	24	22	16	13	58	66	20
Thailand	Males	9	22	14	36	39	38	46	38	40	59	30
1981	Females	11	16	10	10	9	10	14	11	13	27	11
Mexico	Males	48	30	24	92	120	127	135	145	180	348	80
1982	Females	39	21	10	15	16	18	22	31	53	212	20
Costa Rica	Males	22	20	9	28	27	39	48	52	80	274	30
1984	Females	8	10	3	5	7	6	2	5	22	276	9
Sweden	Males	4	5	3	6	13	23	28	37	44	169	28
1984	Females	7	2	1	1	3	3	5	9	20	157	19
United States	Males	20	17	9	22	26	24	27	32	47	145	28
1984	Females	17	11	3	4	5	5	8	11	21	100	13

*a*Excludes motor vehicle fatalities.

SOURCE: Smith and Barss, 1991.

Evidence in Females

Data collected throughout the developed and developing world would appear to indicate that injuries affect males more often than females. If this is the case, why devote space to injuries in a report that focuses on female health in Sub-Saharan Africa? There are several reasons. First, in working or living situations where risks and exposures are shared equally by both sexes, injury rates are similar. As Africa strives for equal treatment of females, it is possible that injury rates will also equalize. Second, although they presently occur at greater rates overall among males, injuries also befall females. Third, strategies to prevent injuries—the leading cause of premature loss of productive life for the young and for adults throughout the world—are similar, whether applied to females or males. Fourth, although injuries befall persons of all ages and of both genders, the young, the elderly, and the socially and economically disadvantaged are most affected as a group. Because women and their children are so often among the most economically and socially disadvantaged groups in any community, they may be at greatest risk of suffering the consequences of injuries. Last, certain injuries predominantly affect females. These injuries—rape and domestic violence—appear to be the direct result of the position of females in society and society's attitudes toward them. Although there are few descriptive studies of the effect of these injuries on females in Africa, media reports and experience in other developing countries indicate that rape and domestic violence occur at rates high enough to have a significant impact on morbidity and disability.

LIFE SPAN APPROACH

Injuries occur differentially throughout the female life span, primarily because of the changing exposure to the risk factors that cause injuries. Box 8-1 illustrates the most prevalent of the injuries seen during a female's life span. The section that follows reviews what is known about these injuries in Sub-Saharan African females.

Motor Vehicle Injuries

Although there are fewer automobiles and miles of roads in developing countries, motor vehicle fatalities are nonetheless the leading cause of injury deaths in most countries, even though motor vehicle fatality rates may vary greatly among countries, and within urban and rural areas in the same country. In Nigeria, Ethiopia, and Kenya,

---

Box 8-1
Prevalent Types of Injuries Throughout the Female Life Span

Prebirth/pregnancy	Selective abortion, battering during pregnancy, mass rape
Infancy	Female infanticide, falls, burns, drowning, poisoning
Adolescence	Child abuse, sexual abuse, rape, falls, burns, motor vehicle injuries (as pedestrian or occupant)
Adulthood	Rape, burns, homicide, suicide, battering, assault
Old age	Suicide, assault, falls, burns

---

for example, rates are higher than those in developed countries (Wintemute, 1985). Most reports of motor vehicle injuries in Africa, however, are only gross estimates, and even motor vehicle fatality reports are often based on unreliable data (Asogwa, 1992).

There is a consistent and direct relationship between socioeconomic development and motor vehicle mortality (Haight, 1980). The *absolute* number of fatalities mounts as the pace of socioeconomic development accelerates, probably as a result of the simultaneous impact of the increased number of motor vehicles and increased reliance on them. Lack of improved roads, driver inexperience, and the mix of road-users (four- and two-wheeled vehicles, nonmotorized transport, and pedestrians) further contribute to increases in the numbers of motor vehicle deaths. As the number of motor vehicles increases, the number of deaths per vehicle and the number of deaths per mile or kilometer—both rate measures—gradually decrease. This is most likely the result of improving road conditions and increasing driving experience in the cohort of motor vehicle operators and pedestrians, as well as a greater number of motor vehicles in the mix of road-users. Still, the number of deaths per 10,000 vehicles in Nigeria, Ethiopia, and Kenya exceeds that in the United States and the United Kingdom by at least 6 times (Jacobs and Sayer, 1983; Figure 8-2).

The profile of motor vehicle injuries in Sub-Saharan Africa differs from those in developed countries in the ways they involve various groups of road-users. There are very few reports that specifically document the road-user group of an injured person, but in a study from Ile-Ife, Nigeria, in 2,667 cases of road traffic accidents (RTA) described during a four-year period, pedestrian casualties accounted for the largest proportion of traffic injuries—28.3 percent (Udoeyop and Iwatt, 1991). In urban areas in the United States and the United Kingdom, that figure is 50 percent. A study in Delhi, India, reported a similar percentage of pedestrian casualties—33 percent of all road traffic fatalities—to that reported for Ile-Ife. In Delhi, only 3 percent of the fatalities were in cars or taxis; in the United States and United Kingdom, between 21 and 40 percent of the fatalities were among motorists. Over 20 percent of fatalities in Delhi were bicyclists, compared with less than 6 percent in the United States and the United Kingdom. Motorcycle fatalities in the developed countries range between 8 and 19 percent of total RTAs; in Delhi, 16 percent of these fatalities were motorcyclists—not so different. In Delhi, however, 11 percent of road crash fatalities were bus commuters, a figure almost negligible in the United Kingdom and United States. The authors concluded that because of the striking variations in the distribution of fatal injuries between road-users in India and those in developed countries, safety countermeasures in Delhi would have to be significantly different from those in more industrialized countries (Mohan and Bawa, 1985). This recommendation may be pertinent in the African context as well.

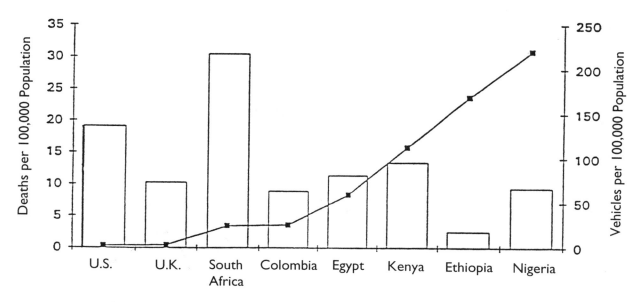

FIGURE 8-2 Motor vehicle fatalities per 100,000 population and per 10,000 vehicles. SOURCE: Trinca et al., 1988.

Implications for Females

In newly motorizing countries, some groups of road-users are at a higher risk than they would be in developed countries. If it is reasonable to extrapolate from the Delhi data, pedestrians and users of public transport are at particular risk. The extent to which females are pedestrians and use such transport in their daily lives will obviously influence their rates of transport injuries. In addition, there are anecdotal reports that morbidity and mortality among pedestrians may be underestimated in developing countries for several reasons. First, real economic and social class differences between a motor vehicle operator and an injured pedestrian may make the authorities reluctant to report a pedestrian injury unless it is severe, or the motorist is also injured. In addition, the involvement of insurance and other kinds of compensatory payment, as well as legal precedents, may discourage official reporting of the injury (Michael Linnan, USAID, personal communication, 1989). Future efforts to survey pedestrian fatalities among females in Sub-Saharan Africa should thus control for biases that could be expected to result in their underenumeration.

Other Unintentional Injuries: Burns, Drowning, Falls, and Unintentional Poisonings

Examination of outpatient or hospital admission records in any urban or rural health clinic reveals a wide range of injuries and a great variety of external causal events. During a three-month period in Alexandria, Egypt, among 10,000 patients seen in trauma units throughout the city, almost 27 percent of the patients were seen for the treatment of injuries that occurred during street fights; the number of male patients in this category was more than twice that of females. Falls comprised 26.6 percent of all recorded visits, and motor vehicle injuries accounted for 11.5 percent. Other frequently reported injuries resulted from fire and chemical burns and unintentional firearm injuries. For females, the principal causes for visits to trauma units were for treatment of injuries that occurred as a result of domestic violence (27.9 percent), falls (24 percent), and cuts (14 percent). All of these injuries occurred in the home (Graitcer et al., 1993).

In a retrospective cohort of 1,134 preschool children in Alexandria, Egypt, 378 children had 429 "significant" injuries during a one-year period. These injuries resulted in permanent disability in 3.7 percent of the children. The male to female ratio was 1.33:1. Most injuries occurred in the home (81 percent), and common causes of injuries were falls, burns, wounds, and poisoning. Children of illiterate mothers and those who lived in large families and in crowded conditions had a higher probability of being injured (Nosseir et al., 1990).

Burns

Because of their exposure to fires used for cooking and heating, females and their children are at greater risk of burns than males. In one series in Alexandria, Egypt, a greater number of females than males were burned, a difference particularly striking in the 16-to-20-year-old age group, which accounted for over 50 percent of all such injuries. Scald burns were more commonly seen in the younger age groups (Etiaba et al., 1984). Between 40 and 62 percent of all burns reported in three Nigerian studies occurred in children less than five years old and were caused either by flames from cooking or lighting or by scalds from oil or water used in cooking. During cooler weather, there was an increase in burns caused by fires, presumably used for heating (Onuba, 1988). Improper storage of kerosene and other flammables in the home was another risk factor associated with fire burns; over 95 percent of the burns in one series were the result of explosions from the use of contaminated kerosene in cookstoves (Datubo-Brown and Kejek, 1989; Grange et al., 1988; Mabogunje and Lawrie, 1988; Sowemimo, 1983). One Nigerian study describes a series of 11 deliberate burns in children and adults. Eight of these were intentional, inflicted during a robbery or a domestic dispute, and four were caused by what the author terms "ignorance": a common folk treatment for treating convulsions in children by holding their feet in a fire (Datubo-Brown, 1989). In rural Egypt, burns among females accounted for 9 percent of the deaths in the group aged 15 to 45, and they were the third leading cause of death after diseases of the circulatory system and complications of pregnancy and childbirth. Of these deaths, 63 percent were associated with burns received from using kerosene or gas cookstoves (Saleh et al., 1986). Ten percent of burn cases in Zaria, Nigeria, involved persons with epilepsy; since the prevalence of epilepsy in Nigeria is unknown, it is not possible to determine whether epileptics are overrepresented in this series.

Drowning

Drowning is often underreported as a cause of injury death. Fatal drownings are often underreported to health authorities, and nonfatal events are rarely reported because they may not require medical treatment. Based on a four-year retrospective study in Cape Town, South Africa, the highest rates of drowning were in white children and adult black males. The majority of the adult drownings were associated with elevated levels of alcohol in the blood. Drownings among black males occurred in an occupational setting, and the majority of drownings among white children were in swimming pools (Davis and Smith, 1985). Another study in South Africa of near-drowning in children found different figures: 46 percent of drownings were in swimming pools, 9 percent in the ocean, and 18 percent in household buckets filled with liquid, the last most prevalent in socially disadvantaged communities (Kibel et al., 1990).

Falls

While there is cause to suspect significant numbers of these events in Sub-Saharan Africa, regional data are virtually nonexistent. In the developed world, outpatient and emergency department case series indicate that falls are one of the leading reasons for visits of both adults and children, but few studies of this topic appear in the developing-world literature. For instance, no data are available that indicate whether falls might be more frequent in young children and in the elderly in developing countries, as they are in the developed world. Anecdotal reports indicate that falls occur both in domestic situations, such as climbing trees or repairing or building roofs, and in occupational settings, such as among climbers of coconut palms in Nigeria (Okonkwo, 1988). There is no quantification of these sorts of events in Sub-Saharan Africa. They are noted here because falls could be a significant cause of morbidity and mortality in the region, although it is not clear that there would be any gender differential in these rates.

Unintentional Poisonings

Similarly, except for reports describing catastrophic or mass poisonings from contaminated bread flour, agricultural pesticides, or adulterated food, there are no studies of unintentional poisoning in Sub-Saharan African populations. Nonetheless, based on the relatively unrestricted availability of a wide variety of insecticides, agricultural chemicals, and medicines in developing countries and the widespread distribution and use of these products, there are undoubtedly sizable numbers of unintentional poisonings, especially among children, their mothers, and agricultural workers, that merit systematic investigation.

VIOLENCE AGAINST FEMALES—A GROWING PUBLIC HEALTH PROBLEM

The intentional injuries of violence, which include homicide, suicide, assault, domestic violence ("battering"), rape, child abuse, and war, are ubiquitous. Violence, particularly violence against females, is universal and respects neither class nor culture (UN, 1991). Although actual levels of violent injuries vary greatly among countries, some developing countries are losing more years of potential life to intentional injuries than to infectious disease (Foege, 1991). Among females subjected to the pressures of economic hardship and racial or social inequities, the prevalence of interpersonal violence is even greater.

Violence against females has been recognized by the Pan American Health Organization (PAHO, 1993) as a health policy issue, but action programs have yet to be developed to address the phenomenon as a public health issue. Although violent injury resulting in death is universally condemned, nonfatal violence—especially when inflicted in a domestic living situation or by a husband or partner—is rarely recognized as either a legitimate health issue or, for that matter, a societal concern (Heise, 1993). Societies have developed mechanisms that legitimize and deny violence, leaving the victims stranded in violent relationships that they and their children cannot escape.

Accurate worldwide and country-specific estimates of the impact of violence on females are not available, largely because there is a social and cultural stigma attached to reporting such violence, especially when it takes place within the confines of a home and is inflicted by a husband or other partner. There is a growing body of well-documented studies and surveys that quantify violence against females (Heise, 1993). It is from this literature that we are able to extrapolate and generalize to different regions, cultures, and socioeconomic situations.

In general, suicide and homicide rates are greater for males than females. Rates of nonfatal intentional injuries, however, prove to be greater for females than for males when violent injuries caused by rape and battering are combined with the other violent injuries that are customarily reported to law enforcement authorities.

Along with gender, race is one risk factor closely associated with increased violence. Butchart and Brown (1991) interviewed nearly 1,600 victims of interpersonal violence seen in hospital emergency rooms in Johannesburg-Soweto. For these victims of nonfatal intentional injuries, the rates averaged 1,380/100,000 residents annually, but they varied greatly by race, ranging from 3,821/100,000 for coloreds, to 1,527 for blacks, 467 for whites, and 433 for Asians. In Cape Town, South Africa, white females were far more likely to die a suicidal, as opposed to homicidal, death. For blacks and coloreds, females were more likely to be victims of homicide than suicide (Lerer, 1992).

Fatal Violent Injuries in Females

Homicide

All available reports indicate that males are murdered at rates that are higher than those for females (Rosenberg and Mercy, 1991), but there are no published national data for African countries (WHO, various years). In like manner, the amount of deliberate murder of female children or discriminatory treatment of female children that results in death is unknown for the Sub-Saharan region. Nevertheless, extrapolating from UNICEF mortality data, the rates for girls under age 4 are higher than for boys in 43 of 45 developing countries for which data are available (UNICEF, 1986), which suggests discriminatory patterns in the treatment of female children for the developing world as a whole. Whether this pattern would hold in the Sub-Saharan countries is an open question. Evidence exists in police records that alcohol may play an important role in the precipitation of a homicidal attack because of the intoxicated behavior of victim and assailant (Muscat and Huncharek, 1991). Lerer (1992) noted that 44 percent of female homicide victims were heavily intoxicated at the time of death, but acute alcohol intoxication did not appear to play a major role in suicide in women in Cape Town.

Suicide

Suicide is the eighth leading cause of death in the United States. Yet even with the sophisticated U.S. health care and data collection systems, it is difficult to accurately determine the number of suicides and suicide attempts in that country. The number of suicides is presumed to be underestimated by 25–50 percent, and the number of suicide attempts that do not lead to death may be still more grossly underestimated. It would be surprising if the underestimation of suicide in the Sub-Saharan region were not at least as severe.

In a six-month prospective study of three main general hospitals in Ibadan, 39 cases of self-inflicted injury were reported out of a total of over 23,000 outpatient visits. Of these cases, more than three-quarters were under 30 years of age. The male-to-female ratio was 1.4:1, and more than half of the cases were students. Most suicide attempts were by ingestion of chemicals and psychotropic drugs (Odejide et al., 1986). In Gabon, males and females committed suicide in equal numbers, but three times as many females as males attempted, but did not complete, suicide. The most common method was ingestion of chemicals, mainly antimalarials (Mboussou and Milebou-Aubusson, 1989). In a review of suicide attempts in Benin City, Nigeria, the crude rate over a four-year period was calculated to be 7/100,000. Over 39 percent of those who made the attempt were between ages 15 and 19, and ingestion of drugs (68 percent) or chemicals (20 percent) were the most common methods. Major disposing factors were mental illness and conflicts with parents (Eferakeya, 1984). Unwanted pregnancy may be also a cause for suicide among unwed women in some Islamic countries (Heise, 1993).

Nonfatal Violent Injuries in Females

Although there is a clear link between domestic violence and subsequent homicide and suicide, injuries from rape and domestic violence are not usually fatal. They do, however, represent a significant cause of nonfatal injuries in females. One study of nonfatal trauma in Johannesburg showed that over 50 percent of injuries were a result of interpersonal violence—in the case of women, often at the hands of spouses and lovers (Butchart et al., 1991).

Domestic Abuse (Battering)

The most common form of violence against females is domestic abuse, also known as battering, or abuse by intimate male partners. A number of studies from both developed and developing countries indicate that between approximately one-quarter and one-half of *all* females report having been physically abused by a present or former partner. In a cluster sample survey in Kenya, 30 percent of all women reported that they were battered, and half of the males and females in this survey reported that their mothers were beaten (Raikes, 1990). In an islandwide national probability sample survey in Barbados, 30 percent of women reported being battered as adults (Handwerker, 1991), and in the United States, 28 percent of females surveyed in a statewide sample in Texas reported at least one episode of physical violence (Grant et al., 1989).

Domestic abuse and assault have entirely different epidemiologic characteristics. For instance, domestic abuse most frequently occurs among females and happens in the home. In a cohort study in South Africa, Butchart and Brown (1991) found that males were most often attacked in the street, females in their homes. The perpetrators are also different. In the same South African study, almost 38 percent of the females were attacked by spouses or lovers, while two-thirds of the males were attacked by strangers. In the case of assaults, causes seem to relate to economic conflicts, although the causes of assaults on females are less likely to be economic (Grant et al., 1989). In rural Ethiopia, about one-third of the cases concerned disputes over land, cattle, and the like; one-third were the result of interpersonal family conflicts; and one-third involved alcohol intoxication. The role of psychiatric disorders in these assaults was minimal (Jacobsson, 1985). One report from Nairobi indicated that 75 percent of the cases of fracture of the mandible were the result of interpersonal violence, only 13.8 percent were the result of motor vehicle crashes, and over eight times as many males as females were seen in the case series as a whole (Mwaniki and Guthar, 1990).

Rape and Sexual Assault

Well-designed studies in the United States, Canada, the United Kingdom, New Zealand, and the Republic of Korea indicate that approximately 7 to 18 percent of females have been raped (Heise, 1993). In addition to these formal studies, throughout history there have been reports by observers and victims indicating that females are particularly vulnerable to rape during times of war or civil insurrection. Recent news reports from Liberia, Uganda, Somalia, and Rwanda seem to confirm that this practice continues. Like homicide, rapes are often committed by a person known to the victim and, like other injuries, youth, lower socioeconomic status, and alcohol are all associated variables.

Implications of Intentional Injury Directed Specifically Toward Females

As we have seen throughout this chapter, most unintentional injuries, homicide, and suicide in Sub-Saharan Africa, as elsewhere in the world, occur more frequently among males than among females. There are several violent injuries that occur almost exclusively in females—domestic assault, rape, and sexual assault. This sort of gender-specific violence is ubiquitous and appears to produce a significant burden of female morbidity and mortality worldwide. That a multitude of cultural, social, and practical constraints have prevented accurate measurement of the actual impact of these injuries on females verges on tragedy. From popular media reports and position papers prepared by various human rights organizations, the concerned researcher and public health worker are left with the impression that while violence is the major injury problem among females, there are few scientific reports to form a basis for valid epidemiologic descriptions of causative risk factors or intervention strategies, not only in Sub-Saharan Africa, but in all regions of the world.

CONCLUSIONS

This chapter has attempted to outline the extent of the impact of injuries on the health and development of developing country populations, with particular emphasis on the effect of injuries on the health of Sub-Saharan females. Unfortunately, for a number of reasons ranging from a lack of data to public attitudes toward injuries, there are few reports to definitively document this impact. Available evidence suggests that injuries occur in developing countries in numbers and at rates comparable to those in the developed world. Of particular concern are the rising rate of injuries associated with motor vehicles and reports that homicide, suicide, and assaults are increasing, especially in African urban areas. These rising rates of injury have special implications for developing countries because they first affect the young and young adults, those who contribute economically to the growth and development of a country.

Table 8-3 indicates the ages at which certain injuries commonly occur in Sub-Saharan African females. What is apparent from the table and from the broader evidence presented in this chapter is that the distribution of injuries in females across their life span is similar to that seen in females in industrialized countries and elsewhere in the developing world. This is, in one sense, good news, because it suggests that injury prevention strategies developed elsewhere in the world may have applicability to the Sub-Saharan African region, and vice-versa.

Other conclusions can be summarized as follows:

TABLE 8-3 Ages of Occurrence of Injuries in Sub-Saharan African Females

In Utero	Infancy/ Early Childhood (birth through age 4)	Childhood (ages 5–14)	Adolescence (ages 15–19)	Adulthood (ages 20–44)	Postmenopause (age 45+)
	Falls	Falls	Falls	Falls	Falls
	Burns	Burns	Burns	Burns	
	Drownings				
	Unintentional poisonings				
		Sexual abuse			
		Rape	Rape		
			Motor vehicle deaths	Motor vehicle deaths	
				Suicide	Suicide (early adulthood)

• Reliable data regarding the target groups, risk factors, and causes of injuries in Sub-Saharan Africa are largely lacking.

• Social and cultural taboos prevent the collection of accurate data on violent injury.

• Evidence from other developing regions suggests that increasing industrialization and development can only drive up rates of injuries in the Sub-Saharan region.

• Little investment has been made in the prevention and control of injuries, primarily because there are data deficiencies, small numbers of trained personnel, and a dearth of policymakers willing to embrace the concept that injuries *are* preventable.

• Nonfatal intentional injuries such as domestic violence and rape are probably as large a public health problem for females in Sub-Saharan Africa as they are for females elsewhere in the world.

RESEARCH NEEDS

Improved Data Sources

• The impact of injuries on females, especially those living in developing countries, is underestimated because of the biases in the delivery of health care services and in society in general. Effective systems for the collection, analysis, and interpretation of data on injuries in Sub-Saharan females must be established. These systems should integrate data from sectors such as the police and health systems and should attempt to use population-based mortality and morbidity information to estimate the total impact of injuries in a community. These data should be disaggregated by gender and age.

• Although falls, burns, and household poisoning cause substantial numbers of injuries, especially in females, there has been little research exploring risk factors for these and other injuries. Instead, injury research has focused on occupational and transport injuries—injuries that primarily affect males. Studies should, therefore, be conducted to identify risk factors for domestic and other injuries in Sub-Saharan females, including burns, falls, nonfatal domestic injuries, intentional and unintentional poisonings, and suicides. A better understanding of risk factors associated with transport injury in females, especially for pedestrian and other nonmotorized road-users, is also needed.

• Violence—especially suicide and nonlethal violence—is underreported in females, and rape and domestic violence may be more severely underreported in certain Sub-Saharan populations because of social, cultural, and religious constraints. The extent to which intentional ("violent") injuries are reported as unintentional injuries—falls, burns, bruises, and poisonings—is unknown and should be determined. To achieve understanding of the causes, risk factors, and strategies required to prevent violence, there is a need for a collaborative approach among a variety of disciplines, including anthropology, law, criminal justice, sociology, psychiatry, rehabilitation, epidemiology, and public health.

• Research exploring the risk and etiologic factors in females should be multidisciplinary, involving in-depth examination of social, economic, and mental health determinants of violence.

Prevention Strategies

• Research on strategies that can prevent and control injuries of importance to females in Sub-Saharan Africa must be undertaken.

• Research to develop effective and appropriate interventions to prevent injury and to control the resulting disability should be undertaken. This research would include examination, based on epidemiologically based priorities, of specific interventions, systems of trauma care, and rehabilitation techniques.

• Research and interventions specifically directed toward the prevention and control of household injuries such as burns, falls, and violence are needed.

REFERENCES

Asogawa, S. E. 1978. Road traffic accidents: a major public health problem. Pub. Hlth. (London) 92:237–245.

Asogwa, S. E. 1992. Road traffic accidents in Nigeria: a review and a reappraisal. Accid. Anal. Prev. 24:149–155.

Butchart, A., and D. S. Brown. 1991. Non-fatal injuries due to interpersonal violence in Johannesburg–Soweto: incidence, determinants and consequences. Forensic Sci. Intl. 52:35–51.

Butchart, A., V. Nell, D. Yach, D. S. O. Brown, A. Anderson, B. Radebe, and K. Johnson. 1991. Epidemiology of non-fatal injuries due to external causes in Johannesburg-Soweto. Part II. Incidence and determinants. S. Afr. Med. J. 79:139–143.

Datubo–Brown, D. O. 1989. Deliberate burns in Nigeria. Trop. Doctor 19:137–140.

Datubo–Brown, D. D., and B. M. Kejek. 1989. Burn injuries in Port Harcourt, Nigeria. Burns 15:152–154.

Davis, L., and L. S. Smith. 1985. The epidemiology of drowning in Cape Town—1980–1983. S. Afr. Med. J. 68:739–742.

Eferakeya, A. E. 1984. Drugs and suicide attempts in Benin City, Nigeria. Brit. J. Psychiat. 145:70–73.

Etiaba, A. H., S I. Fahmy, F. A. Bassiouni, E. A. Kader, and A. S. El Tantawy. 1984. Burns and scalds among school-aged children. Bull. High Inst. Pub. Hlth. 14:227–240.

Fisher, A. J., G. Joubert, and D. Yach. 1992. Mortality from external causes in South African adolescents, 1984–1986. S. Afr. Med. J. 81:77–80.

Foege, W. 1991. Foreword. In Violence in America: A Public Health Approach, M. L. Rosenberg and M. A. Fenley, eds. New York: Oxford University Press.

Graitcer, P. L., H. El-Sayed, R. J. Waxweiler, O. A. Mostafa, I. F. Elias, S. G. Boutros, H. Keladah, M. N. Nassery, A. Hamam, S. Fahmy, L. A. M. Abdel Magid, E. Salem, S. Sallam, Z. Youssef, J. Mercy, and T. Chorbaa. 1993. Injury morbidity and mortality. In Injury in Egypt: Injury as a Public Health Problem, A. Y. Mashaly, R. Graitcer, and Z. Youssef, eds. Cairo: New Press.

Grange, A. O., A. O. Akinsulie, and G. O. Sowemimo. 1988. Flame burn disasters from kerosene appliance explosions in Lagos, Nigeria. Burns 14:147–155.

Grant, R., M. Preda, and J. D. Martin. 1989. Domestic violence in Texas: A study of statewide and rural spouse abuse. Wichita Falls, Tex.: Bureau of Business and Government Research, Midwestern State University.

Gu, X. Y., and M. L. Chen. 1982. Vital statistics of Shanghai County. Am. J. Publ. Hlth. 72 (Suppl.):19–23.

Haight, F. 1980. Traffic safety in developing countries. J. Safety Res. 12:50–55.

Handwerker, P. 1991. Gender power difference may be an STD risk factor for the next generation. Paper presented at the 90th Annual Meeting of the American Anthropological Association, Chicago, Ill.

Heise, L. 1993. Violence against women: the missing agenda. In Women's Health: a Global Perspective, M. A. Koblinsky and G. J. Timyan, eds. Boulder, Colo.: Westview.

Jacobs, G. D., and I. Sayer. 1983. Road accidents in developing countries. Accid. Anal. Prev. 15:337–353.

Jacobsson, L. 1985. Acts of violence in a traditional western Ethiopian society in transition. Acta Psychiatr. Scand. 71:601–607.

Jamison, D. T., W. H. Mosley, A. R. Measham, and J. L. Bobadilla, eds. 1993. Disease Control Priorities in Developing Countries. New York: Oxford University Press for the World Bank.

Kibel, S. M., F. O. Nagel, J. Myers, and S. Cywes. 1990. Childhood near-drowning—a 12-year retrospective review. S. Afr. Med. J. 78(7):418–421.

Lerer, L. B. 1992. Women, homicide and alcohol in Cape Town, South Africa. Forensic Sci. Intl. 55:93–99.

Mabogunje, O. A., and J. H. Lawrie. 1988. Burns in adults in Zaria, Nigeria. Burns 14:308–312.

Mboussou, M., and L. Milebou-Aubusson. 1989. Suicides and attempted suicides at the Jeanne Ebori Foundation, Libreville. Med. Trop. 49:259–264.

Megid, L. 1992. Alexandria Poison Control Center. Photocopy.

Mohan, D., and P. S. Bawa. 1985. An analysis of road traffic fatalities in Delhi, India. Accid. Anal. Prev. 17:33–45.

Mostafa, O. A. 1993. Epidemiology of injuries in rural Egypt. Paper presented at the Second World Conference on Injury Control, CDC, Atlanta, Georgia, May.

Muscat, J. E., and M. S. Huncharek. 1991. Firearms and adult domestic homicides. The role of alcohol and the victim. Am. J. Forensic Med. Pathol. 12:105–110.

Mwaniki, D. L., and S. W. Guthar. 1990. Occurrence and characteristics of mandibular fractures in Nairobi, Kenya. Br. J. Oral Maxiofacial Surg. 28:200–202.

NRC (National Research Council). 1985. Injury in America: A Continuing Health Problem. Washington, D.C.: National Academy Press.

Nosseir, S. A., A. A. Sherif, M. N. Mortada, et al. 1990. A study of accidents among preschool children attending MCH centers in Alexandria. Alex. J. Pediatr. 4:45–48.

Ogba, L. O. 1989. Violence and health in Nigeria. Hlth. Pol. Plan. 4:82–84.

Odejide, A. O., A. O. Williams, J. U. Ohaeri, and B. A. Ikussan. 1986. The epidemiology of deliberate self-harm. The Ibadan experience. Br. J. Psychiat. 149:734–737.

Okonkwo, C. A. 1988. Spinal cord injuries in Enugu, Nigeria–preventable accidents. Paraplegia 26:12–18.

Omram, A. R. 1971. The epidemiologic transition: a theory of the epidemiology of population change. Milbank Mem. Fund Q. 49:509–538.

Onuba, O. 1988. Pattern of burns injury in Nigerian children. Trop. Doctor 18:106–108.

PAHO (Pan American Health Organization). 1990. Violence: a growing public health problem in the Region. Epidemiol. Bull. 11:1–7.

PAHO (Pan American Health Organization). 1993. Resolution XIX, Violence and health. Directing Council, Ninth Plenary Session, October, Washington, D.C.

Raikes, A. 1990. Pregnancy, Birthing and Family Planning in Kenya: Changing Patterns of Behavior: A Health Utilization Study in Kissi District. Copenhagen: Center for Development Research.

Rice, D. P., E. J. MacKenzie, and Associates. 1989. Cost of Injuries in the United States: A Report to Congress. San Francisco, Calif.: Institute for Health & Aging, University of California, and Injury Prevention Center, The Johns Hopkins University.

Rosenberg, M. L., and J. Mercy. 1991. Assaultive violence. In Violence in America: A Public Health Approach, M. L. Rosenberg and M. A. Fenley, eds. New York: Oxford University Press.

Roux, P., and R. M. Fisher. 1992. Chest injuries in children: an analysis of 100 cases of blunt chest trauma from motor vehicle accidents. J. Pediatr. Surg. 27(S):551–555.

Saleh S., S. Gadalla, J. A. Fortney, S. M. Rogers, and D. M. Potts. 1986. Accidental burn deaths to Egyptian women of reproductive age. Burns 12(4):241–245.

Smith, G. S., and P. Barss. 1991. Unintentional injuries in developing countries: the epidemiology of a neglected problem. Epidemiol. Rev. 13:228-266.

Sowemimo, G. O. 1983. Burn injuries in Lagos. Burns 9:280–283.

Stansfield, S. K., G. S. Smith, and W. McGreevey. 1993. Health sector priorities review: injury. In Disease Control Priorities in Developing Countries, D. T. Jamison, W. H. Mosley, A. R. Measham, and J. L. Bobadilla, eds. New York: Oxford University Press for the World Bank.

Trinca, G., I. Johnston, B. Campbell, F. Haight, P. Knight, M. Mackay, J. McLean, and E. Petrucelli. 1988. Reducing Traffic Injury—A Global Challenge. Melbourne: Royal Australian College of Surgeons.

Udoeyop, U. W., and A. R. Iwatt. 1991. Abdominal trauma in southeastern Nigeria. Centr. Afr. J. Med. 37:409–415.

UN (United Nations). 1991. The World's Women 1970–1990, Trends and Statistics. Social Statistics and Indicators, Series K, No. 8. New York.

UNICEF (United Nations Children's Fund). 1986. Statistical Review of the Situation of Children in the World. New York.

Werner, D. 1989. Health for no one by the year 2000: The high cost of placing "national security" before global justice. Presentation at 16th Annual International Health Conference, National Council on International Health, Arlington, Va., June.

Wintemute, G. 1985. Is motor vehicle–related mortality a disease of development? Accid. Anal. Prev. 17:223–245.

WHO (World Health Organization). Various years. World Health Statistics Annual. Geneva.

Zimbabwe Ministry of Health. 1989. Annual Report. Harrare

9

Occupational and Environmental Health

In this chapter an attempt is made to synthesize information on a topic that is elusive when examined from the usual perspective—that is, one that has been heavily skewed toward the developed countries and male subjects. Occupational and environmental health viewed through the prism of female health in Sub-Saharan Africa presents a challenging task of inference from what is known about social, economic, political, labor, and gender relations and the environmental health hazards typical of the region.

As Table 9-1 shows, however, there are already indications of a substantial number of adverse occupational and environmental factors that burden female health status disproportionately in the region. These factors—which include increased exposure to indoor air pollution, toxic wastes, and organic dusts from food processing; job overload; lack of job control; and ergonomic stressors, among others—are discussed in this chapter.

The approach adopted here first attempts to provide a conceptual framework for thinking about female work as a principal source of gendered occupational and environmental health problems. This is followed by a discussion of problems, trends, and emergent issues and their social determinants. The life span perspective is then employed in a systematic examination of the female health hazard profile, which, in turn, is related to adverse health outcomes in the region. Last, public health research implications are drawn from a consideration of the information presented. It must be noted at the outset that there are substantial cross-national differences in most of what is covered in this chapter. The approach adopted will attempt to be as inclusive of these variants as possible.

WOMEN'S WORK IN SUB-SAHARAN AFRICA

Any general consideration of occupational and environmental health is necessarily based on the nature of the work performed in the society at large. Africa, with a few regional exceptions, is a less-developed part of the world. The greater part of agriculture is subsistence farming, and cash crops account for a significant part of the monetary income derived. There is some mining or extractive industry, with petroleum featuring prominently in parts of the continent. Secondary industry is poorly developed, as are governmental and private sector services.

Although the Sub-Saharan region is vast and unevenly developed, it is nevertheless possible to set forth general categories of occupational and environmental hazards. This will allow the reader to combine different categories for any country within the region.

Women play a key role in production in Africa. Before characterizing that role, however, a number of

TABLE 9-1   Adverse Occupational and Environmental Factors in Sub-Saharan Africa: Gender-Related Burden

Problem	Exclusive to Females	Greater for Females than for Males	Burden for Females and Males Comparable, but of Particular Significance for Females
Ergonomic stressors		X	
Exposure to indoor air pollution		X	
Exposure to organic dusts from food processing		X	
Exposure to toxic wastes		X	
Job overload		X	
Lack of job control		X	
Other[a]		X	

NOTE: Significance is defined here as having an impact on health that, for any reason—biological, reproductive, sociocultural, or economic—is different in its implications for females than for males.

[a]Other includes: ill-fitting personal protective equipment designed for men; working under recommended exposure limits for occupational hazards designed for healthy, well-nourished men in the developed countries working an eight-hour day; exposure to malaria prophylaxis and infection that pose serious risks for pregnant women; exposure to uncontrolled chemical and ergonomic hazards that pose risks for the fetus; effects of chemicals, indoor smoke, and injury hazards that extend to infants; work-time requirements that further compromise breastfeeding and infant nutrition; and lack of sufficient "off time" to allow for appropriate rehabilitation from injury or work-related disease, thus exacerbating hazardous exposures or increasing female work loads.

methodological problems require attention. The most salient relates to how women's work in Sub-Saharan Africa is to be conceptualized.

It is tempting to construct a table providing information about where women work by country, region, and sector compared with men. Given the unreliability of currently available information, this would run the risk of reifying such data, thereby allowing facile applications that are unlikely to be meaningful. The available data are not strictly comparable and show such wide variation among countries in Sub-Saharan Africa that they are neither likely nor reasonable on an individual-country basis. Nevertheless, the averages and range of percentages for the region as a whole are significant, and are provided below.

Women's economic participation rates in Sub-Saharan Africa are high, clustering around 50 percent (UN, 1991). Nearly 80 percent of economically active women work in agriculture. About 40 percent of this group work unpaid on family farms, 30 percent are paid agricultural employees, and 30 percent labor on their own farms or in other informal work in the sector. While women make up a little over 40 percent of the agricultural labor force, they produce the bulk of the food in the region (Kerven, 1989). Men's participation in agriculture is restricted to cash-crop production and wage labor on plantations. Agriculture is thus the greatest single component of women's work outside the home.

Women's labor force participation in Sub-Saharan Africa is higher than in most developing countries, and it is growing. This greater involvement of women in economic activities is thought to be a function of both improvements in their educational levels and the global economic crisis, which compels women to work in order to sustain their families (UN, 1991). The mounting proportion of female-headed households in the region also means that these women—up to 66 percent of them—are the main, if not sole, source of sustenance for their families. In some parts of Africa, notably in rural areas that provide male migrants and in periurban shantytowns, this proportion is very high, ranging between 50 and 70 percent of all households (Kerven, 1989). Women and families in both venues are affected by migration: rural families are affected by the emigration of spouses to the urban areas, while women who migrate to urban areas with their families are obliged to participate increasingly in the money economy of those areas, because the requirements of urban living, such as rent and transport, require cash payments.

On average, between 15 and 20 percent of economically active women in Sub-Saharan Africa are in formal employment, with considerable variation across the region (UN, 1991). The overwhelming majority work in services, with very small numbers in manufacturing and other industry. Public and private sector wage labor tends to be monopolized by men.

WOMEN AND WORK IN HISTORICAL CONTEXT

The colonial experience had a substantial impact on the work of women, particularly their role in agricultural production (Gitonga, 1991; Lado, 1992). The social system in much of Sub-Saharan Africa, traditionally patriarchal in the precolonial period, was maintained during the colonial era. The division of labor within the family in much of Africa remains structured according to gender, with women specializing in food farming, processing, and trading outside the home. Land laws in Africa do not permit granting of title to women, even when they cultivate their own land or produce their own crops independently of a spouse. Men are presumed heads of households, and only they can obtain titles to cultivate, own, and occupy land. Sub-Saharan women, therefore, continue to cultivate land owned by men.

During the colonial period, men took over cash-cropping agriculture and participated in the commercial plantation sector, while women remained tied to subsistence farming in ever-greater proportions. This preservation of the traditional exclusion of women from landownership sustained their dependence on men for communal or familial allocation of plots. The best fields went to cash-cropping, while plots for subsistence agriculture were generally more distant, more scattered, and less well prepared. This, in turn, led to production emphasis on crops that demanded less effort, but were also less nutritious, such as cassava, rather than more demanding and more nutritious crops such as yams. Technologies used in the women's agricultural sector have also remained undeveloped, and continue to involve considerable expenditure of human energy and time. The technical innovations that have been introduced have paradoxically expanded women's share of work, while decreasing their income, because of the preferential application of new technologies to cash-cropping and the male monopoly on access to credit and income.

Women's progressive marginalization in the subsistence sector has meant that their productivity and control over resources has been reduced, while their total work burden has increased. This has had severe implications for the nutrition and health of the women and their families. Decrements and losses in women's food production and income have played a large part in the food crisis in Africa, and it is argued that macroeconomic policies are unlikely to be successful unless they explicitly address the role of women in both the subsistence and commercial agricultural sectors (Lado, 1992; Savane, 1980).

The theme of the invisible (female) subsistence sector has been succinctly elucidated by Packard (1989a,b), and constitutes one of the indirect, nonbeneficial effects of industrialization in Africa. One of the major determinants of this invisibility has been the system of migrant labor.

The migrant labor patterns typical of modernization in Sub-Saharan Africa that have resulted in the high proportions of households headed by women, described above, have also affected their children, especially girls. While they are in school, children have reduced economic value in the production of income or labor for family maintenance, and their mother's workload is correspondingly greater in these earlier years. It is not surprising that young girls are pressured to drop out of school at about 12 years of age, or that they are expected to do more housework than boys. Women's work begins at a young age.

These factors have forced many women to engage in informal sector activities in the processing and sale of food products and to participate at high rates in petty commerce, especially in West Africa (Bukh, 1980). The relative absence of a productive, as opposed to a commercial, informal sector in Sub-Saharan Africa is noteworthy when compared with other parts of the world, such as Asia. Work in the informal sector consists of many short tasks that can be performed simultaneously, and it is optimal in a context of constant childcare. Such tasks— whether they are farming, petty trading, processing of crops, or commercial sex work—are typically small-scale activities with no access to capital, and yield little profit. The positive side of women's work, in both the formal and informal sectors, is that in addition to offering more flexibility in childcare, in many cases it affords opportunities for access to resources and allows women control over their own destinies, including economic survival for those fleeing oppressive marriages or without land.

In the service sector in Sub-Saharan Africa, there are proportionately fewer women in clerical and service jobs because men dominate the public and private wage sectors, trade unions, and other employee organizations. This has been the case historically, even for paid domestic work. A higher proportion of the male work force (30 percent) than the female work force (20 percent) is in the service sector (UN, 1991).

Within the manufacturing sector, the picture is similar to that of more developed countries (UN, 1991). There is gender segregation in different occupational groups; within the same occupational group, women's jobs are either less prestigious or less well paid for the same work. The maternity factor continues to discriminate against women in hiring and promotion.

The stabilization and adjustment programs referred to in Chapter 2 have adversely affected women, who have been disproportionately squeezed out of public sector employment. The immediate cause for this diminution has been cuts in government health and social services expenditures. Deregulation has simultaneously accelerated a process, however slightly, of feminization of the wage sector in Sub-Saharan Africa (Standing, 1989). Women in ever-growing numbers may be performing the same work that males performed in the past in the public and private sectors, but do so under worse financial and social security conditions. Finally, the wage freezes associated with regional stabilization programs, combined with the effects of inflation, have driven up the number of working hours necessary to make ends meet.

PROBLEMS OF DEFINITION

There are considerable and overlapping problems of definition involving the nature of work, and whether it is paid or not. For this reason, a rigid, overarching definition of work is not very useful. This chapter employs the categories of formal, informal, domestic, and agricultural food production sectors in dealing with women's work in Africa. The main consequence of definitional fuzziness with respect to women's work is that much of their work is invisible, and this invisibility applies to all categories. Official statistics indicate that this dilemma applies worldwide, but the invisibility phenomenon is likely to be more pronounced in developing countries. The categories selected for discussion here have therefore been determined by their salience for women's work. Paid and unpaid work are, in general, difficult to distinguish in developing countries. Non-market-related unpaid work is almost exclusively the lot of women in Sub-Saharan Africa.

The formal sector is characterized by employment at a wage or salary with Social Security benefits, and it is governed by a legal system of regulation dealing with employment contracts and working conditions. For women in Sub-Saharan Africa, this comprises mainly work in service and, to a lesser extent, clerical work. Women's participation in manufacturing is very low (less than 2 percent of the female work force), and takes place in industries generally perceived to involve "female" work. These include food processing and clothing and textile manufacturing (Naimi, 1991). Private and public sector service work also frequently involve "female" work.

The informal sector is characterized by economically active people working on their own account (self-employed), without employees but with unpaid family workers, in the absence of regulation, including wage contracts (de Soto, 1989; UN, 1991). The growth of this sector is a widespread phenomenon in the developing world, notably in Asia and Latin America. For African women, this sector comprises petty commercial enterprises and small-scale production. It became a major growth sector in the 1980s and now constitutes a major source of women's employment in Africa. Examples include petty trading or home-based industries such as beer-brewing, soap-making, tailoring, and commercial sex work.

The informal sector also makes a major contribution to family income. Women's contributions through this sector in Africa are estimated at around 10 percent for industrial production, and perhaps as high as 90 percent for service provision. Incomes are lower than in the formal sector, although a recent South African study shows that informal sector workers can achieve incomes similar to those of waged domestic workers in the formal sector (Cooper et al., 1991), although informal sector activity is less secure. Low levels of investment in technology, poor economies of scale, high unit prices for raw materials, and limited access to large markets and marketing organizations mean low productivity and returns (UN, 1991). Overall, this is a major labor sector for women, ranking next in importance after domestic work and farm labor.

The domestic sector involves unpaid home provisioning and maintenance activities. These include the preparation, processing, and cooking of food; cleaning; childbearing; childcare; care of the sick and aged; collection and head-portage of water and fuel; and back-portage of children. These tasks all consume large amounts of time and energy and must be constantly balanced against demands on women from other work sectors. As noted earlier, the expansion of women's work loads beyond the domestic sector has served to shift the burden of domestic work to female children.

Because of the dominance of agricultural production in Sub-Saharan Africa, and because women play the largest role in subsistence agriculture, farm labor and food procurement are treated here as a distinct work category—**the agricultural food projection sector**—which includes both formal and informal, or domestic, activity (McGowan and Leslie, 1990; Raikes, 1989).

Up to 80 percent of women work in agricultural production, a sector that can be further broken down into commercial/cash-crop, plantation, and subsistence production. In all three activities, women provide substantial inputs, but the bulk of their activity is on the informal end of the spectrum, in subsistence agriculture; family cash-cropping; and providing unpaid, usually seasonal, assistance for spouses performing wage labor on plantations. Their work also includes preparing, transporting, and marketing agricultural products for sale in the informal sector.

The sum total of these dynamics within the sectors and subsectors described above is that virtually all women's work is effectively unpaid. Women participate little in the formal sector, either in the service or manufacturing industries, but dominate the domestic and agricultural production sectors and, to a lesser extent, commercial and productive activities of the informal sector. The bulk of women's work, then, falls under the rubric of social reproduction of workers in the family unit, as opposed to production. This helps explain its relative invisibility. Failure to take account of that invisible work leads to a serious underestimate of women's contribution to total output. It has been estimated that accounting for that work would have raised the figure for the world's annual recorded production by one-third, or $4 trillion, in 1985 (Sivard, 1985). Not counting women's work is particularly egregious in Sub-Saharan Africa, where women's work hours are extremely long. All over the world, women have been documented as working longer days than men. This distinction is more pronounced in the developing countries, and still more so in Sub-Saharan Africa, where extra hours worked by females have been estimated at 12 to 13 more a week than those worked by males. Time/budget studies have shown that women need to work between 60 and 90 hours a week just to make ends meet (UN, 1991). In some parts of East Africa, women work a total of 16 hours a day doing housework, caring for children, preparing food, and raising between 60 and 80 percent of the food for the family (Fagley, 1976). In Burkina Faso, women have about one hour a day to socialize, participate in community activities, and take care of personal needs (McSweeney, 1979). All of this adds up to a picture of long duration, high-intensity, and exhausting physical labor for women in Sub-Saharan Africa (Lukmanji, 1992).

This has implications for the gendered nature of child labor. Although there is little documentation on child labor in Sub-Saharan Africa, it is clear that, given the nature of production, child labor constitutes a very significant proportion of total labor, and that female children make a disproportionately high contribution because of their involvement in domestic labor.

Finally, the categorization of biological reproduction as a form of work is by no means unwarranted. While turning all aspects of life into work would be detrimental to the understanding and conceptualization of either, women's role in biological (as well as social) reproduction in the family context does free men for visible and paid work. This relationship can at times be brutally direct, as in the case of a woman who is unable to bear children and is forced out of the family to subsist as best she can in the informal sector—through prostitution, for example.

THE NATURE OF OCCUPATIONAL AND ENVIRONMENTAL HEALTH PROBLEMS

There is relatively little in the published literature on environmentally and occupationally related morbidity and mortality in developing countries, least of all for Sub-Saharan Africa. Still, work has been done and serves as a useful indicator of what remains to be done. The topic was substantively reviewed by Packard (1989a) in a seminal article on the broadly conceived health consequences of environmental and occupational exposures in Sub-Saharan Africa. Christiani and colleagues (1990) outlined research needs in the area of occupational health in developing countries more generally; Levy has more recently inventoried ongoing research in environmental and occupational health in the developing countries overall (Levy, 1992a); and a review by Rantanen (1992) emphasizes emerging trends in occupational health. A vigorous debate (Doll, 1992; Landrigan, 1992) has also arisen on the question of health, focusing on the general environment for countries at various levels of development. Finally, there has also been a recent trend toward greater governmental and nongovernmental involvement by the developed countries in developing-country occupational and environmental health issues in the form of the application of modern methods, which promise to provide more reliable data collection and analysis than were hitherto available.

Beyond these studies, perhaps because of the extremely broad range of human conditions and adverse health outcomes encompassed under the rubrics "environmental and occupational health," relevant material is widely dispersed, even in the case of published academic work. Searches of the computerized occupational and environmental health data bases, including Medline and CCInfo-Disc, revealed very few references relating to any two or more of the following terms: Africa, occupational health, environmental health, and women. Not surprisingly, there is very little work, published or unpublished, that looks specifically at women, and most treatments of the subject of work are not differentiated by gender. Thus, ideas about female morbidity and mortality have to be based on inference, and the sources are mainly gender-blind material, on the one hand, and factors arising out of a general analysis of women's work in Africa, on the other. Unpublished work, conference presentations, work published in languages other than English, and internal reports of governmental and nongovernmental agencies have therefore been identified and assembled with more formal publications to permit as full a discussion as possible.

As a result of this paucity of data, the nature of the problem is difficult to articulate succinctly, although it must be of great magnitude if for no other reason than the universal necessity to work in some way to stay alive. For poor people, and for women in particular, work loads, however defined, are extremely heavy and may be expected to give rise to a multiplicity of health effects over the course of a life span and through at least one subsequent generation. Emerging issues and trends must similarly be inferred through extrapolations from known exposures and from general considerations derived from sociodemographic and economic data.

Occupational Injuries

The emerging worldwide pattern of occupational health includes occupational injuries as a serious problem (see Chapter 8). An estimated 100 million occupational injuries, 180,000 occupational fatalities, and 10 million permanent disabilities occur globally each year, and between 70 and 80 percent of these events take place in developing countries (Rantanen, 1992). Rates of injury in those countries are thought to be between three and four times those of developed countries, and the most elevated rates are linked to young and inexperienced workers performing heavy work.

Occupational Diseases

The occurrence of occupational diseases is harder to estimate, but indications that are of increasing importance are noise-induced hearing loss, pneumoconioses, organic-dust-related lung diseases, metal toxicity, musculoskeletal disorders, and infections or infestations from exposure to contaminated water and animals (Rantanen, 1992).

Chemical Hazards

Chemical hazards are major risk factors in developing countries, notably through the penetration of agrochemicals. Poisonings, acute or chronic, are not easily ascertained, but Rantanen (1992) estimates that there are some three million acute episodes of agrochemical poisoning each year, principally from organophosphate insecticides, 99 percent of which are in developing countries, with some 220,000 fatalities annually from this cause alone. Acute poisoning that is work-related becomes relevant for workers and their dependents because storage, distribution, formulation, application, and other handling problems of chemical materials abound, and access is very easy. In addition, containers and packaging are frequently reused in developing countries, where such materials are valuable, and warning labels are useless, either because they are written in foreign languages or because of worker illiteracy. Hazard control of any kind is problematic because engineering methods are generally beyond the means of producers in the developing countries, and the cheaper and easier option of providing personal protective equipment is often impractical. Environmental chemical contamination—especially of water sources—is yet another problem that affects the workplace and the domestic environment.

It may be presumed that heavy work in hot climates engenders significant heat and ergonomic stress. In developed countries, the estimate is that up to 40 percent of all occupational diseases are somehow associated with ergonomic stress; there are no such estimates in developing countries.

Toxic Emissions

The major sources of environmental health problems are indoor air pollution from heating and cooking using biomass and other fuels; general air pollution from motor vehicles in urban areas; point source pollution from production sites such as factories and waste disposal sites; and general chemical contamination from the application of agrochemicals.

Emergent trends show a proliferation in the relocation of hazardous factories to developing countries (LaDou, 1992) and in the export of hazardous waste from developed countries to be dumped in developing countries, especially Africa (Anyinam, 1991). Yet another trend is the export of chemicals, notably agrochemicals that have been banned for use in developed countries (LaDou, 1992). These trends are not well documented by volume, rate, or health effects, yet the evidence is that the international trade in toxic substances is growing much faster than the international monitoring mechanisms and institutions that could manage the problem.

Other naturally occurring toxins are produced by biologic agents such as mycotoxins on stored grains (aflatoxins on peanuts), or exist in a natural state in inadequately prepared food (cassava). These can cause serious liver or nervous system disease, cancers, and birth defects. One example is lathyrism, a central nervous system degenerative disease caused by consumption of grass peas in Ethiopia, which has a community prevalence ranging between 0.5 and 3 percent (Haimanot et al., 1990). Conditions such as esophageal cancer, liver cancer, cardiomyopathies, and other neurological conditions may be partly or wholly attributable to environmental agents or to their synergistic interactions with other causative factors. The amount of thoughtful research required to tease out truly or plausible causal relationships is large. The most efficient resolution would be to extrapolate from known causal relationships in well-analyzed sites in developed countries to comparable situations in developing countries.

LIFE SPAN APPROACH

It is apparent from the age matrix for female health in Sub-Saharan Africa that environmental and occupational hazards produce a variety of effects throughout the life span, with, by definition, the most pronounced effect during the working years, between the ages of 10 and 49.

There are problems with modeling a sequential life span approach quantitatively or epidemiologically because of multiple intermediate variables between initial causes and final outcomes. Analysis of such variables is rather

TABLE 9-2 Environmental Hazards and Typical Outcomes by Phase in the Life Span

Phase	Outcome	Hazards
Intrauterine	Birth defects, prematurity, low birthweight	Hookworm, malaria
Infant/child	Nutrition effects, chemical poisoning, accidents	Pesticides, indoor air pollution
Adolescent	Obstetric problems, infertility, miscarriages	Arduous work, lathyrism
Young adult and middle-age	Acute poisoning, injuries (with breakdown of family life because of migrancy and female-headed households) lead to poverty and overwork with nutrition effects, commercial sex work	Pesticides, indoor air pollution, arduous work, HIV
Old age	Chronic poisoning from toxins interacting with age effects, nervous system and psychiatric problems, infections from children	Childcare

complex, and dependent upon very sophisticated statistical technology, as well as high-quality, plentiful data. These data are generally unavailable, even in developed countries.

Nevertheless, a more qualitative approach may be taken to the life span phases in Table 9-2. There is a degree of reversibility, and some adverse health outcomes in females at selected life phases determine the hazardous exposures health determinants in those in other life phases. It is therefore possible to think of bi-directional effects between the various phases in Table 9-2.

McGowan and Leslie (1990) provide a useful basis for conceptualizing life span/life cycle effects together with some illustrative examples. They deal substantially with the effects of childhood health and nutrition on adult work capacity and the reciprocal effects of adult health, nutrition, and mortality on all aspects of female work.

They note particularly the physical stunting, anemia, and possible mental retardation or visual impairment caused by nutritional deficiency in early life. The impact of these difficulties on work has yet to be adequately studied or documented. There are also consequences of other environmental and occupational exposures on subsequent health status to be considered. These include infections such as polio, chemical poisonings, burns and other disabling injuries, water-related infestations, and blindness from onchocerciasis. The close domestic association between mother and infant leads to chemical and injury exposures both within and outside the home that begin early in life (Gitonga, 1991). For females, the indoor pollution they experience as infants and as children continues into adulthood, and domestic-work-related exposure compounds respiratory problems. Similar considerations may apply to agrochemical exposures.

Reciprocally, adult morbidity and mortality of occupational and environmental causation will adversely affect the nutritional status of younger females and will considerably increase their work load. The effects of adult female morbidity and mortality for those in the informal and agricultural production sectors, as well as for those in female-headed households, have major health implications for female children. Chronic diseases and malnutrition limit work capacity considerably. The most common problems for adult women are anemia, fevers caused by malaria, gastrointestinal disturbances and nutritional depletion from frequent pregnancies, and pregnancy and lactation. All these factors may be considered to be work-related in the sense that they may be caused by biologic agents related to occupation, or work overload in relation to nutritional intakes. Work may thus be thought of as including the physiological work of reproduction and lactation.

NATURE OF THE EVIDENCE

An Occupational and Environmental Health Hazard Profile for Women

Women's very substantial working lives provide a framework for considering a hazard profile for each of the four work sectors.

Injury rates have risen with increasing mechanization and as chemical use has become more widespread (Jinadu, 1987, 1990; Odelowo, 1991; Schmauch, 1991). Mechanized transport is a case in point (Hicks, 1987), but mechanization can also decrease accident rates in the workplace (Asogwa, 1988). An important effect of increased work loads and exhaustion is a higher injury rate. Patriarchal and male dominance and increased pressure for production are likely to lead to domestic violence and to sexual violence at work.

Violence is also related to work in the informal sector such as commercial sex work, home brewing, and running a tavern. Petty trading may also expose women to robbery and criminal violence. Alcohol consumption also plays an important role (Lerer, 1992). Fatal agrochemical poisoning, notably with organophosphates and paraquat (Adebe, 1991; Levin et al., 1979; London, 1992), is increasingly important.

Physical Factors

Given the heavy physical nature of women's work in Sub-Saharan Africa, heat-related illness may be anticipated, ranging from heat rash to heat exhaustion and heat stroke, with possible chronic effects, especially in hot climates. The role of adaptation to heat requires investigation to determine its interaction with the range of heat-related illness. Heavy weights carried while transporting fuel and water require high levels of energy expenditure, energy that is limited by nutritional status, which in turn limits the availability of food at home for those not engaged in work.

Chemical Factors

The nature of work in Sub-Saharan Africa clearly involves substantial exposure to chemical hazards (Institute of Occupational Health Information Office, 1986). Much processing work liberates dust, usually of an organic variety from vegetable and other food products. Indoor smoke pollution from burning biomass fuel for energy constitutes a principal respiratory hazard for women performing domestic work. Smoke particulates have been measured at time-weighted averages well above permissible "nuisance dust" levels in African huts (Grobbelaar and Bateman, 1991) and can cause chronic obstructive pulmonary disease and chronic bronchitis (Myers, 1989). Wet work conditions result in impairment of the integrity and functions of the skin and can enhance the absorption of chemicals, and hence their reactivity. Agricultural water sources are frequently polluted with biologic and chemical agents. The single largest chemical category, however, is agrochemicals, which includes chemicals used as insecticides (including antivector spraying), herbicides, fungicides, nematocides, and avicides. The hazard of acute poisoning by agrochemicals is well known for organophosphate insecticides and for the herbicide paraquat. In addition, chronic toxicity is thought to result from long-term exposure to herbicides containing dioxin and organochlorine and organophosphate insecticides (London, 1992). Apart from the difficulty of ensuring safe work practices with agrochemicals, substantial pollution of water sources is very likely to occur in an environment of poor subsistence farming in the absence of a regulatory system.

Finally, toxic waste—usually heavy metals, organic chemicals, and radioactive materials—has been dumped in increasing quantities in Sub-Saharan Africa. Poor periurban and possibly rural communities may be particularly at risk for exposure. Women searching for fuel, usable garbage, or water are likely to be preferentially exposed.

Biological Factors

Many biologic agents, whether infectious or allergenic, are present in the working environment of women. Their role as informal and formal health care providers involves exposure to a range of infectious agents. These include viruses (HIV and hepatitis B) and bacteria (TB). Those working with livestock are exposed to toxoplasma and brucella. Because much agricultural and domestic work takes place outdoors and involves water, the gamut of water-related infections and infestations pose significant differential risks to women. These include malaria (Kaseje et al., 1987), onchocerciasis, trypanosomiasis, and schistosomiasis. Biological causes of work-related illness are likely to be more prominent here than in developed countries, where they account for only 5 percent of such illness, because immunizations are costly and impractical, and the community prevalence and incidence of hepatitis B infection are much higher. Many poisonous insects, spiders and other arachnids such as scorpions, and snakes pose hazards for agricultural workers.

Women's work as the principal food processors brings them into substantial contact with organic dusts, which are frequently contaminated by fungi and bacteria. Separately or in conjunction with infectious agents, these contaminants may have considerable toxic and allergenic potential for both respiratory and skin problems.

Work Organizational Factors

Psychosocial Organization of Work

Although not proven in the developing countries, Karasek's (1979) job-strain model is useful in conceptualizing the components of hazards related to work organization. In this model stress may be thought of in two dimensions—job load and job control (decision latitude).

Job Load

There are unreasonable male expectations of work from women, including those working full time in the formal sector. Perhaps the most striking aspect of the organization of women's work is the extent of their overload (Lado, 1992; Lukmanji, 1992; McGowan and Leslie, 1990). Overwork comprises two dimensions: intensity and duration. As mentioned above, women frequently work at the extreme limits of their physical capacity in intensity and energy required, while the long hours must inflict substantial physical, mental, emotional, and social wear and tear. Because women have very limited access to other productive resources, their need to increase their production can only take the form of harder work, longer hours of work, or both. Nevertheless, there are absolute limits to an increased work load without the introduction of labor-saving technology in the domestic, subsistence, and informal sectors. Job load or demand is therefore a major and increasing stressor in the context of Sub-Saharan Africa.

Job Control

It is relatively clear from the foregoing that women in Sub-Saharan Africa exercise little control over their work in all four sectors. Decisions about what work they will do, how they will do it, and when it will be done are largely resistant to alteration or choice by women, given the degree of overload. In addition, patriarchal structures do not allow females the autonomy and decision making authority that derive from ownership of land. According to the Karasek model applied in developed country contexts, this combination of high load and low job decision latitude is maximally stressful and might be expected to generate a number of stress-related adverse health outcomes. Other psychological sources of stress include:

- gender discrimination in hiring and promotion affects job satisfaction and strain
- sexual harassment at work
- sexual and other violence at home and at work in the informal sector
- insecurity of job tenure, income, or work conditions in both formal (especially temporary and seasonal work) and informal sectors
- multiple-role-balancing because of multiple responsibilities
- pressure of piecework in cottage industries

- absence of male support in dealing with family or social problems because of migrancy
- worry about childcare for women in the formal sector
- worry about family and individual health problems.

Sources of stress abound in the context of women's work in Sub-Saharan Africa. It has been estimated that up to 20 percent of women have mental health problems requiring expert attention in South Africa (Klugman and Weiner, 1992).

The Physical Organization of Work

Ergonomic stressors are ubiquitous in developing countries (ILO, 1987), but they have not yet been studied to any great extent. Women are subject to such stressors to a considerable degree in the course of their work. These problems originate in their physical size and strength in relation to heavy work and in the protracted periods spent in posturally stressed positions bending over fields; in portage of heavy loads including children, fuel, and water; in extensive distances traveled on foot; and in time spent standing. Formal and informal health care involve them in lifting other people, while work in the manufacturing sector reproduces ergonomic stresses typical of home work, often under less favorable conditions. In the formal manufacturing sector, machinery is usually made to foreign specifications.

Additional Considerations Unique to Women in Sub-Saharan Africa

In addition to a gender-blind consideration of the occupational and environmental health hazard profile in the African setting, special considerations are appropriate for females. Some important gender differences are:

- Personal protective equipment is designed to fit men.
- Recommended exposure limits for occupational hazards are designed for healthy, well-nourished men in the developed countries working an eight-hour day.
- Malaria prophylaxis and infection pose serious risks for pregnant women.
- Uncontrolled chemical and ergonomic hazards pose risks for the fetus, as they would in developed countries.
- The effects of chemicals, indoor smoke, and injury hazards for women extend to their infants.
- Work-time requirements may further compromise breastfeeding and infant nutrition.
- Rehabilitation from injury or work-related disease may be impossible to come by (Burger, 1990; Leger and Arkles, 1989), thus exacerbating hazardous exposures or increasing female work loads.

Adverse Health Outcomes of Occupational and Environmental Hazards

This section needs to be read in conjunction with the life span/life cycle outlined above. Reproductive health is covered in detail in Chapter 4 and will not receive any special emphasis here.

For many years now the approach to occupationally and environmentally caused disease has been limited to a few extreme examples where relatively rare exposures have led to clearly defined adverse health effects that were unlikely to have been caused by other agents. This concept has recently been broadened to encompass direct and indirect determination of health by multiple factors (Schilling and Andersson, 1986). The causative categories are listed in Table 9-3.

Indirect (Group) Health Effects

As Packard (1989a) and Chinemana (1985) point out, this concept needs still further broadening in developing countries to reach beyond the confines of the developed world and its formal employment sector. A broader

TABLE 9-3 Classification of Work-Related Diseases

Cause	Example
Direct	Hut lung and indoor smoke pollution
Contributory	Tuberculosis and overwork or dust
Aggravating	Psoriasis and excessive water contact
Easy access	Acute agrochemical poisoning

approach facilitates a deeper understanding of the panoply of historical and current (direct, or individual, and indirect, or group) effects of environmental and occupational hazards.

Beyond formal sector activity, and the male workers from this sector who are the traditional subjects of study in the developed countries, indirect effects (Packard, 1989a) are borne by those in other employment sectors, who furthermore may not receive much of the benefit from industrialization. Packard provides examples for the most important production sectors in Sub-Saharan Africa. Typical examples are the migratory diseases such as tuberculosis and sexually transmitted diseases, including HIV; the consequences for female subsistence farmers in rural areas of permanent male disability from high-risk mining activities; and increased exposure of women to malaria and schistosomiasis as a result of new irrigation practices used in large-scale agricultural developments.

Other health effects for females may be linked to mining developments, which customarily have been based on forced removal of peasant producers from their land and by the undermining of subsistence production by considering the wage to be a mere supplement. This led to worsening socioeconomic conditions at both poles of the migratory oscillation. Migration facilitated the transmission of infectious disease (Packard, 1989b). The absence of Social Security has meant that the burden of disability from work-related accidents and disease in former miners has been made invisible by relocation to the rural areas (Davies, 1993). Women's work has increased as a consequence. Depending upon the kind of mining operation, additional environmental hazards may ensue. For example, asbestos mining has led to high community prevalences of asbestos-related disease, including cancers (Felix et al., 1990; Myers et al., 1987).

Agricultural developments have led to the recrudescence of malaria and the growth of pesticide-resistant vectors because of irrigation and land use patterns. Economic disruption of communities through the elimination of small producers has led to marginalization and a change in the employment sector mix leading to unemployment, urbanization, and wage dependence.

Developments in manufacturing usually have resulted in draining the rural areas of person power and resources, with consequent transfer of wealth from rural to urban areas.

All these factors are critically important in the consideration of the health of females in Sub-Saharan Africa, because there is a marked female preponderance in the rural areas in countries where the migrant labor system operates.

Direct (Individual) Health Effects

When it comes to occupational and environmental health outcomes in females in Sub-Saharan Africa, there is little documented research (Naimi, 1991; National Workshop on Health and Safety of Women in the Workplace in Zimbabwe, 1988), but it should be borne in mind that even in developed countries female workers are infrequently studied. Health problems in the informal sector have been studied only in India (National Commission on Self-Employed Women and Women in the Informal Sector, 1988). The pattern of disease, however, may be predicted with a fair degree of confidence.

Neurological disease, both central and peripheral, must exist because of the direct effects of acute and chronic poisoning with agrochemicals. The consequences of interactions among toxins, infections, and poor nutrition may be expected to contribute to cancers of the esophagus, liver, and urogenital system. Occupational infections and infestations such as hepatitis B, HIV, TB, brucellosis, toxoplasmosis, fungi, malaria, trypanosomiasis, onchocerciasis, schistosomiasis, hookworm, and guinea worm constitute an important part of the disease spectrum. Protein-energy malnutrition and anemia will compound many health problems.

Overwork and excessive exposure to contact with infectious children and adults may result in lowered resistance to infection. Major cardiovascular diseases in Sub-Saharan cardiomyopathy may have important occupational and environmental etiologies. A wide range of chest conditions constitute important components of female morbidity. Chronic bronchitis, chronic obstructive pulmonary disease, asthma, and restrictive conditions such as anthracosis (Grobbelaar and Bateman, 1991) are known to be particularly prevalent in women. Concomitant tuberculosis is an important aggravating factor.

Dermatoses would be aggravated by domestic and agricultural exposure to water and wet conditions. This would be complicated by contact with allergenic exposures. Based on clinical evidence, Olumide has argued (1987a,b) that domestic water exposure may lead to hardening of the skin, thus offering some protection against other work-related dermatoses. In contrast, evidence from the workplace for women in the food industry, where the prevalence of dermatoses is very high, indicates that this is unlikely to be the case (London et al., 1992a,b,c).

Although undocumented, musculoskeletal disorders, along with venostasis problems that are frequently aggravated by pregnancy, must be an enormous problem. These range from the later effects of bone deformation from poor childhood and adult nutrition, through the consequences of bearing heavy weights from an early age, to the complications of childbirth, to chronic osteoarthritic conditions affecting multiple joints. Work-related musculoskeletal disorders are certain to occur frequently given the nature of women's work, which involves excessive maintenance of unnatural postures with consequent postural stress, the application of considerable force to work movements, and frequent repetition of movements. Postural stress is very likely to involve the lower back, upper limbs, and neck for women in the two most important sectors, domestic work and subsistence agriculture.

Stress-related conditions have been documented for women workers in the developed countries (Doyal, 1990; Hall 1990, 1992). In Sub-Saharan Africa, diabetes, which is thought to be stress-related, has been found to be associated with high work load (McLarty et al., 1990).

Finally, occupational health services provided either directly or by primary health care services are likely to cover only a negligible proportion of women in Sub-Saharan Africa. Rehabilitation services that promote recovery from injuries and occupational disorders are also rare. It is therefore to be expected that there is substantial underassessment of work-related adverse health outcomes.

CONCLUSIONS

In conclusion, the state of occupational and environmental health of females in Sub-Saharan Africa is determined by the major groupings of factors below.

Nature of Women's Work and Problems of Definition

Women are very substantial contributors to the world of work in Sub-Saharan Africa; their efforts are out of proportion with their counterparts in other parts of the world. They contribute equally with men according to official statistics based on visible—and therefore recorded—work. Women's work is not so easily defined, however, and attempts to categorize components run into difficulties with overlaps between paid and unpaid work, formal and informal sector settings, and production sectoral consideration. Since formal sector work for women is limited in Africa to service and clerical work and other "female work," the bulk of women's work falls within the zone of poor visibility or invisibility. Much of women's work is unpaid, whether in agricultural production, domestic work related to social reproduction, or informal sector activities. Informal sector activity has been growing rapidly and makes a very large contribution to provision of services. The increasing number of female-headed households, a product of the very prevalent migrant labor system, intensifies the workload for females further in both rural and urban settings.

There has been a steady increase in women's workload historically. This has been the product of patriarchal relations that put women's agricultural production needs in second place, lack of control over production resources and their own work, and unreasonable male expectations of work from women, including women employed full-time in the formal sector. Other socioeconomic determinants include effects of structural adjustment policies, inflation, and migrant labor. Together these elements led to an inability to cope with the totality of work in all sectors, which resulted in the shifting of the domestic burden to female children, and a consequent intensification of child labor.

Women's resultant overwork has been well quantified as excessive in terms of both duration and intensity.

Morbidity and Mortality

The scant published literature on environmentally and occupationally related morbidity and mortality in Sub-Saharan Africa is gender-blind. Occupational health services provided either directly or by primary care services are likely to cover only a negligible proportion of women in Sub-Saharan Africa. Rehabilitation services that promote recovery from injuries and occupational disorders are also rare. It is therefore to be expected that awareness of environmentally related health problems is low, and that there is substantial underascertainment of work-related adverse health outcomes.

At the same time, given the nature of women's work, the impact of environmental and occupational hazards occurs throughout the life span. As Table 9-4 illustrates, there may be substantial effects of determinants of morbidity and mortality in adult women on children or in the opposite direction. These are especially pronounced in female-headed households. Occupational and environmental exposures to toxic substances or drugs can have devastating effects on the fetus, resulting in either fetal death or long-lasting morbidity or disability in the offspring. Likewise, occupational insults are more likely to occur in younger females (and males), who are in the workforce in greater numbers; these conditions and their sequelae thus can have effects on health status that can extend substantially across the life span. These hazards, in addition, interact with each other and other causes of ill-health to produce a wider range of adverse outcomes. It may be inferred from published work on males that substandard housing, poor nutrition, ubiquitous infectious agents, and overwork, together with other environmental hazards such as chemical toxins, combine to determine a wide range of adverse health outcomes for women. These must include respiratory, dermatologic, neurologic, and work-related musculoskeletal disorders.

TABLE 9-4   Ages of Occurrence of Injuries in Sub-Saharan African Females

In Utero	Infancy/ Early Childhood (birth through age 4)	Childhood (ages 5–14)	Adolescence (ages 15–19)	Adulthood (ages 20–44)	Postmenopause (age 45+)
Maternal exposures to toxic substances	Indoor air pollution	Indoor air pollution	Indoor air pollution	Indoor air pollution	Indoor air pollution
			Job overload	Job overload	Job overload
			Lack of job control	Lack of job control	Lack of job control
			Ergonomic stressors	Ergonomic stressors	Ergonomic stressors
			Other[a]	Other[a]	Other[a]

[a]Other includes: ill-fitting personal protective equipment designed for men; working under recommended exposure limits for occupational hazards designed for healthy, well-nourished men in the developed countries working an eight-hour day; work-time requirements that further compromise breastfeeding and infant nutrition; and lack of sufficient "off time" to allow for appropriate rehabilitation from injury or work-related disease, thus exacerbating hazardous exposures or increasing female work loads.

RESEARCH NEEDS

Because relatively little is known about occupational and environmental health in Sub-Saharan Africa, and even less is known of the status of women, research implications are daunting and somewhat unfocused. This means that the first priority of research is to undertake a substantial body of descriptive work relating to women's work in Sub-Saharan Africa. This may be expected to yield areas that require more in-depth study. The broad components of this descriptive work would involve the study of representative tasks performed by women in all sectors identified above. Work hazard and risk assessment for selected adverse health outcomes should be conducted on this basis.

A mix of in-depth, participant observation, and quantitative methods (Cooper et al., 1990) will be required to adequately characterize environmental and occupational exposures, as well as conditions relevant to health.

Given that most analytic studies have been undertaken in developed countries on male subjects, there is considerable room for attention to female subjects in relation to many exposures and outcomes. Several priority topics are suggested. These include:

• Effects of pesticides and other home chemicals on peasant farmers and on others in plantations and monocropping production. This applies across the life span, and also to the chronic effects that have barely been studied.

• Ergonomic stressors in relation to musculoskeletal disorders, including the impact of bearing heavy weight at different ages and the effects across the life span and life cycle with regard to degenerative osteoarthritic problems.

• Respiratory damage, notably from chronic bronchitis, and reduced lung function across the life span.

• Appropriateness of occupational exposure limits given gender and the multiplicity of other environmental stressors.

• The mental health impact of psychosocial stressors that are related to work and environment. In particular, an examination of the physiological, psychological, and social effects of chronic fatigue arising from the intensity and duration of overwork is required.

• Validation of many routinely used developed country measures (Nell et al.; 1993) for wider application across cultures and across settings (informal versus formal sectors). Many invalid assumptions are made about the utility of research measures across cultures. This is more obvious for neuropsychologic measures, but it applies equally to questionnaires, respiratory function measurements (Myers, 1984), and other seemingly more objective measures (Bachmann et al., 1992).

• Research needed to inform public health policy. Only limited work has been done for developing countries generally (Christiani et al., 1990), for Africa (Khogali, 1982; Levy, 1992a,b; Myers and Macun, 1992), and for women (McGowan and Leslie, 1990).

In addition, it is important in these studies to investigate interactions between exposures related to productive work, the physiologic work of reproduction, and other general determinants of women's health status such as nutrition, anemia, and physical size.

REFERENCES

Adebe, M. 1991. Organophosphate pesticide poisoning in 50 Ethiopian patients. Ethiop. Med. J. 29(3):109–118.

Anyinam, C. A. 1991. Transboundary movements of hazardous wastes: The case of toxic waste dumping in Africa. Intl. J. Hlth. Serv. 21(4):759–777.

Asogwa, S. E. 1988. The health benefits of mechanization at the Nigerian Coal Corporation. Accid. Anal. Prevent. 20(2):103–108.

Bachmann, O. M., J. E. Myers, and B. N. Bezuidenhout. 1992. Quantitative vibration sense testing in workers exposed to acrylamide monomer. Am. J. Indust. Med. 21:217–222.

Bukh, J. 1980. Women in subsistence production in Ghana. Pp. 18–20 in Effects of the Penetration of the Market on Rural Women's Work. Geneva: International Labour Office.

Burger, E. 1990. Rehabilitation of mine injuries. Nursing RSA 5(3):18–21.

Chinemana, F. A. 1985. Effect of work on health—community perceptions in Zimbabwe. J. R. Soc. Hlth. 105(6):216–218.

Christiani, D. C., R. Durvasula, and J. Myers. 1990. Occupational health in developing countries: Review of research needs. Am. J. Indust. Med. 17:393–401.

Cooper, D., W. M. Pick, J. E. Myers, M. Hoffman, and J. M. L. Klopper. 1990. A study of the effects of urbanization on the health of women in Khayelitsha, Cape Town: Rationale and Methods. Department of Community Health, Working Paper No. 1, University of Cape Town.

Cooper, D., W. Pick, J. E. Myers, M. H. Hoffman, A. R. Sayed, and J. M. L. Klopper. 1991. Urbanization and women's health in Khayelitsha—Demographic and socio-economic profile. S. Afr. Med. J. 79:423–427.

Davies, J. C. A. 1993. Occupational lung disease. S. Afr. Med. J. 83(1):64.

de Soto, H. 1989. The Other Path. New York: Harper & Row.

Doll, R. 1992. Health and the environment in the 1990s. Public Health Policy Forum. Am. J. Pub. Hlth. 82(7):933–940.

Doyal, L. 1990. Health at home and in waged work: Part two. Waged work and women's well-being. Women's Stud. Int. Forum 13(6):587–604.

Fagley, R. M. 1976. Easing the burden of women: A 16-hour workday. Assign. Child. 36:9–28.

Felix, M. S., Z. M. Mabitjela, L. Roodt, A. W. J. Carlin, and M. Steinberg. 1990. Aftermath of asbestos mining—health effects of fibers in the environment. In Proceedings of the First International Union for Air Pollution Prevention Associations Regional Conference of Air Pollution, Paper 81, CSIR Pretoria, 2.

Geddes, R. G. 1990. Rehabilitation services for mining injuries. Nursing RSA 5(2):10–13.

Gitonga, L. 1991. Women in African agriculture. Afr. News. Occup. Hlth. Saf. 2:52–53.

Grobbelaar, J. P., and E. D. Bateman. 1991. Hut lung: a domestically acquired pneumoconiosis of mixed aetiology in rural women. Thorax 46:334–340.

Haimanot, R. T., Y. Kidane, E. Wuhib, A. Kalissa, T. Alemu, Z. A. Zein, and P. S. Spencer. 1990. Lathyrism in rural northwestern Ethiopia: A highly prevalent neurotoxic disorder. Int. J. Epidemiol. 19(3):664–672.

Hall, E. M. 1990. Women's Work: An Inquiry into the Health Effects of Invisible and Visible Labor. Baltimore, Md.: The Johns Hopkins University Press.

Hall, E. M. 1992. Double exposure: The combined impact of the home and work environments on psychosomatic strain in Swedish women and men. Int. J. Hlth Serv. 22(2):239–260.

Hicks, A. 1987. Review of accidents happening to employees of a metropolitan bus company in Kenya. E. Afr. Med. J. 64(1):3016.

Institute of Occupational Health Information Office. 1986. International Symposium on Health and Environment in Developing Countries. Section 1: Occupational health and chemical safety. Helsinki.

ILO (International Labour Office). 1987. Ergonomics in Developing Countries: An International Symposium. Geneva.

Jinadu, M. K. 1987. Occupational health and safety in a newly industrializing country. J. R. Soc. Hlth. 107(1):8–10.

Jinadu, M. K. 1990. A case-study of accidents in a wood processing industry in Nigeria. W. Afr. J. Med. 9(1):63–68.

Karasek, R. A., Jr. 1979. Job demands, job decision latitude and mental strain: Implications for job redesign. Administr. Sci. Q. 24.

Kaseje, D. C., E. K. Sempwebwa, and H. C. Spencer. 1987. Malaria chemoprophylaxis to pregnant women provided by the community health workers in Saradidi, Kenya. I. Reasons for non-acceptance. Ann. Trop. Med. Parasitol. 81 (Suppl.) (1):77–82.

Kerven, Izzard. 1989. How poor women earn income in Sub-Saharan Africa and what works against them. World Devel. 17(7):953–963.

Khogali, M. 1982. A new approach for providing occupational health services in developing countries. Scand. J. Work Environ. Hlth. 8(1):152–156.

Klugman, B., and R. Weiner. 1992. Women's health status in South Africa. Centre for Health Policy Women's Health Project, paper 28, Department of Community Health, University of the Witwatersrand, Johannesburg.

Lado, C. 1992. Female labor participation in agricultural production and the implications for nutrition and health in rural Africa. Soc. Aci. Med. 34(7):789–807.

LaDou, J. 1992. Occupational health issues: An international observatory. Transfer of dangerous technology to developing countries. Ramazzini News 1:81–90.

Landrigan, P. J. 1992. Commentary: Environmental disease, a preventable epidemic. Am. J. Pub. Hlth. 82(7)941–943.

Leger, J. P., and R. S. Arkles. 1989. Permanent disability in black mineworkers. A critical analysis. S. Afr. Med. J. 86(10):557–561.

Lerer, L. B. 1992. Women, homicide and alcohol in Cape Town, South Africa. Forensic Sci. Intl. 55:93–99.

Levin, P. J., L. J. Klaff, A. G. Rose, and A. D. Ferguson. 1979. Pulmonary effects of contact exposure to paraquat: a clinical and experimental study. Thorax 34: 150–160.

Levy, B. S. 1992a. Ongoing research in occupational health and environmental epidemiology in developing countries. Arch. Environ. Hlth. 47(3):231–235.

Levy, B. S. 1992b. Occupational health policy issues in Kenya: Considerations for other less developed countries. New Solutions 3(1):55–60.

London, L. 1992. Agrichemical hazards in the South African farming sector. S. Afr. Med. J. 81:560–564.

London, L., G. Joubert, S. I. Manjra, and L. B. Krause. 1992a. Compensatability and contact dermatitis in the canning industry. S. Afr. Med. J. 81:615–617.

London, L., G. Joubert, S. I. Manjra, and L. B. Krause. 1992b. Dermatoses in the canning industry—the roles of glove use and non-occupational exposures. S. Afr. Med. J. 81:612–614.

London, L., G. Joubert, S. I. Manjra, and L. B. Krause. 1992c. Dermatoses—an occupational hazard in the canning industry. S. Afr. Med. J. 81:606–612.

Lukmanji, Z. 1992. Women's workload and its impact on their health and nutritional status. Prog. Food Nutri. Sci. 16(2):163–179.

McGowan, L. A., and J. Leslie. 1990. The linkages between women's work, women's health and economic change: A conceptual framework with implications for policy and research. Paper presented the conference on The Dynamics of Women's Work, Women's Health and Economic Change in West Africa, International Center for Research on Women, Cotonou, Benin, July 23–25, 1990.

McLarty, D. G., L. Kinabo, and A. B. Swai. 1990. Diabetes in tropical Africa: A prospective study, 1981–1987. II. Course and prognosis. Br. Med. J. 300(6732):1107–1110.

McSweeney, B. G. 1979. Collection and analysis of data on rural women's time use. Stud. Fam. Plan. 10:379–383.

Myers, J. 1984. Differential ethnic standards for lung functions, or one standard for all? S. Afr. Med. J. 65: 768–772.

Myers, J. E. 1989. Respiratory health of brickworkers in Cape Town, South Africa: appropriate dust exposure indicators and permissible exposure limits. Scand. J. Work Envir. Hlth. 15(3):198–202.

Myers, J., and I. Macun. 1992. Strategy and policy for occupational health regulation in South Africa. Pp. 189–212 in Protecting Workers' Health in the Third World: National and International Strategies, M. R. Reich and T. Okuba, eds. New York: Auburn House.

Myers, J. E., J. Aron, and I. A. Macun. 1987. Asbestos and asbestos-related disease: The South African Case. Int. J. Hlth. Serv. 17(4):651–666.

Naimi, T. S. 1991. Women and their work: Health risks and realities in Zimbabwe. National Social Security Authority and Zimbabwe Congress of Trade Unions, Harare. Photocopy.

National Commission on Self-Employed Women and Women in the Informal Sector. 1988. Report. New Delhi: Jain.

National Workshop on Health and Safety of Women at the Workplace in Zimbabwe. 1988. Proceedings. Report by the Department of Community Medicine, University of Zimbabwe Medical School, the Ministries of Labour, Manpower Planning, and Social Welfare and the Zimbabwe Congress of Trade Unions, Harare. Photocopy.

Nell, V., J. Myers, M. Colvin, and D. Rees. 1993. Neuropsychological assessment of organic solvent effects in South Africa: Test selection, adaptation, scoring and validation issues. Environ. Res. 63:301–318.

Odelowo, E. O. 1991. The problem of trauma in Nigeria. Pattern as seen in a multicentre study. Trop. Geograph. Med. 43(1–2):80–84.

Olumide, Y. 1987a. Contact dermatitis in Nigeria II. Hand dermatitis in men. Con. Derm. 17(3):136–138.

Olumide, Y. 1987b. Contact dermatitis in Nigeria I. Hand dermatitis in women. Con. Derm. 17(2):85–88.

Packard, R. M. 1989a. Industrial production, health and disease in Sub-Saharan Africa. Soc. Sci. Med. 28(5):475–496.

Packard, R. M. 1989b. White Plague, Black Labor. Berkeley and Los Angeles: University of California Press.

Raikes, A. 1989. Women's health in East Africa. Soc. Sci. Med. 28(5):447–459.

Rantanen, J. 1992. Development of an occupational health and safety program in Third World countries. Pp. 15–40 in Protecting Workers' Health in the Third World, M. R. Reich and T. Okubo, eds. New York: Auburn House.

Savane, M. A. 1980. Women and rural development in Africa. Pp. 26–32 in Women in Rural Development: Critical Issues. Geneva: International Labour Office.

Schilling, R., and N. Anderson. 1986. Occupational epidemiology in developing countries. Occup. Hlth. Saf. Austr. N. Zealand 2(6):468–478.

Schmauch, M. 1991. A fall from a fruit tree—a case for an orthopedist in Mozambique. Lakartidningen 88(4):234–235.

Sivard, R. L. 1985. Women: A World Survey. Washington, D.C.: World Priorities.

Standing, G. 1989. Global feminization through flexible labour. World Devel. 17(7):1077–1095.

UN (United Nations). 1991. The World's Women 1970–1990: Trends and Statistics. 1991 Social Statistics and Indicators Series K, No. 8. New York.

10

Tropical Infectious Diseases

Despite the growing importance of the chronic diseases in the developing world, the infectious and parasitic diseases are still paramount, and the high proportion of deaths in all age groups in the Sub-Saharan African region attributed to them is striking. These diseases account for one-quarter to one-third of the deaths of young adults in the region and figure prominently in Sub-Saharan Africa's persistently high levels of adult mortality, as well as its large burdens of disability. A number of these infections also play a crucial direct or indirect etiologic role in the genesis of some cancers that are of substantial epidemiologic significance in the Sub-Sahara, as well as in the etiology of rheumatic heart disease, hypertension, and diabetes (Feachem and Jamison, 1991; Ofosu-Amaah, 1991; these associations are discussed in Chapter 7).

There were several sets of criteria that might have been used to select, categorize, and prioritize the diseases addressed in this chapter. Among these were other institutional priorities—for instance, the priorities of the WHO Special Programme for Research and Training in Tropical Diseases (TDR), etiologic similarities, and quantitative or qualitative differences in the effects of given diseases on females as compared with males. The final decision was to use the information generated by the WHO/World Bank assessment of the Global Burden of Disease (GBD) and to select and prioritize the diseases addressed here according to the size of their burden as measured in Disability-Adjusted Life Years (DALYs) (Murray and Lopez, 1994). The GBD estimates are based on an extensive analysis of disease-specific epidemiologic studies and all known population studies of mortality and disability available to the authors. As a consequence, the DALY provides a measure of comparability among these diseases that is particularly useful for this chapter.

The chapter discusses the selected diseases in the following order: malaria, schistosomiasis, African trypanosomiasis; trachoma; dracunculiasis; onchocerciasis and lymphatic filariasis; leishmaniasis and leprosy. Although dracunculiasis (Guinea worm disease) was not among the tropical diseases included in the GBD analysis, we considered it a disease of special programmatic interest for this study because it has a particularly deleterious impact on women, and has been targeted for global eradication by the end of 1995.

Table 10-1 presents the burden of infectious and parasitic diseases in males and females in Sub-Saharan Africa compared with males and females in the rest of the world. Diseases are listed in descending order of the size of the burden as measured in DALYs lost. Table 10-2 presents the burden of disease measured in DALYs for Sub-Saharan Africa by sex and age.

Of the tropical infectious diseases discussed in this chapter, five are life-threatening: malaria, schistosomiasis,

TABLE 10-1 Burden of Infectious and Parasitic Disease in Males and Females, Worldwide and in Sub-Saharan Africa, by Cause, 1990 (in hundreds of thousands of DALYs lost)

Disease	Sub-Saharan Africa		Worldwide	
	M	F	M	F
Malaria	161.0	154.1	182.3	175.0
"Tropical cluster"[a]	39.0	25.8	75.0	51.0
Schistosomiasis	23.1	11.8	29.9	15.4
Trypanosomiasis	9.0	8.8	9.0	8.8
Onchocerciasis	3.7	2.7	3.7	2.7
Trachoma	2.1	6.9	9.3	23.7
Leishmaniasis	1.9	2.0	12.0	8.6
Leprosy	1.2	1.1	5.1	5.1
Lymphatic filariasis	1.3	0.5	5.6	2.9

[a]Defined as including: trypanosomiasis, Chagas' disease, schistosomiasis, leishmaniasis, lymphatic filariasis, and onchocerciasis (Murray and Lopez, 1994). Malaria, leprosy, and trachoma are addressed separately in the Global Burden of Disease categorization.

SOURCE: Murray and Lopez, 1994.

African trypanosomiasis, onchocerciasis, and leishmaniasis. Even when episodes of these diseases do not proceed to mortality, they tend to generate considerable morbidity. This is also true for the other four, nonlethal, diseases addressed in this chapter. Thus, it is morbidity, or disability, that has the greatest weight in the total burden of these diseases as a group. Tables 10-3 and 10-4 disaggregate that burden, first in mortality, and second in disability (morbidity).

Finally, Table 10-5 summarizes the gender burden of the tropical infectious diseases in the same fashion as other topics have been presented in each of the chapters of this report: that is, subcategorized by the degree to which the burden of each disease is distinctive for females. Contemplated as a group, the tables indicate that, with little exception, males in Sub-Saharan Africa have higher overall burdens of tropical disease, with higher rates of both mortality and disability, than females experience in the region, although there is significant internal variation.

This general conclusion coincides with several perspectives in the literature that have become almost standard. The first is that the overall worldwide burden of premature mortality and morbidity is higher in males than it is in females, and male life expectancy is correspondingly lower.

The second perspective is that the only noteworthy distinctions between males and females in disease susceptibility and expression lie in their relationship with female reproductive function. One consequence of this viewpoint is that biomedical research on sex differences in infectious disease has focused mainly on that relationship, with emphasis on pregnancy and pregnancy outcomes, placental transmission, and maternally induced protection. Because of these emphases, research into the longitudinal impact of infectious diseases across the female life span, as well as the simultaneous and progressive interactions of those diseases with other maladies and conditions, has been deficient (Feldmeier and Krantz, 1992; Feldmeier et al., 1992; Vlassoff and Bonilla, 1994). Table 10-6, which presents a detailed analysis of the sequelae of the tropical infectious diseases across the female life span, makes it abundantly clear that such a narrow focus does not fit the facts.

The third perspective is that, with the exception of the role of the reproductive factor, any other differences in male/female mortality and disability rates are caused by variations in the nature and degree of exposure and in the social, economic, cultural, and personal factors that influence both exposure and the impact of a given disease (Brabin and Brabin, 1992; Bundy and Medley, 1992).

The present state of the scientific literature offers little justification for disagreeing with any of these perspectives, nor has it offered much basis for expecting either sex to be genetically more predisposed to communicable disease infection. Nevertheless, there is reason begin questioning this assumption. Analysis of the influence of

TABLE 10-2 Burden of Disease Measured in Disability-Adjusted Life Years, by Sex and Age, Sub-Saharan Africa, 1990 (DALYs, in thousands)

| Cause | Both Sexes, All Ages | Males (age group) | | | | | | Females (age group) | | | | | | Differential in Size of Burden, by Gender (%) |
		0–4	5–14	15–44	45–59	60+	All Ages	0–4	5–14	15–44	45–59	60+	All Ages	
Malaria	31,504	12,346	2,372	1,277	78	24	16,096	11,388	2,466	1,428	95	30	15,407	.3
Schistosomiasis	3,490	163	1,675	444	28	6	2,312	79	833	245	17	5	1,178	49.1
Dracunculiasis	—[a]	—	—	—	—	—	—		—	—	—	—	—	
Lymphatic filariasis	—	—	—	90	40	3	132	—	—	—	45	7	51	61.4
Onchocerciasis	641	—	4	176	124	66	370	—	3	128	94	47	272	26.5
African trypanosomiasis	1,782	51	395	362	82	9	899	94	356	371	57	5	883	1.8
Leprosy	227	9	93	9	2	3	116	9	86	10	3	4	111	
Trachoma	901	—	—	168	29	14	210	—	—	558	79		53	690
Leishmaniasis	583	13	186	90	1	—	219	12	188	91	2	—	292	

[a]No data.

SOURCE: Murray and Lopez, 1994.

TABLE 10-3 Estimated Deaths in Sub-Saharan Africa, by Sex and Age, 1990

Cause	Both Sexes	Males (age group)							All Ages	Both Sexes	Females (age group)							All Ages
		0-4	5-14	15-29	30-44	45-59	60-69	70+			0-4	5-14	15-29	30-44	45-59	60-69	70+	
Malaria	805.3	323.5	55.1	19.6	10.0	3.3	1.3	—[a]	413.6	213.2	—	57.5	20.9	13.6	4.1	1.5	1.5	391.7
Schistosomiasis	21.0	—	45.0	4.2	2.1	1.4	—	—	13.6	—	—	1.9	2.3	1.5	—	—	—	7.4
Trypanosomiasis	55.1	1.5	10.2	7.2	3.6	4.8	—	—	28.2	2.7	—	9.1	6.8	4.4	3.2	—	—	26.8
Trachoma	—	—	—	—	—	—	—	—	—	—	—	—	—	—	—	—	—	—
Onchocerciasis	29.1	—	—	2.7	1.4	6.1	4.8	2.4	17.3	—	—	—	1.9	1.2	4.6	2.1	1.7	12.4
Leishmaniasis	10.4	—	3.1	1.0	—	—	—	—	5.0	—	—	3.3	1.1	—	—	—	—	5.4
Leprosy	—	—	—	—	—	—	—	—	—	—	—	—	—	—	—	—	—	—
Lymphatic filariasis	—	—	—	—	—	—	—	—	—	—	—	—	—	—	—	—	—	—

[a] No data.

SOURCE: Murray and Lopez, 1994.

TABLE 10-4 Years Lived with a Disability in Sub-Saharan Africa, by Sex and Age, 1990 (YLDs in thousands)

Cause	Both Sexes, All Ages	Males (age group)						Females (age group)					
		0–4	5–14	15–44	45–59	60+	All Ages	0–4	5–14	15–44	45–59	60+	All Ages
Malaria	4,708	1,576	350	391	29	10	2,356	1,561	347	400	32	13	2,353
Schistosomiasis	2,887	148	1,510	255	2	—[a]	1,916	75	762	133	1	—	971
Dracunculiasis	—	—	—	—	—	—	—	—	—	—	—	—	—
Onchocerciasis	182	—	3	55	34	16	108	—	2	37	23	11	74
African trypanosomiasis	147	2	22	42	12	2	79	3	19	38	7	—	68
Leprosy	209	8	91	7	—	—	107	8	85	7	—	—	102
Trachoma	901	—	—	168	29	14	210	—	—	588	79	53	690
Leishmaniasis	228	2	72	45	—	—	119	2	68	39	—	—[a]	109

[a]No data

SOURCE: Murray and Lopez, 1994.

TABLE 10-5 Tropical Infectious Diseases Adversely Influencing Health in Sub-Saharan Africa: Gender-Related Burden

Problem	Exclusive to Females	Greater for Famales	Burden for Females and Males Comparable, but of Particular Significance for Females
Burkitt's lymphoma		X	
Dracunculiasis		X (pelvic infection)	X
Leishmaniasis			X (stigmatization)
Leprosy		X (in pregnancy)	X (stigmatization)
Malaria		X (in pregnancy)	X
Onchocerciasis			X (stigmatization)
Schistosomiasis		X (ages 15–44)	X
Trachoma	X (neonatal vulvovaginitis)		X
Trypanosomiasis		X (ages 0–4)	X

NOTE: "Significance" is defined here as having an impact on health that, for any reason—biological, reproductive, sociocultural, or economic—is different in its implications for females than for males.

cross-sex disease transmission on mortality suggests the tantalizing possibility that there may be differentials in susceptibility and disease intensity that are biologically based (Aaby, 1992), and not purely derivative of reproductive function.

Exploration of this possibility will demand a much more expansive research framework, since the questions it raises cover broad areas. For example: Are there are genetic, physiologic, or morphologic traits associated with gender that either exacerbate or attenuate disease in males or females? What might those be? How do any such differences vary by disease, and what mechanisms are involved (Aaby, 1992; Michelson, 1992)? Secondary questions would have to do with the ways those fundamental traits play out in mortality, morbidity, and chronic disability throughout either the male or female life span (Mosley and Gray, 1993). Another set of questions—very complicated questions—would have to do with the causal, synergistic, and cumulative roles of comorbidities, an area where research has just begun.

MALARIA

Malaria remains the most important and widespread of the tropical diseases, and levels of malaria transmission are higher in Sub-Saharan Africa than anywhere in the world (Bradley, 1991). The region accounts for over 80 percent of the 110 million clinical cases worldwide each year, 90 percent of the estimated 275 million people in the world who are infected carriers of the parasite, and most of the estimated one to two million deaths that malaria causes annually (Najera et al., 1993; WHO/TDR, 1991a). Yet, although there has been a vast amount of malariological research over the past century, the true magnitude of mortality and morbidity from the disease is still uncertain (Bradley, 1991). Since reporting from tropical Africa has been irregular and fragmentary, reported cases of malaria may represent only 2 to 20 percent of actual cases (Najera et al., 1993).

The disease is transmitted by four species of the parasitic protozoa *Plasmodium*: *P. falciparum, P. vivax, P. ovale, and P. malariae*, each with its own morphology, biology, and clinical characteristics (Miller, 1984). Of

TABLE 10-6 Biological Consequences of Tropical Infectious Diseases for Women[a]

Disease	Infancy/Childhood	Adolescence	Adulthood	Pregnancy
Malaria	*Infancy:* Females are disadvantaged. Fever, weakness, anemia, jaundice, splenomegaly, convulsion, vomiting, diarrhea.	Scant data, only available for pregnant adolescent girls. Clinical signs are similar to signs in childhood.	Anemia, weakness, splenomegaly. Other clinical signs appear to be similar to those in adolescence (more data available for pregnancy).	Hemolytic anemia, cerebral malaria, hypoglycemia, abortion, low birthweight babies, pulmonary edema, placental malaria.
Schistosomiasis				Genital tract involvement (GTI): bladder, ureter
S. haematobium	*Infancy:* Scant data. *Childhood:* Fever, hematuria, weakness, anemia, fatigue, weight loss, muscular pain. In addition, there is lower genital tract disease.	Hematuria, anemia, liver cirrhosis, obstructive uropathy, abortions, delayed menarche, poor growth, delayed puberty, decreased work capacity.	*S. haematobium:* Genital tract involvement, anemia, liver cirrhosis, obstructive uropathy, abortions	*S. mansoni* (no report on GTI in Africa, intestinal polyposis).
S. mansoni			*S. mansoni:* Portal hypertension, obstruction, ascites, gastrointestinal disruption, granulomas	*S. haematobium:* Cancer of the genital tract, bladder and liver; infertility.
Dracunculiasis	*Infancy:* No signs because of length of incubation period. *Childhood:* Blister, itching, severe incapacitation from blisters, Guinea worm ulcer and lesions, tetanus death (from secondary infection).	Blister, fever, localized pain, urticaria. Other symptoms similar to symptoms in childhood.	Severe incapacitation from blisters, depending on location. Tetanus, chronic arthritis (common in women).	Bleeding in pregnancy (rare).
Onchocerciasis	Severe and incessant pruritus, lack of sleep, presence of nodules. Lack of data on the impact of these on the health of the girl child.	Severe and incessant pruritus, loss of restful sleep, presbydermia (premature aging of the skin), ocular lesions, dermal atrophy (lizard skin), severe papular eruption (irreverible and disfiguring lesion).	Blindness (common in savanna), weight loss, poor nutrition status, joint and muscular pains and abscesses, severe dermal atrophy (lizard skin), leopard skin, severe and incessant pruritus, loss of restful sleep, presbydermia (premature aging of the skin).	Exacerbation of skin lesions. Other symptoms in nonpregnant adult women persist and are often exacerbated in pregnancy.

Trypanosomiasis	*T. gambiense:* *Infancy:* Low birthweight, somnolence, fever, hepatosplenomegaly, fetal wastage. *Childhood:* Fever, headache, normochromic anaemia, skin rash, neurologic symptoms, severe mental retardation, death.	Scant data on adolescent females for both types of trypanosomiasis.	*T. gambiense:* Organic dementia, tremors, hypertension *T. rhodesiense:* Early stage fever tremor, hepatocellular jaundice, debility, mild–severe anemia, myocardial involvement.	*T. gambiense:* Increased susceptibility to intrauterine infection, abortion, or sleep and depression, generalized immune depression, cerebral edema.
Trachoma	Maximum active disease.	Repeated infections.	Scarring, disfigurement, blindness.	Pneumonitis, neonatal vulvovaginitis, inclusion conjunctivitis, ophthalmia.
Leishmaniasis	High rate of acquisition.	High rate of acquisition.	High rate of acquisition, severe disfigurement.	
Leprosy	Low birthweight, poor growth, increased susceptibility to infection.	Poor growth, increased susceptibility to infection.	Loss of asymptomatic status/ reactivation/relapse/in pregnancy; nerve damage, blindness.	Reactivation/relapse/nerve damage in pregnancy; impaired placental function.

[a]There are few data on the biological and social consequences of these tropical diseases for postmenopausal and elderly women in Sub-Saharan Africa. For this reason, no separate column has been created for these life span stages.

these, it is *P. falciparum*, the most dangerous, that predominates in Sub-Saharan Africa, followed in frequency by *P. malariae* and *P. ovale* (Miller, 1984). The disease is transmitted through the bite of certain species of mosquitoes of the genus *Anopheles*, which, in Sub-Saharan Africa, includes *An. gambiae* and *An. funestus*, two of the three most efficient malaria vectors in the world. The bite of the female anopheline starts a process of inoculation, proliferation, and red blood cell invasion that, in the case of *P. falciparum*, generates a distinctive pattern of clinical symptoms. It is the high parasitemia of *P. falciparum* that leads to the splenomegaly, severe anemia, renal failure, and cerebral malaria that produce the severe morbidity and mortality associated with this form of the disease.

Malaria in Children

Mortality and morbidity from malaria are highest in infants and in children under age 5. Malaria morbidity accounts for 10 to 80 percent of childhood fevers, for approximately 30 to 35 percent of all presenting cases recorded at the rural dispensaries in the savanna areas of Sub-Saharan Africa (Bradley, 1991), and from 10 to 30 percent of all infant and child deaths in the region (Najera et al., 1993).

Very few malaria studies present data disaggregated by gender, and this has certainly not been done in any extensive or reliable way. This is largely true for all the tropical diseases, and results from the lack of sensitivity to the possibility of gender-specific differences in disease outcomes mentioned above (Vlassoff and Bonilla, 1994) and, in the case of malaria, from overall methodological confusion (Bradley, 1991).

Malaria studies that have produced gender-specific data present a somewhat blurred picture of gender variation in childhood. Two such studies report higher parasite prevalence and densities in infant girls and female children under age 4 (Hendrickse et al., 1971; McGregor, 1964). A third study, from the well-documented and well-executed Garki project in Nigeria, reported prevalence and parasite density rates in male and female children under age 4 that were approximately the same, and rates in females from age 5 years onward that were lower than rates for males of the same ages (Molineaux and Gramiccia, 1980). The more recent GBD data report a DALY burden for males from birth through age 4 that is higher than it is in females, a difference that arises primarily from higher mortality in infant males than in females of the same cohort. Still, the male burden is only about 10 percent higher than the burden for females, and it is succeeded by a shift to a greater burden in females in all subsequent age cohorts (Murray and Lopez, 1994). On the basis of the Garki data, Reubin (1992) has concluded that females are not intrinsically more susceptible to malaria than males, and may actually mount a stronger antibody response. Apart from pregnancy, Reubin attributes any gender differences in malaria infection to a simple differential in exposure. Because the sex difference among all children ages 0 to 4 years is not dramatically large, however, and the female burden overtakes that of males beginning at age 5, well before pregnancy is a factor, any hypothesized female advantage is at least open to question.

Some of the best longitudinal data on malaria prevalence during childhood come from a series of studies in The Gambia, where the disease is hyperendemic and prevalence of falciparum malaria is close to 100 percent throughout childhood, declining gradually through adolescence into adulthood (McGregor and Smith, 1952). Longitudinal mortality data from the same study series show acute malaria exerting its maximum impact during the first and second years of life, when the transient passive placental immunity and levels of antibody titers against falciparum malaria have diminished; the sequelae of the disease during this period are disrupted growth patterns and anemia (McGregor et al., 1956). Morbidity over the longer period from birth to age 5 includes severe anemia; cerebral malaria; and damage to liver, spleen, and kidney, all of which have potential for progressing to mortality. For survivors, the disease appears to have negative effects on growth rates and on mental and motor development. Study of the sequelae of malaria for child development and performance does not seem to be extensive (Pollitt, 1990; UNESCO, 1989), but preschoolers with iron-deficiency anemia, a known sequela of malaria, repeatedly record lower test scores (Levinger, 1992).

Malaria in Adolescent and Adult Females

If females do have any relative advantage in parasite clearance during early childhood, it surely disappears

TABLE 10-7 Prevalence of Malaria (Placental Infection or Parasitemia) among Women in Africa, by Parity at Delivery

Area	Prevalence PG[a]	Percentage MG[b]	Number Examined
West Nigeria	20.2	11.2	451
Nigeria (Ilesha)	62.5	25.3	392
East Nigeria	36.4	16.3	575
Uganda (Kampala)	21.7	14.7	570
Tanzania (Muheza)	37.0	33.0	413
Côte d'Ivoire (Abidjan)	55.0	36.2	192
Gambia, The (rural)	59.1	35.2	1,000[c]
Gambia, The (Banjul)	15.7	8.8	2,765
(Provinces)	46.7	20.4	3,194
Gambia, The (Keneba)	64.0	26.3	532
Nigeria (Lagos)	40.0	8.0	230
Zaire (urban and rural)	38.0	15.0	291

NOTE: All data were collected in hospitals and health clinics. Details on antimalarial therapies/prophylaxis were generally not reported.

[a]PG = Primigravidas.
[b]MG = Multigravidas.
[c]Antenatal parasite prevalence.

SOURCE: Brabin, 1991.

with the onset of the reproductive years, when the changes in immune status that accompany pregnancy dramatically increase female susceptibility to malaria, notably falciparum malaria (McGregor, 1983). A recent study in Nigeria of the prevention and treatment of malaria among 45 pregnant adolescents (mean age, 17.5 years) and a control group of 47 nonpregnant girls of comparable ages found the incidence of malaria parasitemia, anemia, and fever episodes in the study group to be significantly higher (Okonofua et al., 1992). This vulnerability can be especially unfortunate in this early reproductive age group, whose members display low rates of utilization of hospital-level treatment services and health center antenatal care programs.

It is because of this heightened maternal susceptibility, as well as the threat malaria represents for fetal development and survival, that research emphasis on malaria in Sub-Saharan African females has concentrated on its effects on reproductive status, processes, and outcomes. This has provided a window to a better understanding of the functioning of the disease in general, as well as gender-specific understanding that is atypical of most tropical disease research. Nevertheless, questions around differential female burden rates in the nonreproductive years remain unanswered. Because of the behavior of the vector and its complex epidemiology, there is no immediately obvious explanation for these gender differences.

The risks of complications of malaria in pregnancy vary in individual women and appear to be dependent on two factors: parity and maternal immune status. Recrudescence of preexisting malarial infection, placental infection, and frequency of low birthweight infants are all more common in primigravidae than in multigravidae (Hendrickse, 1987), and rates of low birthweights brought about by malaria among primigravidae are particularly high, ranging from 9 to 40 percent (Brabin, 1985; see Tables 10-7 and 10-8). The marked effect of malaria in primiparous women is thought to be the result of "evasion" of host immunity by the parasite (McGregor, 1983) or depressed maternal immunity during the first pregnancy (Brabin, 1985; Oaks et al., 1991).

Of the two factors, it is immune function that appears to be pivotal in the evolution and impact of malaria during pregnancy, and in the higher parasite rates and densities in pregnant women in general. Because of the suppression of cellular immunity in pregnancy, latent malaria has the tendency to develop into acute, overt attacks in pregnant women, with more serious complications than is the case in nonpregnant women. Mortality from

TABLE 10-8 Incidence of Malaria Infection among
570 African Women

Group	Number	Positive	Percentage
Mothers	579	32	5.6
Placentas	570	92	16.1
Neonates	569[a]	1	0.2

[a]One died one hour after birth.

SOURCE: Jelliffe, 1992.

TABLE 10-9 Weights of Female Neonates with Infected and
Noninfected Placentas, by Birth Rank (in grams)

Birth Rank	Infected	Noninfected	Difference
1	2,497 (10)	2,843 (39)	345
2	2,869 (12)	2,933 (33)	64
3	3,074 (11)	3,039 (52)	35
4	2,790 (8)	3,142 (42)	352
5	2,978 (3)	3,061 (31)	83
6	2,721 (7)	3,210 (36)	489

NOTE: Values in parentheses represent the number of subjects in each group.

SOURCE: Jelliffe, 1992.

cerebral malaria during pregnancy has been estimated at 40 percent, and rates of hypoglycemia and pulmonary edema are as high or higher (White and Darrell, 1988). In a study of cellular immune responses to *plasmodium falciparum* antigens in adults in The Gambia, Riley and colleagues (1988) found women of reproductive age (18–45 years) to be less immunologically responsive than men in the same age group, a phenomenon attributed in other studies to suppression of lymphoproliferative responses to the falciparum antigen.

In sum, the nature of the involvement of pregnancy in immunosuppression related to malaria infection remains at the level of theory, and its pathophysiology is still puzzling. Results of studies of *Plasmodium berghei* immunity in pregnant mice (Van Zon et al., 1982) and the higher serum cortisol levels encountered in Tanzanian women with patent malaria infection during pregnancy (Vleugels et al., 1987) have suggested that loss of cell-mediated immunity during pregnancy might be cortisol-related. What is also puzzling is that massive malarial infection can be present in placental blood, even when only a few parasites can be found in the peripheral blood of the mother. The human placenta appears to offer a particularly suitable environment for malaria parasites (Bray and Anderson, 1979; Covell, 1950), with peak frequency and severity of parasitemia at between weeks 13 and 16 of gestation (Brabin, 1985) (see Table 10-9).

The widely held view among Sub-Saharan African women that malaria is responsible for spontaneous abortions, stillbirths, and miscarriages, as well as many other health problems during pregnancy (Kaseje, et al., 1987), is correct. Several studies from Africa have found maternal malaria during pregnancy to be associated with low birthweight (Brabin, 1991; Jelliffe, 1992) and a recent set of hospital and community studies in central Sudan by Taha, Gray, and colleagues (Taha et al., 1993) found significant associations between a maternal history of malaria and low birthweight, a higher risk of low birthweight among primiparous women compared with multiparous women, and increased risk of neonatal mortality associated with malaria during pregnancy. The study also suggests that maternal malaria significantly increases the risk of stillbirth, at least for infections during the first two trimesters. Because malaria treatment, chemoprophylaxis, and use of insecticides are known to decrease the risk of low birthweight, the study authors recommend them as appropriate interventions that should target primigravid women and be initiated early in pregnancy (Taha et al., 1993).

Malaria leads to low birthweight either by premature delivery or by impaired growth *in utero*, because it provides the opportunity for parasites (especially *P. falciparum*) to invade the fetus itself or to impair placental function (McGregor, 1983). Birthweights of female babies born to mothers with infected placentas tend to be significantly lower than birthweights of female babies of noninfected controls. Maternal hematocrits of less than 50 percent are known to be highly correlated with retardation of fetal growth (Harrison, 1976; Harrison and Ibeziako, 1973), and malaria heads a list of causes of anemia in pregnancy, which also includes iron and folate deficiencies, sickle-cell disease, and HIV/AIDS (Fleming, 1989). A likely scenario is that there are synergies among these conditions, as well as between each of them and other parasitic infections (such as schistosomiasis). Anemia in women of reproductive age in Sub-Saharan Africa tends to be multifactorial, reflecting interaction among different causal variables, including comorbidities, malnutrition and malabsorption, and depressed immunity.

Another element of interaction with malaria that could have special programmatic relevance is seasonality. Brabin (1991) has observed seasonal variations in parasite rates in pregnant women, citing six studies from four African countries that reported higher parasite rates in the wet season than in the dry season (see Table 10-10). Her analysis is that since parasitemia persists through the dry season, primigravidas delivering in the late part of the wet season or the early part of the dry season would be at greatest risk for low birthweight, not only because they are primigravidae, but also because they have been, in effect, at risk for malaria throughout most of their pregnancy. Requirements for folate are higher in pregnancy, especially during the last trimester; when hemolysis from malaria stimulates erythroid hyperplasia, demand for folate mounts. When this demand is unmet, the result is the megaloblastic erythropoiesis that is seen in up to 75 percent of severely anemic pregnant women in West Africa.

TABLE 10-10 Parasite Rates in Pregnant Women in the Wet and Dry Seasons (percent)

Area	Parasite Rate		Comment	Number
	Wet	Dry		
Sierra Leone	38.7	22.2	First attendance	1,345
Nigeria (Zaria)	29.8	20.1	First attendance < 24 wks gestation	228
(Asexual forms)	19.2	9.7	(Gametocytes)	
Nigeria (Ibadan)	10.2	8.6	Adego State Hospital and Osegor Health Centre (Placenta)	1,085
Gambia, The (rural)	27.6	26.4	Placental blood	3,500
Senegal	48.8	7.3	First attendance Urban Dakar	866
Senegal	24.1	8.8	Urban Thies (Blood)	444
	7.2	5.2	(Placenta)	443

SOURCE: Brabin, 1991.

Megaloblastic anemia is common at the end of the dry season and during the rainy season because of the heightened prevalence and severity of malaria and consequent iron and folate deficiencies (Fleming et al., 1968). Thus, it would appear that the principal morbidity deriving from malaria during pregnancy may not be from parasite densities *per se*, but rather from the combined effect of persistent parasitemia coupled with the iron and folate deficiencies that are common during the dry season. If this conclusion is correct, it has useful implications for program interventions.

There are interactions of malaria with other conditions that might also merit research attention. Malaria infection has been implicated in three disease syndromes common in Sub-Saharan Africa: Burkitt's lymphoma, quartan malarial nephrotic syndrome, and hyperreactive tropical malarious splenomegaly. There may be some gender-specific differences in the role of malaria in the etiology of Burkitt's lymphoma, a tumor that occurs in areas of Africa that are hyperendemic for *P. falciparum*, and is believed to be an atypical response to Epstein-Barr virus infection. An epidemiologic study in Uganda over the 10-year period between 1959 and 1968 showed median age of onset of lymphoma for both sexes to be under 8 years, but found higher incidence in females under age 5. This may simply be an artifact of differences in prevalence of malaria in the same population, because by the age of 15, the incidence of lymphoma had become higher in males than in females of the same age. Nonetheless, the association has been interesting enough to have evoked research activity that could throw some light on malaria pathology and epidemiology. Hints of some gender differentials in the experience of these syndromes also come from literature outside Africa: Brabin and Brabin (1988) found higher spleen rates in women than in men in Papua New Guinea, where moderate to severe cases of hyperreactive malarious splenomegaly have been reported. There is also some evidence that HIV infection may diminish female capacity, particularly in pregnancy, to control falciparum parasitemia, notably placental infection, with resulting poor fetal growth (Brabin and Brabin, 1992).

SCHISTOSOMIASIS (BILHARZIASIS)

Often referred to as "blood flukes," worms of the genus *Schistosoma* comprise several blood parasites of humans and other animals, of which the three most important are *S. hematobium*, *S. mansoni*, and *S. japonicum*. Each has a slightly different pathway through the human body, and thus produces different patterns of morbidity and mortality. In the case of *S. hematobium*, the pathway is skin, to lungs, to bladder/ureters, with associated hematuria, dysuria, renal failure, and increased risk of cancer of the bladder. The final destination for *S. japonicum* and *S. mansoni* is the human liver, and the sequelae are hepatomegaly, splenomegaly, bleeding esophageal varices, and *cor pulmonale*.

The global area endemic for the three major human schistosomes includes 79 countries with an estimated total population of 3 billion, or approximately 90 percent of the estimated 1980 population of the developing countries (Mahmoud, 1984). Using a prevalence estimate of 21 percent (Iarotski and Davis, 1981), the population at risk in the endemic countries totals approximately 600 million. Current morbidity is estimated at 200 million individuals infected worldwide. Unlike other helminthic infections, which generate mild to severe disability, schistosomiasis produces a substantial burden of mortality, with over 200,000 deaths annually (CDC, 1993; WHO/TDR, 1991a; Walsh, 1990). *S. mansoni* is endemic in much of West and East Africa, overlapping throughout most of that area with *S. hematobium*, whose range extends further to the northeast and southwest. The distribution of both parasites encompasses the limited foci of another schistosome, *S. intercalatum*, in Central and West Africa (Warren et al., 1993).

Schistosomal infection and the patterns of its transmission in endemic communities are powerfully influenced by ecological factors. Thus, there can be considerable variation in disease prevalence and intensity over quite short distances, and the sizes of transmission foci can be quite small (Warren, 1973). The relatively limited sizes of transmission sites, their individual characteristics as habitats for the snail intermediate host, and their proximity to homesteads affect not only the distribution of disease, but also the magnitude of the role of gender in the acquisition and spread of infection. In addition, certain seasons encourage formation of new foci of transmission, and ecological change produced by human activity is a common cause of these new foci.

There are several factors that govern the outcome of the transmission process in endemic areas: a small proportion of snails are infected at any one time, they shed at specific times of the day, cercariae (the infective stage of the parasite) are dispersed in huge bodies of water, and they have limited effective duration of infectivity. Human exposure, susceptibility, and resulting parasite densities respond in some degree to patterns of contact that fit those transmission characteristics (Mahmoud, 1984).

Prevalence and intensity of infection in areas where schistosomiasis is endemic show a characteristic relationship to age and sex (Chandiwana and Christensen, 1988). In most circumstances, both prevalence and intensity (measured by egg count) increase gradually to peak at approximately 10 to 19 years of age, with females in some endemic communities showing slightly less prevalence and intensity than males (Mahmoud, 1984). A cross-sectional study in Machakos, Kenya, identified the pattern of variation more precisely: peak prevalence (98 percent) was found in the age group 10-19 years, with a diminution to 70 percent in older cohorts, and highest egg densities (1,026 eggs/g) were identified in females ages 10-14 and in males ages 20–24 (1,019 eggs/g) (Arap Siongok et al., 1976). Prevalence decreases only moderately by the beginning of the third decade of life, but egg counts decrease dramatically, so that the diagnostic pattern alters with increasing age. Some researchers see this as evidence for accrued immunity, others see changes in patterns of water contact as an equally logical explanation.

The epidemiology and morbidity of schistosomal infection depend on several factors: timing and duration of water contact and exposure, penetration of cercariae, and nutritional status. Of these, it is water contact that heads the list of human activities that determine the intensity of schistosomal infection (Jordan, 1972; Okafor, 1990; Warren, 1973). Although water-contact studies have been relatively few in number, and very few of those have disaggregated their data by gender, the studies that have been carried out have discerned clear patterns: infection rates vary by age and gender in ways that are directly related to water contact. Brabin and Brabin summarize the results of these studies in a recent review (1992) and find two distinct patterns: for males, activities requiring water contact taper off as they get older; for females, those requirements remain constant from early adolescence onward.

Schistosomiasis in Children

The burden of schistosomiasis begins early, because children born to and breastfed by *S. haemotobium*-infected mothers are already at risk of exposure to a circulating schistosome antigen (Camus et al., 1976; Mahmoud, 1984). Risk in communities endemic for *S. mansoni* is especially high. The presence of a thermostable parasite antigen—the "M" antigen—in the milk of mothers with *S. mansoni* infection and its possible transfer to nursing infants may mean that children born to mothers infected with *S. mansoni* will lose their capacity to respond to certain idiotype-induced regulatory stimuli, will be prone to develop hepatosplenic complications, and will be likely to have lower titers of anti-hepatitis B antigens after vaccination (Ghaffar et al., 1989; Santoro et al., 1977).

The role of protective immunity in the epidemiology of urinary schistosome infection is inconclusive (Warren, 1982; Wilkins et al., 1984), so that studies to examine tolerance or sensitization in uninfected children born to infected mothers could be important. Prenatal sensitization would seem to be especially important because it may modify hypersensitivity to both the worm and egg stages of the parasite, and that sensitivity will in turn determine the nature and extent of the morbidity produced by the infection (Warren, 1972).

The two main nutritional consequences of schistosomal infection for very young children are growth faltering and anemia, although other micronutrient deficiencies have been noted. Three channels lead from infection to growth faltering—anorexia, nutrient losses through malabsorption, and decreased nutrient use from impaired liver and spleen function.

Whatever the mechanism, a large and growing literature documents the substantial growth impairment from schistosomiasis (Warren et al., 1993). Given the young age at which the schistosomiasis burden begins to accrue, growth velocities are affected quickly and early. Studies in Kenya, Liberia, Nigeria, Tanzania, and Zimbabwe provide substantial case material to document a frank connection between *S. haematobium* infection and protein-energy malnutrition in children (cf. Burki et al., 1986).

Perhaps because gender roles are not yet as sharply delineated in childhood as they will be later in life, there is no clear picture of gender-related differences in prevalence and intensity of schistosomiasis infection in the early years. In two studies, prevalence was greater in males than in females (El Malatawy et al., 1992; Pugh and Gilles,

1976); in the latter, a study of urinary schistosomiasis, prevalence was four times greater in boys ages 5 to 15 than in girls of those same ages. Studies in Ethiopia also found prevalence declining with age and, again, peaking in the second decade of life, in this case between ages 10 and 14 (Teklehaimanot and Fletcher, 1990). Other studies in Ethiopia also reported increased susceptibility in young boys, adolescent girls, and women ages 15 to 34, and found a clear correlation with the amount of water contact (Hiatt, 1976; Polderman, 1974). Nonetheless, later studies in Mali and The Gambia found that infection rates in males and females were similar, despite apparent differences in exposure patterns (Brinkmann, et al., 1988; Wilkins et al., 1984).

To obscure the picture further, studies carried out in Nigeria found prevalence and intensity of *S. haemotobium* infection to be higher in females, with highest prevalence in the late teen years (Anya and Okafor, 1986). A more recent study in Zanzibar, which measured schistosome-related morbidity in children, found the highest incidences of uropathy and hematuria in girls between birth and age 4; boys had the lowest incidences at those same ages (Hatz et al., 1990). Limited data on seasonal variation in the prevalence and intensity of infection with *S. haematobium* among Gambian children under age 10 (Wilkins and Scott, 1978) suggest that seasonality might be a good place to look for more precise and consistent patterns of etiology.

Schistosomiasis and some other helminthic infections generate very high levels of morbidity in school-age children, but carry relatively low direct consequences for mortality. In the age group 5 to 14 years, the disease has been associated with growth retardation and decreased work capacity (Berkley and Jamison, 1991). Infected children often complain of abdominal pain and other manifestations of infection, including fever, weakness, lassitude, muscular pain, nausea, vomiting, diarrhea, and fatigue (Pollitt, 1990). Research on the effects of schistosomiasis on schooling is scant, but it is extremely likely that such school-related outcomes as academic achievement and school attendance are negatively influenced by schistosomiasis and that girls bear the most severe consequences (Levinger, 1992).

Similar factors—age of exposure, concurrent nutritional deficits, greater prevalence of malaria infection, and longer duration of schistosomal infection—are implicated in schistosomiasis-related morbidity in both school-age children and adolescents. In a study in Kenya, lack of reinfection in 30 percent of 119 school children one year after treatment was classified as resistance to reinfection rather than lack of exposure. Resistance to infection, the authors argued, was an acquired and age-dependent trait, not related to previous egg-induced pathology (Butterworth et al., 1985).

Schistosomiasis and the Adolescent Female

As indicated above, peak prevalence and intensity of urinary and intestinal schistosomiasis generally occur in adolescence—that is, during the second decade of life. By age 15, 37 percent of males and 53.1 percent of females in highly endemic areas in Nigeria (Anya and Okafor, 1986) had urinary schistosomiasis. Earlier observations in northwest Tanzania produced similar findings (Forsyth, 1969). Gender differences would appear to be role-related, since it is in adolescence that girls become more involved in the traditional female responsibilities of fetching water, washing clothing, and helping with agricultural tasks that combine to expose them to infective sites for longer periods than is the case for males.

Schistosomiasis also has severe effects on the female reproductive system, which become manifest in adolescence (see Table 10-11). Primary amenorrhea, delayed menarche, and other menstrual abnormalities have been attributed to ovarian schistosomiasis; later sequelae include risk of ectopic pregnancy, premature birth, and spontaneous abortion. The overall nutritional deficit has made anemia among adolescent females and younger girls of school age a standard feature in Sub-Saharan Africa; the synergy of undernutrition and schistosoma-related hematuria in endemic communities might be expected to generate even higher rates of anemia, but there are no studies that have quantified these putative effects either by gender or age.

Schistosomiasis in Adult Females

Until the advent of ultrasound techniques, egg counts and hematuria and proteinuria detection were the only measures of schistosomiasis-related morbidity (Mott, 1982). A review of these measures by Tanner (1989)

TABLE 10-11   Schistosomiasis and the Female Genital Tract

Organ	Findings	Symptoms, Sequelae	SH	SM	SI
Breast	Granulous, mimicking the mammographic pattern of carcinoma	None	+	0	0
Vulva (vestibule labia)	Ulceration with carcinomatous appearance; granulous, rapidly increasing in size	Irritation/pruritus, secondary infection, destruction of the external meatus	+++	+	0
Vagina, vaginal fornices	Polypoidal granulomas, papillo-matous growth; vesico-vaginal fistulas	Fibrosis	+++	+	0
		Incontinence	+	+	0
Cervix	Erosion, ulceration, polypoidal granuloma, papillomatous growth	Fibrosis; bloody discharge, dyspareunia, intermenstrual bleeding	+++	+	0
Uterus	Endometritis	Lower abdominal pain; menstrual irregularities, menorrhagia	+++	+	0
Fallopian tubes	Salpingitis, granulomas	Chronic backache, lower abdominal pain, dysmenorrhea, menstrual irregularities, sterility, ectopic pregnancy	+++	+	0
Ovaries	Oophoritis	Delayed menarche, primary menorrhea, menstrual irregularity, sterility	+++	+	0

NOTE: + = proven, but rare, +++ = proven, common, 0 = not proven or no data, SH = *S. haematobium*, SI = *S. intercalortium*, and SM = *S. mansoni*.

SOURCE: Feldmeier and Krantz, 1992.

concluded that while examination for hematuria is a reliable and sensitive morbidity indicator, egg count reliability is questionable because of the high day-to-day variability in egg excretion.

The most significant morbidity effects from schistosomal infection are urinary tract sequelae, including calcification in the lower tract, vesico-ureteric reflux, and hydronephrosis from *S. hematobium*. *S. mansoni* infection produces gastrointestinal sequelae, including large gastrointestinal granulomas, obstruction, ascites, esophageal varices, fibrosis, and portal hypertension.

Diagnosis of urinary tract pathology is particularly difficult because of several confounding factors in females: menstruation, since both hematuria and leukocyturia may be complicated by menstrual bleeding; pregnancy, since ultrasound detection may be confounded during that period; and ovarian changes at any point in the life span (Poggensee, 1992).

While schistosomiasis is debilitating for both adult males and females, the complications of chronic disease—including anemia, genital involvement, hepatosplenomegaly, and obstructive uropathy—affect women of reproductive age most severely. Several studies (McMeeley et al., 1988; Parker, 1992) note that, as in the case of malaria, pregnancy is a time of particular vulnerability both to schistosomal infection and the troublesome sequelae that derive from the disease; the condition is thus, by definition, one of high risk. Pregnancy is, however, not the only time of risk: the ova of *S. hematobium* may migrate to the female genital tract at any time, and frequently do; potential sequelae are sterility; infertility; and, later in life, cancer.

AFRICAN TRYPANOSOMIASIS

An estimated 25,000 new cases of African trypanosomiasis occur each year, there are an estimated 20,000 trypanosomiasis-related deaths annually, and approximately 50 million individuals in 36 Sub-Saharan African countries are at risk of infection (WHO/TDR, 1991a). Of the six major parasitic diseases, it is the only one that is exclusive to Sub-Saharan Africa, and its range on that continent is confined to a third of the Sub-Saharan belt, with some patchy distribution in eastern, east-central, and western Africa.

African trypanosomiasis is caused by two morphologically identical subspecies of *Trypanosoma brucei*, which are transmitted by the tsetse fly *Glossina*. The first is *T. brucei gambiense*, the classic African sleeping sickness. It has a gradual course, sometimes lasting for years before onset of the typical sleeping sickness syndrome preceding its terminal phase, and occurs largely in the western, west-central, and northern regions of Sub-Saharan Africa. The second is *T. brucei rhodesiense*, which has an acute and rapid clinical course, typically ends in cardiac failure as the cause of death, and occurs mainly in eastern and southern Africa. Cattle and other mammals are important reservoir hosts for these diseases, as well as being vulnerable themselves to a third trypanosome, *T. brucei brucei*; cattle mortality from *T. brucei brucei* has important consequences for local economies and human nutrition (Hajduk, et al., 1984).

While each disease form manifests differently, in general the early stage of the disease, when the trypanosomes are in the human peripheral blood system, is either asymptomatic or characterized by vague symptoms of malaise, lassitude, and irregular fevers. These are classically followed by a range of symptoms including headache, anemia, sensory disturbances, nausea, disturbed circadian rhythms, joint pains, and swollen tissues. Symptoms become progressively worse as the parasite passes into the central nervous system (CNS) (much more quickly in the case of Rhodesian trypanosomiasis) and precipitates the late stage of immune suppression, cardiac involvement, general deterioration, coma, and death (Buyst, 1977; WHO/TDR, 1991a).

Early treatment of trypanosomiasis, before there is CNS invasion and before epidemic situations can develop, is crucial (WHO, 1979). Yet males, females, and entire communities are affected by difficulties in diagnosis that are peculiar to the disease, whose variable and unspecific symptoms are easily confused with the fever, headache, and general body and joint pains typical of malaria. Currently available diagnostic tools are insufficiently sensitive and primary health care personnel are not trained for even reasonably reliable diagnosis of presumptive symptoms. The effectiveness of vector management programs has been limited by the wide distribution of the flies, the presence of animal reservoirs, the underground habitat of their pupal stages, and uneven success in motivating adequate levels of community participation (Hajduk et al., 1984). Prospects for a vaccine seem remote, and research has been focused on understanding the causes of disease pathology, vector control measures, and therapies that are effective and free from the high toxicity and teratogenicity of currently available treatments (WHO/TDR, 1991a). FDA approval in 1990 of a new trypanocidal drug, eflornithine (trade name, Ornidyl), will be very helpful in treating late-stage gambiense infections, but it must be administered intravenously in hospital and its cost (US$140 per adult dose) is high, even though its producer, Marion Merrell Dow, has been providing the drug for several years at lower than production costs and will eventually donate all patient rights, licensing agreements, and the like to WHO (WHO/TDR, 1991b). Beyond eflornithine, the most promising intervention so far appears to be development of new diagnostics with high specificity and sensitivity (WHO/TDR, 1991a).

As in the case of so many tropical infectious diseases, exposure to the infective vectors of African trypanosomiasis is closely related to individual and community behavior, notably the work patterns of males and females and the different age groups (Robertson, 1963). Duration of exposure to tsetse fly bites is a major contributory factor to infection for individuals of any age and either gender. Thus, the division of family labor that is performed in fly-dense areas becomes pivotal.

African Trypanosomiasis in Children

The greatest overall burden of African trypanosomiasis, as measured in DALYs, is borne by individuals of both sexes between the ages of 5 and 44. The highest rates of mortality occur in the cohort aged 5–14, and are somewhat lower between ages 15 and 29; the cohort with the highest rates of disability is between the ages 15 and 44 (Murray and Lopez, 1994). Transition from asymptomatic status—that is, change from early-stage, peripheral-blood-system involvement to late-stage CNS invasion—can occur in early childhood (Brabin and Brabin, 1992), although the mechanism precipitating transition remains obscure (WHO/TDR, 1991a). Preschool children who experience transition and survive may be severely disabled, sometimes severely mentally retarded. Good information on the epidemiology of these different sequelae is nonexistent.

Similarly, the epidemiologic picture of prevalence of the African trypanosomiases by sex is extremely unclear, partly because of the wide divergences between results from parasitological and serological studies, and partly because of the mysteries around transition from asymptomatic status. For example, in areas of endemic rhodesiense sleeping sickness where prevalence is high (for example, The Gambia and southeast Uganda), males have been reported to be at greater risk than females (Mulligan and Potts, 1970; Robertson, 1963; Scott, 1970). Yet in a study in northeast Zambia, where a higher proportion (66.7 percent) of all children under 10 had rhodesiense trypanosomes in their cerebrospinal fluid compared with older subjects (39.2 percent), females under age 10 displayed higher infection rates than boys of the same ages (Boatin et al., 1986). And again, in a study in Zaire based on parasitologically diagnosed cases of gambiense sleeping sickness, infection rates were found to be higher in females under age 10 than in boys of the same ages (Henry et al., 1982).

African Trypanosomiasis in Adolescent and Adult Females

Under the kinds of epidemic conditions that have prevailed in the past—for instance, in Zaire and several other countries of the region between 1920 and 1981—both male and female adults are, theoretically, at equal risk of infection (Morris, 1960; Robertson and Baker, 1958). Under "nonepidemic" conditions, risk of infection derives primarily from regular patterns of exposure and sex differences in those exposures, most significantly involvement in farm work. Until relatively recently, the theory has been that since males bore the greatest responsibility for on-farm labor, their exposure and infection rates would be considerably greater than those of the female members of the family, whose role was seen as largely confined to the home site. That contention now seems inaccurate or, at best, not widely applicable.

First of all, the epidemiologic data do not support this view. Although the distribution of the burden of African trypanosomiasis does not differ dramatically when aggregated for all ages for each sex (899,000 DALYs for males, compared with 883,000 for females), the burden of trypanosomiasis in females between ages 15 and 44 is higher than it is for males (see Table 10-2). Individual studies would seem to corroborate these aggregate data. Household surveys in Zaire (Henry et al., 1982) and Côte d'Ivoire (Felgner et al., 1981) show higher rates of trypanosomiasis in females under age 30 than in males of the same ages. Of 3,500 Ivoiriens studied, higher percentages of females than males tested positive for *T. gambiense* infection in almost all age groups, with women ages 20–29 having the highest infection rate. And, in the 1964 epidemic in Central Nyanza, Kenya, while both sexes were equally infected, peak prevalence was found in women aged 20 through 29 (Willett, 1965). That same female cohort has been implicated in other studies, including two predicated on serological surveys, one in the Congo (Frezil, 1981) and another in Nigeria (Edeghere et al., 1989). In a recent review, Brabin and Brabin (1992) suggest that the observed sex differences in these cohorts are attributable either to increased susceptibility to disease in women of reproductive age or to loss of asymptomatic status during pregnancy.

Patterns of historical change are also highly explanatory. Data from a study of rural women's economic roles in Kenya, collected between 1974 and 1976 (Smock, 1979); from time allocation studies in Burkina Faso and Zaire (Carael and Stanbury, 1983; McSweeney, 1979); and from a 1984 review by the Food and Agriculture Organization (FAO) all concluded that it is adolescent and adult females, rather than males of those ages, who are the greatest contributors to agricultural production. As Chapter 2 explained, the introduction of cash-crop farming in central and southern Africa led to the recruitment of men from rural areas for work on large plantations and in the mines; other waves of males have flowed out of rural areas in more recent decades in search of white- and blue-collar job opportunities in urban areas. Thus, large populations of adult males have been cumulatively removed from the tsetse fly belt, leaving women with the major responsibility for subsistence farming and family welfare, and exposure of adult females to the infective bites of the *Glossina* vectors of *T. brucei gambiense* and *T.*

TABLE 10-12   Typical Workday for Zambian Women during the Planting Season

Task	Percentage of Time Spent	Waking Hours
Walking to the field with baby on back	30 min	3.2
Plowing, planting, hoeing	9 hrs, 30 mins	59.4
Collecting firewood and carrying it home	1 hr	6.2
Pounding or grinding grain or legumes	1 hr, 30 mins	9.4
Fetching water	45 mins	4.7
Lighting fire and cooking meal for family	1 hr	6.2
Serving food, eating	1 hr	6.2
Washing children, self, clothes	45 mins	4.7
Total	16 hrs	100.0

NOTE: Percentage of workday spent outdoors away from the family compound is 71.9.

SOURCE: Modified from Sadic, 1995.

rhodesiense increased strikingly, particularly during the planting period, which coincides with the rainy season when rates of tsetse fly infectivity peak. Females of all age groups were also left with their traditional responsibilities for water and fuelwood collection (UN/ECA, 1974) (see Table 10-12), leading to even greater exposure in areas of high fly density.

Unfortunately, these historical changes are not reflected in numbers of trypanosomiasis cases reported at the hospital level, where women do not appear to present for treatment in numbers commensurate with presumed morbidity rates. The theory has been advanced that this stems from the cultural requirement that women seek medical help only with a husband's permission and only when clinical signs and symptoms are obvious and severe. Because at least some males are absent, as noted above, this theory is open to question.

African Trypanosomiasis and Pregnancy

Like malaria, African trypanosomiasis has special impact on women during pregnancy. First, and perhaps most important, there appears to be generalized immunosuppression in women already suffering from trypanosomiasis, and loss of asymptomatic status during pregnancy. Even when infected females remain asymptomatic for longer periods than men during infancy and adolescence, pregnancy appears to reverse this gender-related advantage (Goodwin et al., 1972). In pregnancy, infection with *T. gambiense* can convert from its typically slow course, become acute, and lead to spontaneous abortion, stillbirth (Duboz, 1984), greater maternal morbidity, and possibly mortality. Data on the speed and timing of this process, as well as the factors that precipitate it, do not exist.

The other possibility is that the infection will *not* convert and will remain subclinical, with subsequent intrauterine transmission of the infection to the fetus, which will not manifest until later in the infant's lifetime (Olowe, 1975). One case report, by Woodruff and colleagues (1982), underscores the implications of this slower, occult course of the disease: a "healthy carrier" mother, asymptomatic for over three years following infection in an area endemic for gambiense trypanosomiasis, gave birth and remained asymptomatic for yet another 39 months, at which time her child was found to have been infected *in utero*. Rhodesiense trypanosomiasis can also be congenitally transmitted (Boatin et al., 1986; Brabin and Brabin, 1992; Henry et al., 1982; Lowenthal, 1971; Morris, 1960; Robertson and Baker, 1958; Traub et al., 1978; Willett, 1965).

While such cases are not uncommon, we do not know how common they are, nor do we understand the mechanism of transplacental transmission in either type of trypanosomiasis. Given the high prevalence of the disease in women ages 20–29, and given the sequelae of the disease for both mother and child, further research would seem to be merited. Brabin and Brabin (1992) comment on the direction such research should take: "To concentrate attention on classification of cases is likely to obscure the public health significance of asymptomatically infected mothers, who give birth to apparently normal babies in whom neurological sequelae and illness may not develop until the second year of life."

TRACHOMA

Trachoma is a chlamydial infection that occurs epidemically in many developing areas. The current annual toll of trachoma worldwide is 500 million cases, which include 6 to 8 million individuals in whom it has caused blindness (CDC, 1993). Although the disease is not fatal, it generates a huge burden of disability and ranks fourth among all the tropical infectious diseases included in the GBD calculations. The total burden of DALYs from trachoma in Sub-Saharan Africa for both sexes of all ages was 901,000 in 1990; still, that burden is half the 1.8 million DALY burden produced by the third-ranked disease, African trypanosomiasis.

The ubiquitous etiologic agent of trachoma is *Chlamydia*, a genus of nonmotile, gram-negative, small coccoid bacterial parasite that causes infection in birds, humans, and other mammals. *Chlamydia trachomatis* includes human pathogens and is separated into three biovars on the basis of their behavior in laboratory animals and in cell culture: trachoma, lymphogranuloma venereum (LGV), and one mouse pneumonitis strain.

Trachoma is not one of the WHO/TDR priority diseases, perhaps because its incidence and severity have decreased greatly over recent decades in areas with improving hygienic conditions and living standards. Although there are still pockets of the disease somewhere on virtually every continent, its main foci are in North and Sub-Saharan Africa and the Middle East, where its presence was first recorded in 1500 B.C., and where it is still the major cause of preventable blindness. The *C. trachomatis* biovar in these areas causes trachoma, inclusion conjunctivitis, and eye infection and respiratory infection (pneumonitis) in the newborn. Clinical trachoma is rare in Europe and North America, where the *C. trachomatis* biovar is, instead, the most common cause of sexually transmitted disease, with highest incidence in young adults during the period of maximum sexual activity (Grayston and Kuo, 1984). This sexually transmitted form of the biovar is also present in much of the developing world, including Africa, where it is the cause of several acute diseases (urethritis, cervicitis, salpingitis), pregnancy-associated conditions (ophthalmia and pneumonia in the newborn; postpartum endometritis in the mother), and chronic conditions (infertility, ectopic pregnancy) (Germain et al., 1992).

In endemic areas, trachoma is a chronic, familiar disease perpetuated by eye-to-eye transmission. Overcrowding, close family grouping, inadequate water supply, and low standards of hygiene increase frequency of reinfection and enhance severity. Under these conditions, where a "pool" of infection is established and maintained, the disease usually runs a course of recurrence and remission, with repeated scarring and deformation of the conjunctiva, which may eventuate in blindness. Chronic or latent infections occur frequently, immunity produced in the host is usually incomplete and short-lived, and drug administration may fail to eradicate the infecting agent, so that prolonged antimicrobial therapy with a long period of patient observation is desirable. Because of the high risk of familial and community reinfection, the best course is simultaneous antibiotic treatment of all active cases in household units, and even entire communities (Grayston and Kuo, 1984; Taylor et al., 1989).

Trachoma in Children

In trachoma-endemic areas, the highest rate of active infection is found among children under 10 years of age. The disease is perpetuated in the family by infection of susceptible young children, so that almost all the older children and adults in the family will almost inevitably reacquire active disease because of their exposure to the younger children. There are no data on differential rates of infection by gender (and, indeed, there is no reason to suspect any at this early age).

The disease can also be contracted during delivery through the birth canal of a mother with *C. trachomatis* genital infection. Again, there would seem to be no reason to suspect that either sex of newborn would be at differential risk in this mode of transmission. There is, however, some variation in site of infection in newborns infected in the birth process. While the primary infection site for both male and female newborns is ocular, there may also be some vulvovaginitis in baby girls. This seems to subside after an acute phase, although there seem to be no data from Africa on whether this infective manifestation has any further sequelae of significance. There are some clues, nonetheless, that might justify further inquiry. Episodes of inclusion conjunctivitis after infancy are transmitted by autotransfer or heterotransfer of genitourinary material to the eye, and the sequelae of transmission can be either ocular or genitourinary.

Infants are also at risk of *C. trachomatis* pneumonia, a distinctive respiratory syndrome in infants less than 6 months of age that is acquired from the infected cervix of its mother during delivery. Eyes and nasopharynx are the initial colonization sites, and diagnosis is aided by a positive maternal history of sexually transmitted disease, as well as by isolation cultures (Grayston and Kuo, 1984).

Trachoma in Adolescent and Adult Females

For both males and females, by far the greatest burden of disability from trachoma occurs between ages 15 and 44—that is, their most economically productive years and the reproductive years of females (Murray and Lopez, 1994). This is not in itself surprising, since the principal disabilities caused by the disease are progressive. Although the disease is initially acquired in early childhood, deteriorated vision, disfigurement, and, ultimately, blindness do not occur until the adult years, after a cumulative process of reexposure, repeated infection, scarring, and distortion of the upper eyelid. While the accumulation of scars can be halted with appropriate interventions, changes that have already taken place cannot be reversed (Taylor et al., 1989).

The special relevance of trachoma to this volume is the stunningly large burden of the disease it produces in Sub-Saharan African women. In 1990, that burden amounted to 690,000 DALYs, over three times the burden of 210,000 DALYs produced by trachoma in males. It is somewhat surprising that this large gender differentiation appears to have been noted only relatively recently (cf. Congdon et al., 1993). The range of sequelae produced by trachoma, from cosmetic disfigurement to total blindness, are highly likely to have more severe implications for females than for males: that is, exclusion from marriage possibilities, social isolation, dependency, neglect, or any or all of these events.

In addition, the pattern of transmission for the disease is such that adult females who care for young children in domestic environments are at distinctively high risk. A meticulous study in Tanzania provides evidence that close physical contact with preschool children, especially preschool children with trachoma, is associated with an increased odds ratio for active trachoma in women and may also be associated with development of chronic sequelae (Congdon et al., 1993). The researchers raise the question of whether the mothers were the source of infection for their children, rather than the converse, but since other epidemiologic data suggest that preschool children are the reservoir of active trachoma in village environments, and men have much lower rates of active disease, the conclusion is that women are the recipients of infection within the family, not its source. These data underscore the need for intervention strategies that interrupt transmission at the household level and programs of antibiotic therapy that are aimed both at children and their caretakers.

DRACUNCULIASIS (GUINEA WORM)

Dracunculiasis is a helminthic infection caused by the nematode parasite *Dracunculus medinensis*. A communicable disease, it is acquired solely through ingestion of water contaminated with tiny crustaceans called copepods, or "water fleas," that act as intermediate hosts of the organism and harbor infective larvae. When the ingested copepods are killed by the digestive juices in the stomach, the larvae are released and move to the small intestine. They penetrate the intestinal wall and migrate to the connective tissues of the thorax, where male and female larvae mature and mate 60 to 90 days after infection. Over the next year, female worms grow to maturity, reach a length of 2 to 3 feet, and slowly migrate to the surface of the body, where they form burrows in subcutaneous tissues. When they reach maturity, a blister is formed, which eventually ruptures, exposing the worm. Shortly before the skin lesion forms, pronounced systemic symptoms may occur, including intense itching and pain, nausea, vomiting, diarrhea, and dizziness. Worms emerge from the lower extremities in about 90 percent of cases, but can also appear in the upper extremities, trunk, buttocks, genitalia, or other parts of the body (Ruiz-Tiben et al., 1995).

Dracunculiasis is endemic in areas of severe poverty in India, Africa, and the Middle East. Its transmission is limited to periurban and rural communities lacking any form of public drinking water supply, and where water for household use is consequently drawn from artificial ponds and bodies of stagnant water (Muller, 1984). About 120 million people are at risk of dracunculiasis in 17 African countries; in 1986, there were an estimated 3.32 million cases of the disease in the Sub-Saharan region (Hopkins, 1987).

Guinea worm infection is seldom fatal, but it is typically debilitating, often frankly crippling for long periods, and complications are common. As the worm emerges through the skin lesion, the affected person pulls it out slowly and carefully, usually by winding a few centimeters each day on a stick, a very painful process that may last many weeks (Ruiz-Tiben et al., 1995). In about 50 percent of cases, there is secondary bacterial infection of the worm track, which also provides entry for tetanus spores and possible process to mortality (Muller, 1984). In addition, over the time it takes for an entire worm to be expelled, numerous ulcers may be formed, some of which may become chronic. Other possible chronic sequelae include fibrous ankylosis of joints, tendon contraction, arthritis, and synovitis. In addition, since each worm is the result of a separate infection event and immunity does not seem to be acquired, each year may bring dracunculiasis reinfection, for which there is no cure.

Infected individuals are also carriers: when they wade or bathe, the immature forms of the worms they carry enter the water source to continue the cycle. It is also the case that some proportion of a population at risk will never become infected; one explanation is that high gastric acidity, which kills the larvae when they reach the stomach, confers protection in such individuals (Muller, 1984).

Dracunculiasis in Children and Adolescents

The picture of age and sex differences in Guinea worm infection, like every other tropical disease, is spotty. Information about the disease in infancy is slight, except for published epidemiologic surveys that show dracunculiasis infection to be rare in the first year of life. The average 12-month incubation period of the disease means that any infection acquired during the neonatal period is unlikely to become patent until after the first year of life (Kale, 1977).

There is some limited information concerning Guinea worm infection in children under age 5. In a recent survey of 501 households ($n = 6,527$ persons) in Nigeria, incidence of dracunculiasis was higher in girls under age 5 (12.8 percent) and between ages 5 and 15 (32 percent) than it was among boys in those same cohorts (6.5 percent and 25.9 percent, respectively). In contrast, rates in males over age 15 were higher than in females at the same age (Ilegbodu et al., 1991).

The impact of dracunculiasis on school-age children has been demonstrated in a number of studies in Nigeria, and elevated absenteeism and dropout rates have been reported among infected children (Edungbola, 1983; Edungbola and Watts, 1984; Ivoke, 1990; Nwosu et al., 1982), but the data are not disaggregated by gender. These appear to be the only studies that take adolescents as a group specifically into account.

Generally there is a high correlation between rates of school absenteeism and infection (Edungbola, 1983; Nwosu et al., 1982). Ivoke (1990) examined monthly variations in absenteeism among 617 children in 14 primary schools in Nigeria's Imo State, and encountered the highest rate of absenteeism (35 percent) in March, the peak month for farming activities; 17 pupils missed the promotion examinations in November because they were incapacitated by dracunculiasis. Ilegbodu and colleagues (1986) studied the impact of Guinea worm disease on 727 school-age children in southwestern Nigeria and found that infected children were absent from school for about 25 percent of schooldays, and noninfected children were absent only 2.5 percent of schooldays, while almost 6 percent of children dropped out of school because of dracunculiasis. (See Figure 10-1.)

For girls, an unknown proportion of this absenteeism may also be attributable to their mothers' disability

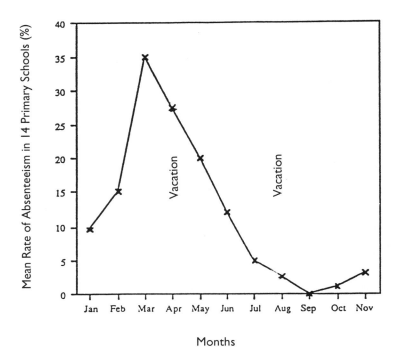

FIGURE 10-1   Absenteeism caused by dracunculiasis-induced incapacitation in 14 primary schools in Imo State, Nigeria. SOURCE: Ivoke, 1990.

rather than their own, and the resulting need to stay at home to take care of domestic responsibilities. The disability inflicted by the disease on adult women requires them to depend on family members and friends for help with their customary responsibilities, typically on another woman, generally a relative or neighbor. If there is an adolescent female in the family, it is often she who must take on household chores and childcare; this means either that she must abandon her schooling or enter the informal sector of the labor force to support the family financially (Ivoke, 1990; Nwosu et al., 1982).

Dracunculiasis in Adult Females

The highest rates of Guinea worm infection occur in adults between ages 15 and 45 (Belcher et al., 1975). In an exhaustive review, Muller (1971) found infection rates for males and females in most surveys to be approximately the same, suggesting comparable exposures for both sexes. In a study in Imo State, Nigeria, in four of six communities studied ($n = 6,539$), infection rates were similar for both sexes; in the remaining two communities, prevalence rates were higher in males (26.5 percent) than in females (15 percent) (Ivoke, 1990).

The importance of dracunculiasis resides not in mortality rates, but in the prolonged disability it produces in infected men and women and its consequences for the individual, family, and community. Three factors influence the degree of disability: worm burden, location of the lesions produced by the infection, and the nature of clinical complications.

Duration of disability varies widely and depends on age, the site of the lesion, initial degree of disability, and treatment effectiveness. According to several studies, average duration of incapacitation for effective work is between 90 and 100 days; the mean is three months, but disability sometimes extends for as long as 30 weeks (Kale, 1977; Smith et al., 1989). Although a number of studies report differences in prevalence rates by sex, none compares duration of disability by gender.

Epidemiologic surveys conclude that gender differences in Guinea worm infection are primarily dependent on exposure to infection foci; that is, the quantity of infected water consumed during the peak period of transmission, which invariably coincides with peak agricultural activity (Kale, 1985) and/or with the secondary rainy season (Petit et al., 1988). Because dracunculiasis-endemic villages tend to be farming communities, and peaks of agricultural demand coincide with the peak periods of disease transmission, in effect, whole villages can become disabled. In such cases, there are few alternative labor sources to replace ailing agricultural workers, and there is a marked reduction in agricultural output; the socioeconomic consequences can be severe (Ivoke, 1990; Kale, 1985; UNICEF, 1987). In southern Ghana, average work loss in untreated adults with Guinea worm disease was over five weeks (Belcher et al., 1975). According to a UNICEF report (1987), dracunculiasis was responsible for significant reductions in person-days of rice production in four Nigerian states. Another study in Nigeria, utilizing interviews with 20 male and female farmers incapacitated by infection, found a total income loss for the group of 25,590 *naira* (approximately US$1,163.18) because of their inability to plant their crops (Brieger and Guyer, 1990). Disability in this group lasted from one to seven months, and all crops were affected. In a study in Burkina Faso, agricultural loss attributable to dracunculiasis was estimated at an equivalent of 8 percent of all annual grain imports to the country (Guiguemde et al., 1984).

None of these studies disaggregates findings by gender. For the most part, epidemiologic research on Guinea worm disease has addressed its prevalence in the general population and in the agricultural labor force as a whole, so that its economic impact on women in particular is largely a matter of hypothesis.

Guinea worm infection of the pelvis affects both men and women but, at least in West Africa, is more common in women, for whom it has obstetric and gynecologic implications (Scott, 1960). St. George (1975) reported bleeding during pregnancy caused by retroplacental worm location, as well as a pattern of repeated spontaneous abortions of uncertain etiology in a very short time period, a pattern terminated successfully by worm removal.

The debilitation produced by Guinea worm infection makes itself felt across much of the female life span. The best documentation of its serial effects to date comes from a 1988 study in Nigeria sponsored by the Water and Sanitation for Health (WASH) Project. A total of 42 mothers of children 24 months of age and younger were interviewed, using focus group and in-depth techniques, and mothers' morbidity histories were analyzed through four variables—self-care functions, childcare duties, domestic activities, and economic pursuits (USAID, 1988).

According to the report, over one-quarter of the sample had experienced an episode of Guinea worm at some point during their most recent pregnancy; 76.9 percent of this subgroup reported that pain from Guinea worm had worsened during the pregnancy itself, and 13.5 percent had experienced a worm attack during the postnatal period. The entire sample reported anorexia and consequent reduction in food intake; arrested breastfeeding because of fever and pain; and inability to care for themselves or their new babies. Brieger and colleagues (1989a,b) observed that disability from dracunculiasis had been responsible for 50 percent of child immunization defaults in two Nigerian communities and had also kept women from making adequate use of antenatal services and engaging in regular trading activities. Incapacitation was so severe in some cases that women ate and drank sparingly simply to avoid the need to go outside to defecate (Watts et al., 1989).

In another Nigerian site (Idere), 21.3 percent of mothers interviewed had developed dracunculiasis during their last pregnancy or since the most recent birth. Average number of sick weeks for the total sample was 6.1, 96.9 percent had worms in their legs, and 45 percent had secondary infections that had produced further incapacitation (Brieger et al., 1989b). Of the 53 mothers who experienced the disease during pregnancy, over two-thirds had been unable to continue with family care and domestic chores.

Dracunculiasis has especially severe implications for female-headed households. These women report being unable to work and earn money to send children to school, and in cases where they are the principal agricultural laborers, their exposure is the same as similarly employed males, but their vulnerability as the sole providers of family income is considerably greater.

Prospects for eliminating this burden of disease from the lives of Sub-Saharan African women are more promising than for any other tropical infectious disease. Dracunculiasis has been the subject of a global eradication campaign initiated at the U.S. Centers for Disease Control in 1980 in connection with the beginning of the International Drinking Water Supply and Sanitation Decade (1981–1990). The eradication effort was first endorsed by the World Health Assembly (WHA) in 1986; in 1991, the WHA officially set the global target of

TABLE 10-13 Changes in the Status of Dracunculiasis Eradication, 1990–1994

Dracunculiasis Cases Reported, 1990[a]		Dracunculiasis Cases Reported, 1994[b]	
Country	Number of Cases	Country	Number of Cases
Nigeria	394,082	Sudan	53,092
Ghana	117,034	Nigeria	39,774
Burkina Faso	42,187	Niger	23,568
Benin	37,414	Uganda	10,409
Mauritania	8,036	Ghana	8,432
India	4,798	Burkina Faso	6,859
Togo	3,042	Mali	5,396
Cameroon	742	Togo	5,045
Pakistan	160	Mauritania	5,029
Chad	N.A.	Côte d'Ivoire	4,700
Côte d'Ivoire	N.A.	Benin	3,440
Ethiopia	N.A.	Ethiopia	1,252
Kenya	N.A.	Chad	640
Mali	N.A.	India	371
Niger	N.A.	Senegal	186
Senegal	N.A.	Yemen	74
Sudan	N.A.	Kenya	37
Uganda	N.A.	Cameroon	30
Yemen	N.A.	Pakistan	0

NOTE: N.A. = No information available at this time.

[a]Cases reported to the World Health Organization from countries completing national case searches or from active village-based surveillance.

[b]Provisional data reported to the World Health Organization from countries completing national case searches or from active village-based surveillance. Sudan's report to WHO includes cases reported by the Passive Surveillance System.

SOURCE: Ruiz-Tiben et al., 1995.

achieving eradication by the end of 1995—a target that African ministers of health in almost all the dracunculiasis-endemic countries had already set for themselves as of 1988 (Hopkins and Ruiz-Tiben, 1990).

Guinea worm is eradicable for several reasons. There is no human carrier beyond the one-year incubation period and there is no known animal reservoir, detection of patient infections is easy, transmission is markedly seasonal, control methods are simple, and the disease is well recognized by local populations in endemic areas (Ruiz-Tiben et al., 1995). The simple, economical procedure of filtering drinking water through a cloth to remove the crustacean intermediate host seems to be a culturally acceptable and effective control intervention in many endemic areas, and is the method of choice for controlling this helminthiasis until enclosed water supplies are available. Provision of such supplies, combined with health education, has been shown to eradicate the disease within three years (Edungbola et al., 1988; Edungbola and Watts, 1990).

Table 10-13 displays the changes in the status of dracunculiasis eradication in Africa between 1990 and 1994. It is clear that progress has been significant, but success has been mixed. Two major challenges remain. The first is to complete implementation of the case-containment strategy and other control interventions, such as insecticide use, in villages of all affected countries. The second is to mobilize greater public support in those countries; the initiative still has to deal with lack of public and political awareness and inadequate funding (CDC, 1993), as well as the characteristic difficulties of changing human behavior.

The countries that pose the greatest eradication challenge are Sudan, Niger, and Nigeria. One Nigerian study reported that over two decades of health education activities concerning communicable diseases, disseminated through the satellite facility of the University of Ibadan Medical School, had made little or no difference in the behavior of residents of Idere village, only 5 kilometers from the university. Lack of response in this instance was attributed to a belief that the disease was in the blood of the members of this particular village, sent by God, and unique to them (Ilegbodu et al., 1991). Success appears to be associated with instances where villagers have come to appreciate the link between Guinea worm infection and the water supply and have responded with such village-based preventive measures as well-digging (Edungbola and Watts, 1990). Yet even countries with the fewest cases will require markedly tighter control measures to completely interrupt dracunculiasis transmission by the end of 1995. This will depend, in turn, on the continued support of national and international entities (Ruiz-Tiben et al., 1995).

ONCHOCERCIASIS AND LYMPHATIC FILARIASIS

Both onchocerciasis and lymphatic filariasis result from infection by parasitic nematode worms of the family filariidae. Four species are of particular importance: *Onchocerca volvulus*, which causes onchocerciasis and is transmitted by *Simulium* blackflies; and *Wucheria bancrofti*, *Brugia malayi*, and *Brucheria timori*, all responsible for lymphatic filariasis transmitted by various species of mosquito. Infection with *W. bancrofti* leads to the most severe form of lymphatic filariasis, affecting breasts, genitalia, and all limbs; it can also induce tropical pulmonary eosinophilia. There are two subspecies of *O. volvulus*, identical under the microscope but with different vectors and ecological niches, one of which causes savanna onchocerciasis, the other forest onchocerciasis. Its *Simulium* vector breeds on objects in freely flowing streams and rivers, thus the name "river blindness."

The different types of filariasis are rarely life-threatening in themselves, but all cause chronic suffering and disability. Lymphatic filariasis can lead to hugely swollen limbs (a condition known as elephantiasis), produced an estimated 90 million cases in 1991, and currently affects 76 countries with a total of 905 million people at risk. Onchocerciasis is one of the four leading causes of blindness worldwide, and it produced an estimated 17.6 million cases of disease, including 326,000 people blinded; it currently affects 34 countries, with 90 million people at risk. Over 95 percent of all the world's cases of onchocerciasis are found in the Sub-Saharan region, most in equatorial Africa.

Onchocerciasis begins with inoculation of infective larvae into the human skin by the blackfly bite. The larvae develop into adult worms over several months, and then coil into subcutaneous nodules containing males and females, which subsequently mate. Gravid females release large numbers of microfilariae, which migrate out of the nodule and throughout human host tissues. Transmission of infection to other individuals is initiated by the bite of a female fly, which ingests microfilariae from the host skin along with a blood meal. The pathology of onchocerciasis is manifested primarily in the skin, lymph nodes, and eyes, leading to intense itching and disfiguring dermatitis, and damage to the eyes, including blindness.

Over 60 percent of the *W. bancrofti* parasites originate—in ever-increasing numbers as the cities of the developing world swell in size—in the pools of stagnant, polluted water common in poor urban areas, ideal breeding sites for the parasite's vector, the female *Culex quinquefasciatus* mosquito. The bite of the vector releases infective larvae into the human body. Once matured, the adult worms make their home in the lymphatic system, in some sites for many years. The resulting systemic damage causes buildup of lymph fluid in the limbs, with subsequent edema and the painful and disfiguring swelling of the limbs typical of late-stage disease (Greene, 1984; WHO/TDR, 1991a).

Onchocerciasis in Sub-Saharan Africa produces a much larger burden in DALYs than does lymphatic filariasis: a total of 641,000 DALYs from onchocerciasis as of 1990, compared with 184,000 from lymphatic filariasis. In both instances, males bear the largest burdens compared with females; in the case of lymphatic filariasis, the burden of DALYs for males of all ages totals 132,000, compared with 51,000 for females; in the case of onchocerciasis, the DALY burden for males is 370,000; for females, 272,000. Because of the substantial difference in burden for the two diseases in Sub-Saharan Africa, this discussion will focus largely on onchocerciasis.

There are important differences in the epidemiology of onchocerciasis that warrant attention before proceeding further. The frequency of the various sequelae of the disease varies not only according to duration and intensity of exposure, as might be expected, but by geographic location. For the same degree of filarial and microfilarial load, the savanna form of the disease causes at least three times more blindness than the forest form (WHO/TDR, 1991a), and, while blinding onchocerciasis occurs in over 10 percent of the population in savanna areas (Remme et al., 1989), it is quite rare in rainforest zones. Nevertheless, males and females in rainforest areas suffer from severe and irreversible skin lesions, including pronounced atrophy and depigmentation (Anderson et al., 1974; Greene, 1984); the manifestations are both less frequent and less severe in many instances in savanna zones, and prevalence is much lower (McMahon et al., 1988).

The reasons for the differences in the transmission, clinical patterns, and severity of the disease between the two zones have a complex and not clearly understood etiology. This is partly the result of the distinct nature of both parasite and vector populations in each zone (Anderson and Fulsang, 1977; Duke et al., 1966; Lobos and Weiss, 1985). In addition, intensity of antiparasite reactions in victims is quite various, almost individualized; this suggests considerable complexity in host-parasite interactions in filarial infections (Ottesen, 1984), perhaps attributable to differences in host immune responses (Anderson and Fulsang, 1977; Remme et al., 1989). Finally, because onchocerciasis occurs in foci that are determined by the relation of the population to *Simulium* breeding sites, levels of endemicity vary according to distance from larval and pupal habitats; hyperendemic areas are those closest to a given focus (Greene, 1984).

Onchocerciasis in Children

The epidemiology of *O. volvulus* infection indicates that prevalence is age-specific, rising progressively after the first few years of life to almost 100 percent by the age of 30 to 40 years in hyperendemic areas (Anderson et al., 1974). Prevalence of both ocular and dermal onchocerciasis also rises steadily, to almost 100 percent by the fifth decade of life.

Still, prevalence rates may be misleading, and microfilarial density is now considered a better measure. The risk of ocular complications actually relates more closely to intensity of infection than it does to prevalence. Risk of transmission in any area is determined by the number of fly bites and the proportion of flies harboring infective larvae (Greene, 1984). Even though the adult worms of *O. volvulus* do not multiply in the human host, 'with repeated exposure and reinfection in hyperendemic areas, human adult worm burdens and microfilaria counts mount over the years (Brabin and Brabin, 1992; Greene, 1984), and there is no persuasive evidence for development of protective immunity with age.

Because onchocerciasis is a cumulative disease, morbidity in early childhood is typically limited to mild systemic effects from early infections, such as slight pruritus. Although congenital infection has been reported from early studies in Ghana (Brinkmann et al., 1976), we found no subsequent studies that address this subject specifically. As for gender differences, where onchocerciasis is hyperendemic, microfilarial densities in females are lower than they are in males beginning in early childhood; in hypoendemic areas, densities are similar for both sexes (Brabin and Brabin, 1992).

Effects on older children can be substantial. In a study of 2,876 persons in Taraba River Valley, Nigeria, the effects of eye lesions on visual acuity were assessed using the "tumbling E" method. The striking result from this study was that, in children under age 10, particularly those with head nodules, serious and irreversible eye lesions were already present and visual acuity was significantly affected (Akogun, 1992). No differences were reported by gender.

Onchocerciasis in Adolescents

In general, males are 1.5 times as likely to be blind as females of the same age with the same level of microfilariae, and greater frequency of onchocercal eye lesions, particularly lesions of the posterior segment of the eye, is reported for males (Ottesen, 1984). Yet the Taraba River Valley study cited above reported that all forms of visual impairment increased with age in a similar fashion for both males and females, and in a study in the Onchocerciasis Control Programme area, the only significant differences in ocular lesions were found in individuals with lesions of the posterior segment of the eye, a condition more typical of male symptomatology (Remme et al., 1989). Given the present state of knowledge, the hypothesis must be that any gender-specific differences in symptomatology and microfilarial densities derive from differences in exposure rather than from any inherent sex differences (Brabin, 1990).

At the same time, the social consequences of the skin lesions produced by onchocerciasis can be particularly significant, if not devastating, for girls as they enter marriageable age in cultures where marriage and children are the source of identity and self-esteem. Browne (1960) observed that while blindness may be of greater clinical and economic importance than chronic lesions, the implications of lesions are far from negligible. Recent studies in forest areas of Nigeria show that cosmetic impairment from severe onchocercal dermatitis stigmatizes adolescent girls and affects their life chances (Amazigo, 1994). Girls of marriageable age with severe skin lesions are usually avoided and will not be viewed as eligible until there is evidence of at least partial cure. While young males and females with severe lesions may both feel the effects of stigma, girls with cosmetically disfiguring lesions attempt to conceal them and tend to withdraw from social activities in the community and at school (Amazigo and Obikeze, 1991).

Onchocerciasis in Adult Females

The skin lesions produced by *O. volvulus* may begin as early as age 5, and continue to be produced into adulthood; after age 40, the number of exposed persons with different forms of onchocercal lesions is significantly higher than those who will eventually become blind. The most acute onchocercal lesions are marked hypo- and hyperpigmentation, skin atrophy, and excoriation, alone or in combination. Pruritus, caused by dead filariae left under the skin after invasion by the live parasite, commonly produces incessant scratching, acute papular skin eruptions, and great discomfort. After prolonged infection and the lesions of fibrosis, irreversible atrophy, pigmentary changes, and extreme scarring of dermal tissue, there is little or no potential for clinical improvement with even the most effective filaricidal treatment (Duke, 1990). It is rare that the pruritus from onchocerciasis has no sequelae: a study of 452 individuals in western Ethiopia found onchocercal dermatitis of the typical maculo-papular type, often with excoriation, in 54 percent of 150 persons clinically examined, a percentage corresponding exactly to the proportion of individuals complaining of pruritus (Woodruff et al., 1977).

The spectrum of the clinicopathological features of the dermatologic sequelae of *O. volvulus* has been studied for some time (cf. Cannon et al., 1970; Connor et al., 1983; Edungbola et al., 1983; Gibson and Connor, 1978; Shafi-Mohammed, 1931). While acute lesions may be more prevalent in males (Edungbola et al., 1983), this may be a function of the unwillingness of females to present themselves in a clinical setting with an acute lesion. There do appear to be pathologies that are particular to females, such as the hanging pouch of lymphadenomatous skin produced by advanced dermatitis that is often seen in women (Connor and Palmieri, 1985).

The systemic effects of onchocerciasis can also produce substantial morbidity in women, as measured by parasitological diagnostic techniques that use shallow skin biopsy samples to take microfilarial counts. In a study of subjective complaints and measurable morbidity, Burnham (1990) found that of 5,653 subjects examined in Malawi, 57 percent of those with positive skin snips complained of itching, a frequency of subjective complaints from persons with positive skin snips that was significantly higher than in subjects with negative skin snips, and reports of dizziness, backache, joint and generalized body aches and pains, pruritus, and poor vision that corresponded to higher microfilarial counts. Women with onchocerciasis-caused blindness weighed 6.8 kilograms less than normally sighted women, and bilateral blindness was correlated with an 11 percent decrease in body mass. Even women who were sighted but had positive skin snips weighed 1.6 kg less than those with negative skin snips. All correlations were statistically significant. A very few other studies report on symptoms that are generally found in females. In an early study in Tanzania, Gabuthuler and Gabuthuler (1947) implicated onchocerciasis as a cause of muscular abscesses in women.

Onchocerciasis also affects reproductive processes. An observation in Nigeria indicates that in pregnant women infected with the disease, there is severe and rapid exacerbation of skin lesions with increased gestational age, as well as deterioration of papular and pustular eruptions by 24 weeks of gestation (Amazigo, 1994). This may be the result of hormonal changes or immunosuppression. More generally, morbidity in women of reproductive age from hypergic onchocerciasis may also have something to do with lack of immune tolerance and onchocercal lymphadenopathy. Rainforest onchocerciasis may have especially adverse consequences for women's reproductive health, and studies in Tanzania, Mali, and Nigeria report that women in those zones do hold onchocerciasis responsible for a number of reproductive health problems, including infertility, sterility, abortion, and stillbirth (Brieger et al., 1987; Gabuthuler and Gabuthuler, 1947; Hielscher and Sommerfeld, 1985). To date, none of these subject areas has received research attention.

Finally, onchocerciasis may have direct health effects that go beyond the immediate victim. In a preliminary study to explore the effects of onchocercal pruritus on breastfeeding, 73 percent of 75 women with positive microfilariae in skin biopsies experienced itching and other associated morbidity that were linked with early weaning of infants by 26 percent of the positive sample (Amazigo, 1994).

The relationship between onchocerciasis and mortality is not clear. Measured in DALYs, the burden of estimated mortality from the disease is much smaller than its burden of morbidity. For males of all ages in Sub-Saharan Africa, estimated deaths account for 17,300 DALYs, but years lived with a disability (YLD) amount to 108,000. For females, those figures are 12,400 and 74,000, respectively (Murray and Lopez, 1994).

Clinical analysis would also suggest a relatively modest direct connection between the disease and mortality. Some heavily infected individuals show wasting and generalized weakness, with loss of adipose tissue and muscle mass, and such persons may be at increased risk of other infections, such as tuberculosis. Although microfilariae have been found in most major internal organs at autopsy, there is no convincing evidence that significant organ dysfunction occurs as a result of widespread infestation (Greene, 1984). An additional puzzle is that, while excess mortality is found among males with high microfilarial loads, it is not seen among females with comparable loads (Brabin and Brabin, 1992).

The relationship among general disease pathology, mortality, and the blindness that is the most severe complication of the savanna form of onchocerciasis is also unclear. Using weight/height as an index of nutritional status, Kirkwood and colleagues (1983) found that the nutritional status of blind or visually impaired subjects was lower than that of subjects with normal vision; that mortality was three to four times higher among blind onchocerciasis sufferers than among those with no visual damage; and that onchocerciasis-related mortality was, overall, most meaningfully correlated with microfilarial load. Prost and Vaugelade (1981) suggest that increased mortality among the blind is indirect, and is primarily attributable to high accident rates or to social and economic conditions resulting from blindness, rather than to any systemic effects of the disability. Studies of the burden of blindness in adult populations in Burkina Faso have determined that the average life span after the onset of blindness is between seven and nine years (Prost and Paris, 1983); absent additional data on age of all subjects, it is difficult to interpret the meaning of this information.

Reported prevalence of blindness in a given village at any one time may misrepresent the true magnitude of the burden that onchocercal blindness places on the population at large, especially in the productive age group (Prost, 1986). According to Prost's study, in hyperendemic villages with an annual incidence of blindness of 5.7 percent, the real probability was that more than 46 percent of the males in those villages who were age 15 at the time of the study would become blind in adulthood. Although the proportion of females between ages 20 and 40 with some visual impairment was higher at the time of the study, a smaller proportion—35 percent—would proceed to blindness. The study provides no further information on blindness in women or its impact on them, nor does any other that the authors of this chapter have been able to identify.

LEISHMANIASIS AND LEPROSY

Four of the six major tropical diseases that produce visible disfigurement have already been discussed in this chapter: schistosomiasis, dracunculiasis, onchocerciasis, and lymphatic filariasis. Two remain: leprosy and leishmaniasis.

Epidemiological data on these diseases are generally recognized as poor, primarily because of their low case-fatality rates. Leishmaniasis is not among the reportable diseases in many countries, and the World Health Organization has estimated that two-thirds of the leprosy cases in the world are still unregistered (Htoon et al., 1993).

The best estimates are that 350 million individuals in 80 countries are considered at risk of leishmaniasis, with 12 million individuals infected and 400,000 new cases yearly (WHO, 1990). Even in countries where leishmaniasis is reportable, the actual number of cases is estimated to be three to five times higher, because the disease typically occurs in remote areas where people live within zoonotic foci and in poor countries where other health problems are of higher priority (WHO/TDR, 1991a). Leishmaniasis ranks sixth in DALY burden in Sub-Saharan Africa, following not far behind onchocerciasis. The DALY burden for all Sub-Saharan African males in 1990 was 291,000; for all females it was 292,000. The burden in all cohorts for both sexes is virtually the same, with the greatest weight borne by individuals in the cohort ages 5–14, followed at some distance by the older cohorts, ages 15–44 (Murray and Lopez, 1994). The mortality component of the burden is relatively small, since just one of its three forms—the visceral form known in Africa as *kala-azar*—can proceed to fatality (CDC, 1993). It is the visceral form that is most prevalent in Africa (Sudan, Kenya, Uganda, Ethiopia, Central African Republic, Chad, Gabon, The Gambia, and Somalia) (Wyler and Marsden, 1984). In some countries of the region (Ethiopia, Kenya), epidemics of visceral leishmaniasis have been responsible for tens of thousands of deaths, because the disease is usually lethal if untreated (WHO/TDR, 1991a).

As for leprosy, the number of officially registered cases was 3.7 million in 1990, plus an estimated 2 million additional undetected, partially disabled patients. Ninety-three countries were affected, with a prevalence of at least one per 10,000 population. There were 2.46 million people living in leprosy-endemic countries, defined as those having a prevalence rate of at least one per 10,000 population (WHO/TDR, 1991a). It is estimated that 250,000 of those with leprosy are blind, a figure that is greater if visual acuity is less strictly defined (Htoon et al., 1993). Leprosy ranks seventh in DALYs, well behind leishmaniasis and, again, the burdens for males and females are almost the same (Murray and Lopez, 1994).

While the two diseases are similar in producing equivalent burdens of disability in both males and females, the number of registered cases of leprosy began a noteworthy decline in 1985, perhaps because of the implementation of multidrug therapy and the consequent release of large numbers of patients from treatment (Htoon et al., 1993). This advance might now be slowed, if not halted, as resistance of leprosy bacilli to chemotherapeutic drugs increases (CDC, 1993).

In contrast, there is no reason to expect diminution in the overall prevalence of leishmaniasis unless an effective vaccine is developed (Wyler and Marsden, 1984; WHO/TDR, 1991a). Controlling transmission of the disease is complicated by a number of powerful epidemiological and ecological factors. The parasite can be transmitted by over 50 species of its sandfly vector, whose breeding and resting sites are diverse and widespread, and the life cycles of the various leishmanias also involve a variety of zoonotic reservoirs. The disease also flourishes under the sorts of environmental transformations that accompany certain kinds of socioeconomic and demographic change, including large-scale migrations of nonimmune individuals into leishmania-endemic regions. An additional element of complexity is that both malaria and kala-azar coexist in similar geographic areas; they may present similar symptoms, be diagnostically confused at a certain stage, and may also interact and complicate each other (Cox, 1987; Kaendi, 1992; Southgate, 1981).

Unlike malaria, which is relatively even-handed in the distribution of its burden across all age groups, the heaviest burden of leishmaniasis in Sub-Saharan Africa falls upon children ages 5–14, followed at some distance by the burden on the late teenage and adult years, from ages 15 to 44 (Murray and Lopez, 1994). Until recently, leishmaniasis was thought to affect males more than females, at least in part because of occupational demands—for instance, herding and work in forest environments. The sandfly vector has been found to be peridomestic as well, however, which obviously changes the gender equation (Mutinga, 1984; Wyler and Marsden, 1984). A reasonable hypothesis is that there is no immediately obvious reason why, overall, male and female exposures should not be comparable. There is reason to expect some difference in the male and female experience, which would derive from heightened vulnerability of pregnant females to the sequelae of malaria and consequent or preexisting anemia. Any of these could produce synergy in susceptibility to visceral leishmaniasis or to more intense and threatening episodes of the disease, although this is highly speculative. What is not speculative is that the scarring from the lesions of cutaneous leishmaniasis will be disfiguring, always more of a liability for females than it is for males.

Disfigurement is also a historical and well-understood sequela of leprosy. Until now, both the prevalence and incidence of leprosy in endemic countries has generally been understood to be higher in males than in females. That higher occurrence has been attributed to the greater mobility of males and their increased opportunity for exposure and contact with infectious cases. It may also be a product of the failure to detect disease in females because of social attitudes, which result in less thorough examination of females by health workers (Htoon et al.,

1993; Ulrich et al., 1992). To what extent this traditional pattern prevails today is unclear, but the GBD analysis would indicate some change.

Again, there is differential experience of the disease by gender. Because of maternal immunosuppression during pregnancy, disease in a leprous mother may become overt, relapse if previously cured, or deteriorate during pregnancy and puerperium. Especially during pregnancy and lactation, there is increased likelihood of development of erythema nodosum leprosum (ENL), a painful immune complex disease. There may also be reversal reaction during lactation, with additional progressive nerve damage and corresponding sensory and motor loss. The babies of infected mothers tend to have smaller placentae, lower birth weights and slower growth rates, increased susceptibility to infection, and higher mortality in the first year of life than offspring of healthy mothers. These sequelae are all most marked in mothers with the most severe form of the disease, lepromatous leprosy (Duncan, 1992), which is characterized by heavy bacillary load, greater infectivity, tendency to relapse even after prolonged drug treatment, and marked host cellular immunodeficiency, considered the main reason for progression of the disease into this form (Harboe, 1984).

Recent studies have raised more questions about the interactions of leprosy and the reproductive processes than they have answered. All of these suggest directions for further fundamental and operational research, particularly in development of a vaccine and therapeutic drugs, prevention and treatment of disability, aspects of case management, and education at the household and community levels (Htoon et al., 1993).

CONCLUSIONS

It is clear that the tropical infectious diseases are closely associated with deprivation: with poverty; isolation, and powerlessness; with lack of clean water, sanitation, and effective vector control; and with unavailability of adequate preventive and curative medical response. It is also clear that vulnerability to infection is closely associated with exposure and, in turn, the socioeconomic and cultural factors that shape the timing, duration, and intensity of that exposure. It is less clear that there are genetic and biological factors that influence susceptibility and physiological response to parasitic infection by age, sex, and individual.

In addition, there is no period in the female life cycle where these diseases do not threaten—episodically, because of the additional risk they impose on pregnancy and childbearing, or because of the cumulative burdens they generate across the life span. These effects are displayed in Table 10-14.

The very best way of dealing with these diseases would be to eradicate them, so that they threatened no one, or to control them so they threatened far fewer. Thus, the list of research needs that follows deliberately excludes concepts of eradication or control; these are considered gender-free goods, to be desired and sought for all affected groups, males and females of all ages. Vector control is an essential element for all these diseases, although more feasible and cost-effective for some than for others. Other strategies include: for malaria, reduction of breeding sites, bednets and curtains impregnated with synthetic pyrethroids and use of soap containing pyrethrin, use of repellents, and chemoprophylaxis where this is not problematic; for dracunculiasis, provision of safe water and treatment of secondary infection; for onchocerciasis, mass treatment with ivermectin and use of repellents; and for trypanosomiasis, avoidance of infection loci and eflornithine treatment. Because of the extent of their exposure and their pivotal role in the household and community, Sub-Saharan African women will be crucial in the success of any efforts to conceptualize and carry out activities that contribute to eradication and control; any such effort that excludes them should be considered benighted.

That said, there are some generic statements that can be made about the parasitic infections in the context of female health and well-being. First, despite the tendency to view these infections as episodic, the burden they produce is one of enormous and persistent disability. Furthermore, these diseases act synergistically with one another and with other, nonparasitic diseases, and produce more severe disability and, in some cases, mortality where it might not otherwise occur.

Second, the epidemiologic burden of these diseases, once seen to be especially heavy for males, appears to have shifted, and it is now to be more equitably distributed between the sexes. Migration and changes in distribution of labor by geography and gender appear to lead the list of factors contributing to this shift. Documenting this conclusion will require solid longitudinal data.

The third conclusion has to do with the traditional biomedical perspective that the only interesting distinctions between male and female susceptibility to the tropical infectious diseases lie in their relationship with female reproductive function. For that reason, where there has been any biomedical research on sex differences in manifestations of disease, it has focused on that relationship, principally in terms of pregnancy and pregnancy outcomes, placental transmission, and maternally induced protection in the neonate. This approach has excluded understanding of nonreproductive effects and limited gender-relevant research to the diseases that produce these effects. It is true that science must often proceed narrowly to achieve depth of understanding, and this sort of research—for instance, malariological research—has provided insights into the workings of all parasitic diseases that have great value. It is time to broaden that focus.

Fourth, there is another, environmental perspective that produces its own biases. While it is certain that differential exposure is a dominant factor in infection, there are tantalizing clues in research on nonparasitic infections that there may be genetic and sex-specific differences in response to infection that may not be linked to reproductive function *per se*. Such findings as the sex differences in the incidence of uropathy and hematuria in children between birth and age 4 are provocative; their meaning and the possibility of other such differences in additional tropical infectious diseases are unknown and could be relevant to understanding of those diseases. In addition, research on cross-sex transmission of measles raises some profound questions about the existence of genetic, physiologic, or morphologic traits associated with sex that either exacerbate or attenuate diseases in males and females. This raises questions about basic mechanisms at the cellular level and about the relative biological strength of the sexes that might have consequences for research on sex and on infection, and ultimately lead to improved control of severe and potentially fatal infections in general.

Finally, there are what might be called "nonbiological" effects of these diseases that must be taken into account in research. While there is growing knowledge about the impact of the parasitic diseases in general on the abilities to learn in school and to produce in the world of work, there is little knowledge about other effects of those diseases. For example, their ability to produce physical disfigurement is appalling. This chapter has suggested that such disfigurement is particularly difficult for females, especially females of marriageable age for whom it has large social, and even economic, implications. In societies where marriage and children are crucial to societal worth, the absence of those can be crushing, yet there are indications that young females conceal or do not report signs and symptoms of such diseases as urinary schistosomiasis or leprosy for fear of losing those options, apprehension about more general stigma, and shame. We do not know this in a quantified way, but it would be possible to find out, in zones of high endemicity, what proportion of reported cases were timely and what proportion of cases identified in the population at large had not been reported at all. It may be that in the cases of diseases for which there are effective therapies, earlier reporting might obviate the disfigurement and stigma women want so desperately to avoid. It is true that control and eradication of these diseases are desirable enough in themselves; it might also be true that until these goals are realized, more investment in methods of palliating the physical and social pain they produce would be well placed.

RESEARCH NEEDS

- As in virtually every other chapter in this report, this review of tropical infectious diseases in Sub-Saharan African females argues for the need for consistent longitudinal data on the incidence and prevalence of those diseases by sex. These data are not only necessary to knowing what the larger trends are, but are central to keeping track of their processes in populations and individual human beings. Where these data have been collected, they are inevitably gathered among both males and females so that, for the most part, the challenge is at the level of analyzing or reanalyzing data that already exist. Nevertheless, there is now enough evidence of significant variation between the effects of these diseases in males and in females across the life span that all future data-gathering and analysis should account for both sex and age in their design and analysis.

- Human immunodeficiency virus (HIV) infection appears to diminish a woman's capacity, particularly in pregnancy, to control *falciparum* parasitemia; placental infection, with subsequent severe impact on fetal growth, seems to worsen in the presence of HIV, but the mechanisms of these effects, not only in the case of malaria but in connection with other tropical infectious diseases, have not commanded research interest. This is understand-

TABLE 10-14 Ages of Occurrence of Tropical Infectious Diseases and their Adverse Health Effects in Sub-Saharan African Females

In Utero	Infancy/ Early Childhood (birth through age 4)	Childhood (ages 5–14)	Adolescence (ages 15–19)	Adulthood (ages 20–44)	Postmenopause (age 45+)
Malaria (fetal wastage)	Malaria (low birthweight, birth defects)	Malaria (anemia, cerebral malaria)	Malaria (severe anemia, pulmonary edema, splenomegaly)	Malaria severe anemia, pulmonary edema, splenomegaly)	
Schistosomiasis (fetal wastage)		Schistosomiasis (anemia, weight loss, lower genital tract disease)	Schistosomiasis (delayed menarche, spontaneous abortions, liver cirrhosis, disfigurement)	Schistosomiasis (infertility, cerebral edema in pregnancy, liver cirrhosis, disfigurement)	Schistosomiasis (chronic backache, cancer of genital tract/bladder/liver, disfigurement)
			Dracunculiasis (disfigurement)	Dracunculiasis (disfigurement, chronic arthritis)	Dracunculiasis (disfigurement, chronic arthritis)
		Onchocerciasis (severe pruritus, sleep loss)	Onchocerciasis (deterioration of lesions in pregnancy, disfigurement)	Onchocerciasis (blindness, disfigurement)	Onchocerciasis (blindness, disfigurement)

Trypanosomiasis (fetal wastage)	Trypanosomiasis (low birthweight)	Trypanosomiasis (loss of asymptomatic status, mental retardation, anemia, myocardial involvement)	Trypanosomiasis (loss of asymptomatic status)	Trypanosomiasis (loss of asymptomatic status, organic dementia, anemia, myocardial involvement)	Trypanosomiasis (loss of asymptomatic status, organic dementia, myocardial involvement)
	Trachoma (pneumonitis, neonatal vulvovaginitis, inclusion disease) conjunctivitis, ophthalmia	Trachoma (maximum active disease)	Trachoma (repeated infections)	Trachoma (scarring, disfigurement, blindness)	Trachoma (scarring, disfigurement, blindness)
		Leishmaniasis (high rate of acquisition)	Leishmaniasis (high rate of acquisition)	Leishmaniasis (severe disfigurement)	Leishmaniasis (severe disfigurement)
Leprosy (impaired placental function, low birth weight)	Leprosy (poor growth, increased susceptibility to infection)		Leprosy (loss of asymptomatic status, reactivation/ nerve damage in pregnancy)	Leprosy (reactivation/relapse/ nerve damage in pregnancy, blindness, nerve damage, disfigurement)	Leprosy (blindness, nerve damage, disfigurement)

able because of the justifiable urgency of understanding the HIV infections in themselves.   Research into the effects of co-infection and comorbidity with all the tropical infectious diseases, however, might provide illumination on disease mechanisms that could be helpful. If there is no reason to think this is the case, then it would perhaps be a misguided investment of increasingly scarce funds for biomedical research, but the question should at least be raised.

• Work in parasitic diseases, notably malaria, schistosomiasis, and dracunculiasis, reflects differences between Western biomedical and indigenous concepts in perceptions of the meaning and management of the tropical infectious diseases. These differences must be highly relevant to the proper design of health education and preventive interventions, but the findings from that work and experience with their applications remain largely unanalyzed, and certainly undisseminated. A thoughtful synthesis of this work, including material from unpublished documentation, would not be overly costly, and could be very useful. Lessons that have application beyond a particular disease or setting have special value.

• Early treatment of trypanosomiasis, before there is central nervous system involvement and before epidemic situations can develop, is crucial. Yet males, females, and entire communities are affected by difficulties in diagnosis that are peculiar to the disease, which has symptoms that are easily confused with those of other diseases, including the fever, headache, and general joint pains typical of malaria. Similar confusion seems to prevail in connection with leishmaniasis (kala-azar), which also can complicate cases of malaria. All three diseases interact deleteriously with pregnancy and anemia. The testing capability required for accurate diagnosis of most tropical diseases is not available at the primary care levels typical of most rural environments. Furthermore, primary health care personnel have inadequate training for making even reasonably reliable diagnoses of presumptive symptoms, although creation of such capability is within the realm of possibility. A workable scoring system using signs and symptoms for diagnosis by rural health workers was developed as part of a study in northeast Zambia and could be adapted for use elsewhere, but to our knowledge, this has not been replicated. The analysis that could promote its replication is a research need.

• The size of the burden of trachoma on Sub-Saharan African females—close to twice that in males when calculated in Disability-Adjusted Life Years (DALYs)—was one of the surprises that emerged during the preparation of this report. While the DALY calculations are constrained by the data base beneath them, the size of the total burden and the size of the differential would seem to be too great to be wrong in a relative sense. The hypothesis is that females, as primary child caretakers, are most exposed to the pool of domestic infection. This sounds reasonable, but search for additional support for that hypothesis and consideration of its public health and educational implications would be a worthy focus of research.

• The role of shame or fear of losing marriage chances in late reporting or nonreporting of tropical infectious diseases for which there are early-stage remedies seems important. There are other factors in the delay in health-seeking and in compliance with therapeutic regimens. All these delay factors, including the usual factors such as distance, cost, and availability of time for health-seeking, can be important in effective treatment. For example, the progression of damage from onchocerciasis may not be reversible, but it can be halted, so that early recognition and reporting are crucial. At present, the information about the behavioral aspects of individual and household management of cases of tropical infection are known largely at the level of ethnographic anecdote, and "vertically" by disease. Compilation of what is known about how younger and older females manage their experience of the tropical infectious diseases, as a basis for integrating that knowledge into case management and public education, could be very useful. The role of Sub-Saharan African women's groups at different levels—for example, university and community—in compiling this information and developing public health interventions could be pivotal.

• Dracunculiasis is one of the diseases in the world that has the potential for actual eradication in the near future, and its target year is approaching. Any investment in new applied research or analysis and synthesis of existing research that would hasten the successful attainment of that goal should receive priority research investment. Again, this is not necessarily costly, but it is urgent.

• Differential physiologic manifestations of disease by sex and age, and the analysis of earlier research on cross-sex transmission, raise questions about the possibility of genetic, physiologic, or morphologic traits associated with sex that either exacerbate or attenuate diseases in males and females, as well as about the relative biological strength of the sexes. Pursuit of answers to such questions might lead to fuller understanding of basic mechanisms at the cellular level and, ultimately, to improved control of severe and potentially fatal infections in general.

• Life span analysis makes it clear that there are significant differences over time and by gender in the biology and behavioral management of the tropical diseases in Sub-Saharan Africa. This suggests that most research should have some dimensions that are integrated and interdisciplinary. From scientists at the bench, who now can work with epidemiological and clinical findings that suggest illuminating differences between the sexes at a very fundamental level, to the conceptualizers of public health interventions, who must educate populations who experience a number of these diseases over a lifetime, ongoing integrated and interdisciplinary "cross-referencing" to one another's learning will be essential for a long time to come. The guidelines for all research in tropical medicine can only profit from a gender approach in which women are involved, as persons with more than biological needs and as primary providers of health within the African family and society.

REFERENCES

Aaby, P. 1992. Influence of cross-sex transmission on measles mortality in rural Senegal. Lancet 340:388–391.

Agyepong, I. A. 1992a. Medical, economic, and sociocultural issues in malaria infection among adolescent girls in rural Ghana. Paper presented at WHO/TDR Meeting on Women and Tropical Diseases, Oslo, April 1992.

Agyepong, I. A. 1992b. Women and malaria: social, economic, cultural and behavioural determinants of malaria. In Women and Tropical Diseases, P. Wijeyaratne, E. M. Rathgeber, and E. St.-Onge, eds. Ottawa: International Development Research Centre.

Akogun, O. B. 1992. Eye lesions, blindness and visual impairment in the Taraba valley, Nigeria, and their relation to onchocercal microfilariae in skin. Acta Trop. 51:143–149.

Alonso, P. L., et al. 1991. The effect of insecticide-treated bed nets on mortality of Gambian children. Lancet 337:1499–1502.

Amazigo, U. 1992. Gender and tropical diseases in Nigeria: a neglected dimension. In Women and Tropical Diseases, P. Wijeyaratne, E. M. Rathgeber, and E. St.-Onge, eds. Ottawa: International Development Research Centre.

Amazigo, U. O. 1993. Traditional and Western attitudes towards the care of tropical diseases: the case of onchocerciasis. J. Seizon Life Sci. 4:239–251.

Amazigo, U. O. 1994. Detrimental effects of onchocerciasis on marriage age and breastfeeding. Trop. Geogr. Med. 46:322–325.

Amazigo, U. O., and D. S. Obikeze. 1991. Socio-cultural factors associated with prevalence and intensity of onchocerciasis and onchodermatitis among adolescent girls in rural Nigeria. SER/TDR Project Report. Geneva: World Health Organization.

Anderson, J., and H. Fulsang. 1977. Ocular onchocerciasis. Trop. Dis. Bull. 74:257–272.

Anderson, J., H. Fulgsang, P. J. S. Hamilton, and T. FdeC. Marshall. 1974. Studies of onchocerciasis in the United Cameroon Republic: 1. Comparison of populations with and without onchocerca volvulus. R. Soc. Trop. Med. Hyg. 68:209–222.

Anya, A. O., and F. C. Okafor. 1986. Prevalence of Schistosoma haematobium infections in Anambra State, Nigeria. Bull. FLFANT 46 (9A):3–4.

Anyangwe, S., and O. M. Njikain. 1992. Urinary schistosomiasis in women: an anthropological and descriptive study of a holoendemic focus in Cameroon. Paper presented at the WHO/TDR Meeting on Women and Tropical Diseases, Oslo, April 1992.

Anyangwe, S., O. Njikam, et al. 1994. Gender issues in the control and prevention of malaria and urinary schistosomiasis in endemic foci in Cameroon. In Gender, Health, and Sustainable Development: Proceedings of a Workshop in Nairobi, Kenya, 5–8 October 1993, P. Wijeyaratne, L. J. Arsenault, J. H. Roberts, and J. Kitts, eds. Ottawa: International Development Research Centre.

Apted, F. I. C. 1972. Review of: Trypanosomiasis successfully treated in pregnant women, M. N. Lowenthal. Trop. Dis. Bull. 69:496.

Arap Siongok, T. K. A., A. A. F. Mahmoud, et al. 1976. Morbidity in schistosomiasis in relation to intensity of infection: study of a community in Machakos, Kenya. Am. J. Trop. Med. Hyg. 25:273–284.

Archibald, H. M., and L. S. Bruce-Chwatt. 1956. Suppression of malaria with pyrimethamine in Nigerian school children. Bull. WHO 15:775–784.

Ballard, J., E. E. Sutter, and P. Fotheringham. 1978. Trachoma in a rural South African community. Am. Trop. Med. Hyg. 27:11120.

Belcher, D. W., F. K. Wurapa, et al. 1975. Guinea worm in southern Ghana: its epidemiology and impacts on agricultural productivity. Am. J. Trop. Med. Hyg. 24:243–249.

Benton, B., and E. Skinner. 1990. Cost-benefit of onchocerciasis control. Acta Leid. 59:405–411.

Berkley, S., and D. Jamison. 1991. Conference on the Health of School-age Children. Rockefeller Foundation, Bellagio, Italy. August 12–16, 1991.

Boatin, B. A., G. B. Wyatt, F. K. Wnrapa, and M. K. Bulsara. 1986. Use of symptoms and signs for diagnosing trypanosoma in rhodesiense trypanosomiasis by rural health personnel. Bull. WHO 64:389–395.

Boserup, E. 1970. Women's Role in Economic Development. London: George, Allen and Unwin.

Brabin, B. J. 1985. Epidemiology of infection in pregnancy. Rev. Infect. Dis. 7:579–603.

Brabin, B. J. 1991. The risks and severity of malaria in pregnant women. Applied Field Research in Malaria Reports, No. 1. Geneva: WHO/TDR.

Brabin, B. J., and L. Brabin. 1988. Splenomegaly in pregnancy in a malaria-endemic area of Papua, New Guinea. Trans. R. Soc. Trop. Med. Hyg. 82:677–682.

Brabin L. 1990. Sex differentials in susceptibility to lymphatic filariasis and implications for maternal child immunity. Epidemiol. Infect. 105:335–353.

Brabin, L., and B. J. Brabin. 1992. Parasitic infections in women and their consequences. Parasitol. 31:1–81.

Bradley, D. J. 1991. Malaria. In Disease and Mortality in Sub-Saharan Africa, R. G. Feachem and D. Jamison, eds. New York: Oxford University Press for the World Bank.

Bray, R. S., and M. J. Anderson. 1979. Falciparum malaria in pregnancy. Trans. R. Soc. Trop. Med. Hyg. 73:427–431.

Brieger, W. R., and J. Guyer. 1990. Farmer's loss due to Guinea worm disease: a pilot study. J. Trop. Med. Hyg. 93(2):106–111.

Brieger, W. R., J. Ramakrishna, J. D. Adeniyi, C. A. Pearson, and O. O. Kale. 1987. Onchocerciasis and pregnancy: traditional beliefs of Yoruba women in Nigeria. Trop. Doctor 17:171–174.

Brieger, W. R., E. Engel, et al. 1989a. Maternal health and Guinea worm: the Idere experience. Poster Exhibition, University of Ibadan Conference.

Brieger, W. R., S. Watts, and M. Yacoob. 1989b. Guinea worm, maternal morbidity and child health. J. Trop. Paediatr. 35:285–288.

Brinkmann, U. K., P. Kramer, et al. 1976. Transmission *in utero* of microfilaria of *Onchocerca volvulus*. Bull. WHO 54:708–709.

Brinkmann, U. K., C. Werler, et al. 1988. Experiences with mass chemotherapy in the control of schistosomiasis in Mali. Trop. Med. Parasitol. 39:167–174.

Browne, S. G. 1960. Onchocercal depigmentation. Trans. R. Soc. Trop. Med. Hyg. 54:325–334.

Buckley, A. D. 1985. Yoruba Medicine. London: Oxford University Press.

Bundy, D. A. 1988. Gender-dependent patterns of infection and disease. Parasitol. Today 4:186–189.

Bundy, D. A., and G. F. Medley. 1992. Immuno-epidemiology of human geohelminthiasis: ecological and immunological determinants of worm burden. Parasitology 104 (Suppl.):S105–119.

Burki, A., M. Tanner, et al. 1986. Comparison of ultrasonography, intravenous pyelography and cystoscopy in detection of urinary tract lesions due to *Schistosoma haematobium*. Acta Tropica 43:139–151.

Burnham, G. E. 1990. Onchocerciasis in Malawi. 2. Subjective complaints and decreased weight in persons infected with *Onchocerca volvulus* in the Thyolo highlands. Trans. R. Soc. Trop. Med. Hyg. 85:493–496.

Butterworth A. E., M. Capron, J. S. Cordingley, et al. 1985. Immunity after treatment of human *schistosomiasis mansoni*. II. Identification of resistant individuals, and analysis of their immune response. Trans. R. Soc. Trop. Med. Hyg. 796:393–408.

Buyst, H. 1977. Sleeping sickness in children. Ann. Soc. Belge Med. Trop. 57:201–211.

Camus, D., Y. Carlier, J. C. Bina, R. Borojevic, A. Prata, and A. Capron. 1976. Sensitization of *S. mansoni* antigen in uninfected children born to infected mothers. J. Infect. Dis. 134:405–408.

Cannon, D. H., N. E. Morrison, F. Kerdel-Vegas, H. A. Berkoff, F. Johnson, R. Tunnicliffe, et. al. 1970. Onchocerciasis. Onchocercal dermatitis, lymphadenitis and elephantiasis in the Ubangi territory. Hum. Pathol. 1:553–597.

Carael, M., and J. B. Stanbury. 1983. Promotion of birth spacing in Idjwi Island, Zaire. Stud. Fam. Plan. 14(5):134–142.

CDC (Centers for Disease Control). 1993. Recommendations of the International Task Force for Disease Eradication. Morbidity and Mortality Weekly Report RR-16 (December 31):42.

Chandiwana, S. K., and N. O. Christensen. 1988. Analysis of the dynamics of transmission of human schistosomiasis in the high veldt region of Zimbabwe: a review. Trop. Med. Parasitol. 39:187–193.

Chandler, J. W., E. R. Alexander, T. A. Pheiffer, et al. 1977. Ophthalmia neonatorum associated with maternal chlamydial infection. Trans. Am. Acad. Ophthalmol. Otolaryngol. 83:302–308.

Cherfas, J. 1991. New hope for vaccine against schistosomiasis. Science 215:631.

Congdon, N., S. West, S. Vitale, et al. 1993. Exposure to children and risk of active trachoma in Tanzanian women. Am. J. Epidemiol. 137:366–372.

Connor, D. H., and J. R. Palmieri. 1985. Blackfly bites. Onchocerciasis and leopard skin. Trans. R. Soc. Trop. Med. Hyg. 79:415–417.

Connor. D. H., D. W. Gibson, R. C. Neafie, B. Merighi, and A. A. Buck. 1983. Onchocerciasis in North Yemen: a clinicopathologic study of 18 patients. Am. J. Trop. Med. Hyg. 32:123–137.

Covell, G. 1950. Congenital malaria. Trop. Dis. Bull. 47:1147–1167.

Cox, F. G. 1987. Interactions between malaria and leishmaniasis. In Leishmaniasis: Current Status and New Strategies of Control, D. T. Hart et al., eds. NATO ASI Series. New York: Plenum.

Curtis, C. F., J. D. Lines, et al. 1990. Impregnated bednets and curtains against malaria mosquitoes. In Appropriate Technology in Vector Control, C. F. Curtis, ed. Boca Raton, Fla.: C.R.C.

Dadzie, Key, J. Remme, A. Rolland, and B. Thylefors. 1989. Ocular onchocerciasis and intensity of infection in the community. II. West African rainforest foci of the vector *Simulium yahense*. Trop. Med. Parasitol. 40:343–354.

Dawson, C. R., B. R. Jones, and M. L. Tarizzo. 1981. Guide to Trachoma Control. Geneva: WHO.

Duboz, P. 1984. L'homme et la trypanosomiase en République du Congo. Etude demographique de la structure de la population et fécondité des femmes. Cahiers ORSTOM, Ser. Entomol. Med. Parasitol. 22:289–301.

Duke, B. O. L. 1990. Human onchocerciasis: an overview of the disease. Acta Leid. 59:924.

Duke, B. O. L., D. J. Lewis, and P. J. Moore. 1966. Onchocerca-Simulium complexes: transmission of forest and Sudan-savannah strains of *onchocerca volvulus* from Cameroon by *Simulium damnosum* from various West African bioclimatic zones. Ann. Trop. Med. Parasitol. 60:318–336.

Duncan, M. E. 1992. Leprosy. In Women and Tropical Diseases, P. Wijeyaratne, E. M. Rathgeber, and E. St.-Onge, eds. Ottawa: International Development Research Centre.

Edeghere, H., P. O. Olise, and O. S. Olatunde. 1989. Human African trypanosomiasis: sleeping sickness: new endemic foci in Bendel State, Nigeria. Trop. Parasitol. 40:16–20.

Edungbola, L. D. 1983. Babana parasitic diseases project. II. Prevalence and impact of dracontiasis on Babana District, Kwara State, Nigeria. Trans. R. Soc. Trop. Med. Hyg. 77:310-314.

Edungbola, L. D. 1984. Dracunculiasis in Igbon, Oyo State, Nigeria. J. Trop. Med. Hyg. 87:153–158.

Edungbola, L. D., and S. Watts. 1984. An outbreak of dracunculiasis in a peri-urban community of Ilorin, Kwara State, Nigeria. Acta Trop. 4:155–163.

Edungbola, L. D., and S. J. Watts. 1990. The elimination of dracunculiasis in Igbon, Oyo State, Nigeria: the success of self-help activities. J. Trop. Med. Hyg. 93:1–6.

Edungbola, L. D., G. A. Oni, and B. A. Aiyedun. 1983. Babana parasitic diseases project. I. The study area and a preliminary assessment of onchocercal endemicity based on the prevalence of "leopard skin." Trans. R. Soc. Trop. Med. Hyg. 77:303–309.

Edungbola, L. D., S. J. Watts, T. O. Alabi, and A. B. Bello. 1988. The impact of a UNICEF-assisted rural water project on the prevalence of Guinea worm disease in Asa, Kwara State, Nigeria. Am. J. Trop. Med. Hyg. 39:79–85.

El Malatawy, A., A. Habasky, et al. 1992. Selective population chemotherapy among school children in Beheiva governorate: the UNICEF/Arab Republic of Egypt/WHO Schistosomiasis Control Project. Bull. WHO 70(1):47–56.

Fauveau, V., M. A. Koenig, and B. Wojtyniak. Excess female deaths among rural Bangladeshi children: an examination of cause-specific mortality and morbidity. Intl. J. Epidemiol. 20(3):729–735.

Feachem, R. G., and D. T. Jamison. 1991. Disease and Mortality in Sub-Saharan Africa. New York: Oxford University Press for the World Bank.

Feldmeier, H., and I. Krantz. 1992. A synoptic inventory of needs for research on women and tropical parasitic diseases. I. Application to urinary and intestinal schistosomiasis. Acta Trop. 55(3):117–138.

Feldmeier, H., I. Krantz, and G. Poggensee. 1992. A synoptic inventory of needs for research on women and tropical parasitic diseases. II. Gender-related biases in the diagnosis and morbidity assessment of schistosomiasis in women. Acta Trop. 55(3):139–169.

Felgner, P., U. Brinkmann, U., Zillman, D. Mehlitz, and S. Abu-Ishira. 1981. Epidemiological studies on the animal reservoir of Gambiense sleeping sickness. Part II. Parasitological and immunodiagnostic examination of the human population. Trop. Parasitol. 32:134–140.

Fleming, A. F. 1989. Tropical obstetrics and gynecology. I. Anaemia in pregnancy in tropical Africa. Trans. R. Soc. Trop. Med. Hyg. 83:444–448.

Fleming, A. F., J. P. de V. Hendrickse, and N. C. Allan. 1968. The prevention of megaloblastic anaemia in pregnancy in Nigeria. J. Obstet. Gynacol. Br. Com. 75:425–432.

FAO (Food and Agriculture Organization). 1984. Economic change and the outlook for nutrition. Food. Nutr. 10:71–79.

Forsyth, D. M. 1969. A longitudinal study of endemic urinary schistosomiasis in a small East African community. Bull. WHO 40:771–783.

Frezil, J. 1981. Le Trypanosomiase Humaine en République Populaire de Congo, Paris: ORSTOM.

Gabuthuler, M. J., and A. W. Gabuthuler. 1947. Report of onchocerciasis in the Ulanga District. E. Afr. Med. J. May:189–195.

Germain, A., K. K. Holmes, P. Piot, and J. N. Wasserheit, eds. 1992. Reproductive Tract Infections: Global Impact and Priorities for Women's Reproductive Health. New York: Plenum.

Ghaffar, Y. A., M. K. el Sobky, A. A. Rauof, and L. S. Dorgham. 1989. Mother to child transmission of hepatitis B virus in a semirural population in Egypt. J. Trop. Med. Hyg. 92(1):20–26.

Gibson, D. W., and D. H. Connor. 1978. Onchocercas lymphademtis: clinicopathologic study of 34 patients. Trans. R. Soc. Trop. Med. Hyg. 72:137–154.

Goodwin, L. G., D. G. Green, M. W. Guy, and A. Voller. 1972. Immunosuppression during trypanosomiasis. Br. J. Exp. Path. 53:40–43.

Grayston, J. T., and C. Kuo. 1984. Chlamydia. In Tropical and Geographical Medicine, K. S. Warren and A. A. F. Mahmoud, eds. New York: McGraw-Hill.

Greene, B. M. 1984. Onchorcerciasis. In Tropical and Geographical Medicine., K. S. Warren and A. A. F. Mahmoud, eds. New York: McGraw-Hill.

Guiguemde, T. R., K. Steib, T. Compaore, et al. 1984. Epidemiological studies and control of dracontiasis in a humid savanna zone (southwest Burkina Faso). III. The socioeconomic consequences of dracontiasis: outline of a method for evaluation of the economic cost of the disease. OCCGE Inform. 12(89):73–90.

Hajduk, S. L., P. T. Englund, A. A. F. Mahmoud, and K. S. Warren. 1984. African trypanosomiasis. In Tropical and Geographical Medicine, K. S. Warren and A. A. F. Mahmoud, eds. New York: McGraw-Hill.

Harboe, M. 1984. Leprosy. In Tropical and Geographical Medicine, K. S. Warren and A. A. F. Mahmoud, eds. New York: McGraw-Hill.

Harrison, K. A. 1976. Sickle cell disease in pregnancy. Trop. Doctor 6:74–79.

Harrison, K. A., and P. A. Ibeziako. 1973. Maternal anaemia and fetal birthweight. J. Obstet. Gynecol. Br. Comm. 80:798–804.

Hatz, C., L. Sarioli, C. Mayombana, J. Dhunputh, et al. 1990. Measurement of schistosomiasis-related morbidity at community level in areas of different endemicity. Bull. WHO 68:777–787.

Hendrickse, R. G. 1987. Malaria and child health. Ann. Trop. Med. Parasitol. 81(5):499–509.

Hendrickse, R. G., A. H. Hasan, L. O. Olumide, and A. Akinkunmi. 1971. Malaria in early childhood: an investigation of 500 seriously ill children in whom a clinical diagnosis of malaria was made on admission to the Children's Emergency Room at University College Hospital, Ibadan. Ann. Trop. Med. Parasitol. 65(1):1–20.

Henry, M. C., J. F. Ruppol, and H. Bruneel. 1982. Distribution de l'infection par Trypanosoma brucei gambiense dans une population du Bandundu en République du Zaire. Ann. Soc. Belge Med. Trop. 62:301–313.

Hiatt, R. A. 1976. Morbidity from *Schistosoma mansoni* infections: an epidemiologic study based on quantitative analysis of egg excretion in two highland Ethiopian villages. Am. J. Trop. Med. Hyg. 25:808.

Hielscher, S., and J. Sommerfeld. 1985. Concepts of illness and the utilization of health care services in a rural Malian village. Soc. Sci. Med. 21(4):469–481.

Hill, K., and L. Brown. 1992. Gender differences in child health: evidence from the Demographic and Health Surveys. Paper presented at the World Bank Consultation on Women's Health, Windsor, Ontario.

Hopkins, D. R. 1987. Dracunculiasis eradication: a mid-decade status report. Am. J. Trop. Med. Hyg. 37(1):115–118.

Hopkins, D. R., and E. Ruiz-Tiben. 1990. Dracunculiasis eradication: target 1995. Am. J. Trop. Med. Hyg. 43:296–300.

Htoon, M. T., J. Bertolli, and L. D. Kosasih. 1993. Leprosy. In Disease Control Priorities in Developing Countries, D. T. Jamison, W. H. Mosley, A. R. Measham, and J. L. Bobadilla, eds. New York: Oxford University Press.

Huttly, S. R. A., D. Blum, et al. 1990. The Imo State (Nigeria) drinking water supply and sanitation project. II. Impact on dracunculiasis, diarrhoea, and nutritional status. Trans. R. Soc. Trop. Med. Hyg. 84:316–321.

Iarotski, L. S., and A. Davis. 1981. The schistosomiasis problem in the world: results of a WHO questionnaire survey. Bull. WHO 59:114–127.

Ilegbodu, V. A., O. O. Kale, R. A. Wise, B. L. Christensen, J. H. Steel, and L. A. Chambers. 1986. Impact of Guinea worm disease on children in Nigeria. Am. J. Trop. Med. Hyg. 35(5):962–964.

Ilegbodu, V. A., A. E. Ilegbodu, R. A. Wise, B. L. Christensen, and O. O. Kale. 1991. Clinical manifestations, disability and use of folk medicine in dracunculus infections in Nigeria. J. Trop. Med. Hyg. 94:35–41.

Ivoke, N. 1990. Studies of some aspects of the epidemiology and ecology of dracunculiasis in northeastern Imo State, Nigeria. Ph.D. dissertation, Department of Zoology, University of Nigeria, Nsukka.

Jelliffe, E. F. P. 1992. Materno-fetal malaria: multiple dyadic dilemmas. In Women and Tropical Diseases, P. Wijeyaratne, E. M. Rathgeber, and E. St.-Onge, eds. Ottawa: International Development Research Centre.

Jones, B. R. 1980. Changing concepts of trachoma and its control. Trans. Ophthalmol. Soc. UK 100:225–229.

Jordan, P. 1972. Epidemiology and control of schistosomiasis. Br. Med. Bull. 28:55–59.

Kaendi, J. M. 1992. Gender issues in the prevention and control of visceral leishmaniasis (Kala-azar) and malaria. In Women and Tropical Diseases, P. Wijeyaratne, E. M. Rathgeber, and E. St.-Onge, eds. Ottawa: International Development Research Centre.

Kale, O. O. 1977. The clinico-epidemiological profile of Guinea worm in the Ibadan District of Nigeria. Am. J. Trop. Med. Hyg. 26:208–214.

Kale, O. O. 1985. Clinical and therapeutic aspects of Guinea worm disease. Proceedings of the First National Conference on Dracunculiasis in Nigeria, Ilorin, Kwara State, Nigeria.

Kaseje, D. C., E. K. Sempebwa, and H. C. Spencer. 1987. Malaria chemoprophylaxis to pregnant women provided by community health workers in Saradidi, Kenya. I. Reasons for nonacceptance. Ann. Trop. Med. Parasitol. 81(Suppl.1):77–82.

Khan, M. E., and L. Manderson. 1992. Focus groups in tropical disease research. Hlth. Pol. Plan. 7(1):56–66.

Kirkwood, B., P. Smith, T. Marshall, and A. Prost. 1983. Relationships between mortality, visual acuity and microfilarial load in the area of the Onchocerciasis Control Programme. Trans. R. Soc. Trop. Med. Hyg. 77(6):862–868.

Lancet. 1992. Editorial: Guinea worm: good news from Ghana. Lancet 340:1322–1323.

Levinger, B. 1992. Nutrition, health and learning: current issues and trends. Network Monograph Series #1. Paper delivered at the Meeting of the International Task Force on School Health and Nutrition, Rome, December 1992.

Lilio, M. S. 1992. Gender and acceptance of technologies for tropical disease: Impregnated mosquito bednets for malaria control. In Women and Tropical Diseases, P. Wijeyaratne, E. M. Rathgeber, and E. St.-Onge, eds. Ottawa: International Development Research Centre.

Lobos, E., and N. Weiss. 1985. Immunochemical comparison between worm extracts of *Onchocera volvulus*. Trop. Med. Parasitol. 7:333–347.

Lowenthal, M. N. 1971. Trypanosomiasis successfully treated in a pregnant woman. Med. J. Zambia 5:175–178.

Mahmoud, A. A. F. 1984. Schistosomiasis. In Tropical and Geographical Medicine, K. S. Warren and A. A. F. Mahmoud, eds. New York: McGraw-Hill.

Malaty, R., S. Zaki, M. E. Said, et al. 1981. Extraocular infections in children in areas with endemic trachoma. J. Infect. Dis. 143:835.

Manderson L., and P. Aaby. 1992. Can rapid anthropological procedures be applied to tropical diseases? Hlth. Pol. Plan. 7:46–55.

McGregor, I. A. 1964. Studies on the acquisition of immunity to *Plasmodium falciparum* infection in Africa. Trans. R. Soc. Trop. Med. Hyg. 58(1):80–92.

McGregor, I. A. 1983. Current concepts concerning man's resistance to infection with malaria. Bull. Soc. Pathol. Exotiq. Filiales. 76:433–435.

McGregor, I. A., and D. A. Smith. 1952. A health, nutrition and parasitological survey in a rural village (Keneba) in West Kiang, Gambia. Trans. R. Soc. Trop. Med. Hyg. 46(4):403–427.

McGregor, I. A., H. M. Gilles, J. H. Walters, A. H. Danies, and F. A. Pearson. 1956. Effects of heavy and repeated malarial infection on Gambian infants and children, effects of erythrocytic parasitization. Br. Med. J. ii:686–692.

McMahon, J. M., S. I. C. Sowa, G. N. Maude, and B. R. Kirkwood. 1988. Onchocerciasis in Sierra Leone. II: A comparison of forest and savannah villages. Trans. R. Soc. Trop. Med. Hyg. 82:595–600.

McMeeley, D. F., and M. R. Nazu. 1988. Schistosomiasis. In Parasite Infections in Pregnancy and the Newborn, C. L. McLeod, ed. Oxford, U. K.: Oxford University Press.

McSweeney, B. G. 1979. Collection and analysis of data on rural women's time use. Stud. Fam. Plan. 10:379–382.

Michelson, E. H. 1992. Adam's rib awry: women and schistosomiasis. In Women and Tropical Diseases, P. Wijeyaratne, E. M. Rathgeber, E. St–Onge, eds. Ottawa. International Development Research Centre.

Miller, L. H. 1984. Malaria. In Tropical and Geographic Medicine, K. S. Warren and A. A. F. Mahmoud, eds. New York: McGraw-Hill.

Miller, M. S. 1958. Observations on the natural history of malaria in the semi-resistant West Africa. Trans. R. Soc. Trop. Med. Hyg. 52:152–168.

Molineaux, L., and G. Gramiccia. 1980. The Garki Project: Research on the Epidemiology and Control of Malaria in the Sudan savannah of West Africa. Geneva: World Health Organization.

Morris, K. R. S. 1960. Studies on the epidemiology of sleeping sickness in East Africa. Trans. R. Soc. Trop. Med. Hyg. 54:212–224.

Mosley, W. H., and R. Gray. 1993. Childhood precursors of adult morbidity and mortality in developing countries: implications for health programs. In The Epidemiological Transition: Policy and Planning Implications for Developing Countries, J. N. Gribble and S. H. Preston, eds. Washington, D.C.: National Academy Press.

Mott, K. E. 1982. Control of schistosomiasis morbidity, reduction and chemotherapy. Acta Leiden. 49:101–111.

Muller, R. 1971. Dracunculus and dracunculiasis. Adv. Parasitol. 9:73–151.

Muller, R. 1984. Dracunculiasis. In Tropical and Geographical Medicine, K. S. Warren and A. A. F. Mahmoud, eds. New York: McGraw-Hill.

Mulligan, H. W., and W. H. Potts. 1970. The African Trypanosomiases. London: George, Allen and Unwin.

Murray, C. J. L., and A. Lopez, eds. 1994. Global Comparative Assessments in the Health Sector: Disease Burden, Expenditures and Intervention Packages. Geneva: World Health Organization.

Mutinga, J. M., et al. 1984. Epidemiological investigations of visceral leishmanisis in West Pokot District, Kenya. Insect Sci. Appl. 5(6).

Najera, J. A., B. H. Liese, and J. Hammer. 1993. Malaria. In Disease Control Priorities in Developing Countries, D. T. Jamison, W. H. Mosley, A. R. Measham, and J. L. Bobadilla, eds. New York: Oxford University Press.

Nwaorgu, O. C. 1992. Schistosomiasis and women in Amagunze, southeastern Nigeria. Paper presented at the WHO/TDR Meeting on Women and Tropical Disease, Oslo, April 1992.

Nwosu, A. B. C., E. O. Ifezulike, and O. A. Anya. 1982. Endemic dracontiasis in Anambra State, Nigeria: geographical distribution, clinical features, epidemiology and socioeconomic impact of the disease. Ann. Trop. Med. Parasitol. 76:187–200.

Oaks, S. C., Jr., V. S. Mitchell, G. W. Pearson, and C. C. J. Carpenter. 1991. Malaria: Obstacles and Opportunities. Washington, D.C.: Institute of Medicine, National Academy Press.

Ofosu-Amaah, S. 1991. Disease in Sub-Saharan Africa: an overview. In Disease and Mortality in Sub-Saharan Africa, R. Feachem and D. Jamison, eds. New York: Oxford University Press for the World Bank.

Okafor, F. C. 1990. *Schistosoma haematobium* cercariae transmission in freshwater systems of Anambra State, Nigeria. Ann. Parasitol. 31:159–166.

Okonofua, F. E., B. J. Feyisetan, A. Davies-Adetugbo, and Y. O. Sanusi. 1992. Influence of socioeconomic factors on the treatment and prevention of malaria in pregnant and nonpregnant adolescent girls in Nigeria. J. Trop. Med. Hyg. 95:309–315.

Olowe, S. A. 1975. A case of congenital trypanosomiasis in Lagos. Trans. R. Soc. Trop. Med. Hyg. 69:57–59.

Ottesen, E. A. 1984. Immunological aspects of lymphatic filariasis and onchocerciasis in man. Trans. R. Soc. Trop. Med. Hyg. 78 (Suppl.):9–18.

Parker, M. 1992. Does schistosomiasis infection impair the health of women? In Women and Tropical Disease, P. Wijeyaratne, E. M. Rathgeber, and E. St-Onge eds. Ottawa: International Development Research Centre.

Petit, M. M., M. Deniau, C. Tourte-Scgaeferm, and K. Amegbo. 1988. Etude épidémiologique longitudinal dans le sud du Togo. Bull. Soc. Pathol. Exotic. Filiales. 82:520–530.

Poggensee, G. 1992. Urinary schistosomiasis. Paper presented at the WHO/TDR Meeting on Women in Tropical Diseases, Oslo, April 1992.

Polderman, A. M. 1974. The transmission of intestinal schistosomiasis in Begender Province, Ethiopia. Acta Leidensia. 42:1.

Pollitt, E. 1990. Malnutrition and Infection in the Classroom. Paris: UNESCO.

Prost, A. 1986. The burden of blindness in adult males in the savannah villages of West Africa exposed to onchocerciasis. Trans. R. Soc. Trop. Med. Hyg. 80:525–527.

Prost, A., and F. Paris. 1983. L'incidence de la cécité et ses aspects épidémiologiques dans une région rurale de l'Afrique de l'Ouest. Bull. WHO 61:491–499.

Prost, A., and J. Vaugelade. 1981. La surmortalité des aveugles en zone de savane ouest-africaine. Bull. WHO 59:773–776.

Pugh, R. N. H., and H. M. Gilles. 1976. Malumfashi Endemic Diseases Research Project. 3. Urinary schistosomiasis: a longitudinal study. Ann. Trop. Med. Parasitol. 2:471–482.

Remme, J., K. Y. Dadzie, A. Rolland, and B. Thylefors. 1989. Ocular onchocerciasis and intensity of infection in the community. I. West African savanna. Trop. Med. Parasitol. 40:340–347.

Reubin, R. 1992. Women and malaria. In Women and Tropical Diseases, P. Wijeyaratne, E. M. Rathgeber, and E. St.-Onge, eds. Ottawa: International Development Research Centre.

Riley, E. M., S. Jepsen, G. Anderson, L. N. Otoo, and B. M. Greenwood. 1988. Cell-mediated immune responses to *Plasmodium falciparum* antigens in adult Gambians. Clin. Exp. Immunol. 71:377–382.

Robertson, D. H. H. 1963. Human trypanosomiasis in southeast Uganda. Bull. WHO 28:627–643.

Robertson, D. H., and J. R. Baker. 1958. Human trypanosomiasis in southeast Uganda. Trans. R. Soc. Trop. Hyg. 52:337–348.

Ruiz-Tiben, E., D. R. Hopkins, T. K. Ruebush, and R. L. Kaiser. 1995. Progress toward the eradication of dracunculiasis (Guinea worm disease):1994. Emerg. Infect. Dis. 1(2):58–62.

Rutabanizbwa-Ngaiza, J., K. Heggenhougen, and G. Walt. 1985. Women and health: a review of parts of Sub-Saharan Africa, with a selected annotated bibliography, G. Walt, ed. EPC Publication No. 6.

Sadic, N. 1995. The State of World Population 1995: Decisions for Development—Women, Empowerment and Reproductive Health. New York: New York United Nations Population Fund.

Santoro, F., Y. Carlier, R., Borojeric, D. Bout, P. Tachon, and A. Capron. 1977. Parasite 'M' antigen in milk from mothers infected with *schistosoma mansoni*. Ann. Trop. Med. Parasitol. 71(1).

Schachter, J., and C. R. Dawson. 1981. Chlamydial infections, a worldwide problem: epidemiology and implications for trachoma therapy. Sex. Trans. Dis. 8:167–1174.

Scott, D. 1960. An epidemiological note on Guinea worm infection in northwest Ashanti, Ghana. Ann. Trop. Med. Parasitol. 45:32–43.

Scott, D. 1970. The epidemiology of Gambian sleeping sickness. In African Trypanosomiasis, H. W. Mulligan and W. H. Potts, eds. London: George, Allen and Unwin.

Scrimshaw, S. C. M., and E. Hurtado. 1987. Rapid Assessment Procedures for Nutrition and Primary Health Care. Tokyo: United Nations University.

Shafi-Mohammed, A. 1931. Contribution to the study of the pathology and morbid histology of human and bovine onchocerciasis. Ann. Trop. Med. Parasitol. 25:215–298.

Smith, P. G., and R. H. Morrow, eds. 1991. Methods for Field Trials of Interventions Against Tropical Diseases: A "Toolbox." Oxford, U.K.: Oxford University Press.

Smith, G. S., D. Blum, et al. 1989. Disability from dracunculiasis: effect on mobility. Ann. Trop. Med. Parasitol. 83:151–158.

Smock, A. C. 1979. Measuring rural women's economic roles and contributions in Kenya. Stud. Fam. Plan. 10:385–390.

Southgate, B. A. 1981. Insect-borne diseases: filarial infections and kala-azar. In Seasonal Dimensions to Rural Poverty, R. Chambers et al., eds. Allanheld: Osmum.

Spencer, H. C., D. C. Kaseje, J. M. Roberts, and A. Y. Houng. 1987. Symptoms associated with common diseases in Saradidi, Kenya. Ann. Trop. Med. Parasitol. 81 (Suppl.):128–131.

St. George, J. 1975. Bleeding in pregnancy due to retroplacental situation of guinea worm. Ann. Trop. Med. Parasitol. 69(3):383–386.

Taha, E. T., R. H. Gray, and A. A. Mohamedani. 1993. Malaria and low birthweight in central Sudan. Am. J. Epidemiol. 138(5):318–325.

Tanner, M. 1989. Evaluation and monitoring of schistosomiasis control. Trop. Med. Parasitol. 40:207–213.

Taylor, H. R., S. K. West, B. B. O. Mmbaga, et al. 1989. Hygiene factors and increased risk of trachoma in central Tanzania. Arch. Ophthalmol. 107:1821–1824.

Tayo, M., R. N. H. Pugh, and A. K. Bradley. 1980. Water contact activities in the schistosomiasis study area. Ann. Trop. Med. Parasitol. 74:374–354.

Teklehaimanot, A., and M. Fletcher. 1990. A parasitological and malacological survey of *schistosomiasis mansoni* in the Beles Valley, Northwestern Ethiopia. J. Trop. Med. Hyg. 93:12–21.

Tielsch, J. M., K. P. West, J. Katz, et al. 1988. The epidemiology of trachoma in southern Malawi. Am. J. Trop. Med. Hyg. 38:392–399.

Traub, N., P. R. Hira, C. Chintu, and C. Mhango. 1978. Congenital trypanosomiasis: Report of a case due to *trypanosoma brucei rhodesiense*. E. Afr. Med. J. 55:477–481.

Ulrich, M., A. M. Zulueta, Gisela Caceres-Dittmar, et al. 1992. Leprosy in women: characteristics and repercussions. In Women and Tropical Diseases, P. Wijeyaratne, E. M. Rathgeber, and E. St.-Onge, eds. Ottawa: Intronational Developement Centre.

UNICEF (United Nations Children's Fund). 1987. Guinea Worm Control as a Major Contributor to Self-Sufficiency in Rice Production in Nigeria. UNICEF/WATSAN/NIG/GW/2/87. New York.

UNESCO (United Nations Education, Scientific and Cultural Organization). 1989. Report of the First Technical Meeting of the New UNESCO Project to Improve Primary School Performance through Improved Nutrition and Health. ED-89/WS/101, Nutrition Education Series, Issue 18. Paris.

UN/ECA (United Nations/Economic Commission for Africa). 1974. Africa's Food Producers: The Impact of Change on Rural Women. Women's Programme, Human Resources Development Division. Addis Ababa.

USAID (United States Agency for International Development). 1988. Nigeria Maternal Morbidity from Guinea Worm and Child Survival. WASH Field Report. No. 232, Bureau for Science and Technology, USAID, WASH Activity No. 424. Washington, D.C.

Van Zon, A. A. J. C., W. M. C. Eling, C. C. Hermsen, and A. G. M. Koekkoek. 1982. Corticosteroid regulation of the effector function of malaria immunity during pregnancy. Infect. Immunol. 36:484–491.

Veatch, E. P. 1946. Human trypanosomiasis and tsetse flies in Liberia. Am. J. Trop. Med. 26 (Suppl.):5–52.

Vlassoff, C., and E. Bonilla. 1994. Gender-related differences in the impact of tropical diseases on women: what do we know? J. Biosoc. Sci. 26:37–53.

Vleugels, M. P. H., W. M. C. Eling, R. Rolland, and R. de Graaf. 1987. Cortisol and loss of malarial immunity in human pregnancy. Br. J. Obstet. Gynaecol. 94:758–765.

Walsh, J. A. 1990. Estimating the burden of illness in the tropics. In Tropical and Geographical Medicine, K. S. Warren and A. A. F. Mahmoud, eds. New York: McGraw-Hill.

Warren, K. S. 1972. The immunopathogenesis of schistosomiasis: a multidisciplinary approach. Trans. R. Soc. Trop. Med. Hyg. 66:414–434.

Warren, K. S. 1973. Regulation of the prevalence and intensity of schistosomiasis in man: immunology or ecology? J. Infect. Dis. 127:595–609.

Warren, K. S., and A. A. F. Mahmoud, eds. 1984. Tropical and Geographical Medicine. New York: McGraw-Hill.

Warren, K. S., D. A. P. Bundy, R. M. Anderson, et al. 1993. Helminth infection. In Disease Control Priorities in Developing Countries, D. T. Jamison, W. H. Mosley, A. R. Measham, and J. L. Bobadilla, eds. New York: Oxford University Press for the World Bank.

Warren, K. W. 1982. Selective primary health care: Strategies for control of disease in the developing world. I. Schistosomiasis. Rev. Infect. Dis. 4:715–726.

Watts, S. T. 1986. Human behavior and the transmission of dracunculiasis: a case study from the Ilorin area of Nigeria. Intl. J. Epidemiol. 15:252–265.

Watts, S. J., W. R. Brieger, and M. Yacoob. 1989. Guinea worm: an in-depth study of what happens to mothers, families and communities. Soc. Sci. Med. 29(a):1043–1049.

West, S. K., B. Munoz, V. Turner, et al. 1991a. The epidemiology of trachoma in central Tanzania. Intl. J. Epidemiol. 20:1088–1992.

West, S. K., N. G. Congdon, S. Katala, et al. 1991b. Facial cleanliness and risk of trachoma in families. Arch. Ophthalmol. 109:855–857.

White, N. J., and D. A. Darrell. 1988. The management of severe malaria. In Malaria: Principles and Practice of Malariology, Vol. 1, W. H. Wernsdorfer and I. A. McGregor, eds. Edinburgh: Churchill.

Wilkins, H. A., and A. Scott. 1978. Variation and stability in *Schistosoma Haematobium* egg counts: a four-year study of Gambian children. Trans. R. Soc. Trop. Med. Hyg. 72:397–404.

Wilkins, H. A., P. H. Goll, T. F. Marshall, and P. J. Moore. 1984. Dynamics of *Schistosoma Haematobium* infection in a Gambian community. I. The pattern of infection in the study area. Trans. R. Soc. Trop. Med. Hyg. 78:216–221.

Willett, K. C. 1965. Some observations on the recent epidemiology of sleeping sickness in Nyanza Region, Kenya, and its relationship to general epidemiology of Gambian and Rhodesian sleeping sickness in Africa. Trans. R. Soc. Trop. Med. Hyg. 59:374–394.

Woodruff, A. W., D. A. Evans, and N. O. Owino. 1982. A healthy carrier of African trypanosomiasis. J. Infect. 5:89–92.

Woodruff, A. W., J. Anderson, L. E. Pettit, M. Tukur, and A. H. W. Woodruff. 1977. Some aspects of onchocerciasis in Sudan savanna and rain forest. J. Trop. Med. Hyg. 80:68–73.

World Bank. 1993. World Development Report 1993: Investing in Health. New York: Oxford University Press for the World Bank.

WHO (World Health Organization). 1979. The African Trypanosomiases: Report of a Joint WHO Expert Committee and FAO Expert Consultation. Technical Report, Series N, 635. Geneva.

WHO (World Health Organization). 1990. The control of leishmaniases. Report of a WHO Expert Committee, Technical Report Series No. 793. Geneva.

WHO/TDR (World Health Organization, Special Programme for Research and Training in Tropical Diseases). 1991a. Tropical Diseases: Progress in Research, 1989–1990. Tenth Programme Report of the UNDP/World Bank/WHO Special Programme for Research and Training in Tropical Diseases (TDR). Geneva.

WHO/TDR (World Health Organization, Special Programme for Research and Training in Tropical Diseases). 1991b. Sleeping Sickness. "Resurrection" Drug Approved. TDR News 34:1–2.

Wyler, D. J., and P. D. Marsden. 1984. Leishmaniasis. In Tropical and Geographical Medicine, K. S. Warren and A. A. F. Mahmoud, eds. New York: McGraw-Hill.

11

Sexually Transmitted Diseases and HIV Infection

In Sub-Saharan Africa, sexually transmitted diseases (STDs) are among the most common reasons that adults, as a group, seek health care (Hira et al., 1992b; Meheus et al., 1990; Zimbabwe, 1989). Yet this statistic refers primarily to males. Most women with STDs will not seek medical care at all, or will only present late for treatment, when complications have already developed, complications that have devastating physical, psychological, and social consequences, particularly for women and their children (Carty et al., 1972; Latif, 1981). These consequences for individuals, in turn, have serious repercussions for the societies of which they are part.

Human immunodeficiency virus (HIV) infection is considered by many to be the most serious STD because of its multiple debilitating manifestations, its high fatality rate, and the severe stigma and discrimination that surround it in communities around the globe. In Sub-Saharan Africa, where the infection is acquired sexually in most cases, HIV seriously affects, and will spread among, the very same women and men who already have very high rates of other STDs.

Table 11-1 depicts the gender-related burden of HIV infection and the STDs reviewed in this chapter. As the table indicates, both are of unique significance to female health because of their capacity for transmission from mother to offspring during pregnancy and birth and, in the case of HIV infection, through breast milk. In contrast to HIV infection, which in Sub-Saharan Africa is a disease of both women and men, the other STDs disproportionately affect women, who bear 80 percent of the disability-adjusted life years (DALYs) lost to these diseases (World Bank, 1993). In addition, compared with HIV infection, which has stimulated extensive research, including research related to the women of Sub-Saharan Africa (de Bruyn, 1992; Mane et al., 1994; Mann et al., 1992; Orubuloye et al., 1993; Temmerman et al., 1994; Ulin, 1992; WHO, 1993, 1994), relatively little attention has been paid to the other STDs. We therefore choose to consider HIV and other STDs together, and to place greater emphasis on non-HIV STDs.

This chapter first provides a conceptual framework for thinking about STDs and HIV infection. It then highlights the gender differences that make all STDs a critical women's health concern and examines special issues that are unique to the different stages of women's lives. Next, the chapter describes the magnitude of the problem in Sub-Saharan Africa and, analyzing existing data, explores the geographic distribution and clustering of five common STDs, including HIV infection. The chapter proceeds to an examination of societal factors that may influence STD and HIV prevalence, and closes with a discussion of implications for research, policy, and programs.

TABLE 11-1 HIV Infection and Other Sexually Transmitted Diseases in Sub-Saharan Africa: Gender-Related Burden

Disorder	Exclusive to Females	Greater for Females than for Males	Burden for Females and Males Comparable, but of Particular Significance for Females
HIV infection	X[a]		
Other STDs		X[a]	

NOTE: Significance is defined here as having impact on health that, for any reason—biological, reproductive, sociocultural, or economic—is different in its implications for females than for males.

[a]Both HIV infection and other STDs have the capacity to be passed on from an infected mother to her offspring through congenital, perinatal, or neonatal transmission.

OVERVIEW

STDs, Including HIV Infection, and Their Complications

One of the simplest and most useful ways to classify STDs is based on their two most common syndromes: genital discharge and genital lesions. STDs such as gonorrhea, chlamydia, and trichomoniasis cause genital discharge. Others cause genital lesions that can be further categorized as ulcerative diseases such as syphilis, chancroid, and genital herpes, or as nonulcerative diseases such as genital warts. In addition, a few STDs, such as human immunodeficiency virus (HIV) infection, do not fit this syndromic classification. The final stage of HIV infection, acquired immunodeficiency syndrome (AIDS), develops after a variable period of time, with onset generally following initial infection within approximately 10 years, during which it remains largely asymptomatic. The symptomatic stages of AIDS are characterized by the onset of opportunistic infections or cancers, some of which, such as cervical cancer, affect the genital tract.

This chapter refers to studies from Africa whenever they are available. When African data do not exist, or when comparison is appropriate, data are presented from other countries, particularly Sweden, which has accumulated a substantial and unique body of data on STDs in women.

Complications of STDs

Untreated or inappropriately treated, STDs may lead to severe complications, which account for most of their morbidity. Such complications occur most frequently in populations that lack ready access to effective treatment. Furthermore, both the anatomy of the female genital tract—prone to ascending infections—and reproductive events and related medical procedures—childbirth, stillbirth, abortion, uterine curettage, and intrauterine device insertion—are additional risk factors for STD complications particular to women (Meheus et al., 1990). The main STD complications include pelvic inflammatory disease (PID) and its sequelae, and the most important of these are impaired fertility and adverse pregnancy outcomes, enhanced HIV transmission, and cervical cancer.

The clinical manifestations associated with HIV infection depend on several factors, including the pathogens to which an individual has been exposed; the susceptibility of the host; possibly, the strain of HIV; and access to medical care. Most studies have not highlighted significant gender differences in disease progression. In the United States, however, one study indicated that, compared with men, HIV-infected women were at increased risk of death, which may reflect differential access to health care or different socioeconomic status and social support for women compared with men (Melnick et al., 1994). In Africa, little information is available on the natural history of HIV infection, particularly among women. The clinical picture of HIV infection in Sub-Saharan Africa

TABLE 11-2 Sexually Transmitted Diseases in Women

		Potential Complications			
Syndrome	Etiology	Infertility/ Ectopic Pregnancy[a]	Adverse Pregnancy Outcome[a]	Cervical Cancer[a]	Enhanced HIV[a] Transmission
Discharge	Chlamydia	X	X		X
	Gonorrhea	X	X		X
	Trichomonas		X		X
Lesions Genital ulcers					
	Syphilis		X		X
	Chancroid				X
	Herpes		X		X
Other					
	HPV infection and genital warts		X	X	

[a]Potentially fatal.

appears to be dominated by dermatological and gastrointestinal manifestations and by tuberculosis (De Cock et al., 1993; Kreiss and Castro, 1990).

A recent study strongly suggests that a sexually transmitted herpes virus causes Kaposi's sarcoma, one of the clinical manifestation of AIDS (Chang, 1994). In Africa, while this cancer has always been endemic, predominantly affecting men, with the spread of HIV its incidence has risen notably, and it is affecting an increasing number of women. In Zambia, the proportion of women among persons with Kaposi's sarcoma increased from 9 percent in 1983 to 30 percent in 1990–1992 (Ebrahim et al., 1993).

The onset of AIDS may be delayed by antiretroviral drugs. Because of their high cost, however, it is unlikely that these drugs will become widely available in the near future in Sub-Saharan Africa. Most important, several AIDS-indicative diseases may be prevented. Indeed, some opportunistic infections can be prevented by the use of chemoprophylaxis, and invasive cervical cancer can be prevented by proper recognition and treatment of cervical dysplasia or early cervical cancer.

The syndromic classification of STDs described above also suggests the kinds of complications that may occur. For example, fertility impairment is primarily associated with the genital discharge syndromes, and both genital discharges and genital ulcers may be prodromal to poor pregnancy outcomes and enhanced risk of sexual HIV transmission (Table 11-2).

In men, STD complications do not have the frequency, severity, or consequences they have in women. They result mainly from urethral infections, and include urethral strictures and epididymitis, an inflammation of the excretory duct of the testicle and the leading cause of male infertility in parts of Sub-Saharan Africa (Berger, 1990).

Pelvic Inflammatory Disease and Its Sequelae In women, pathogens that cause genital discharge, such as gonococci and chlamydiae, tend to rise into the upper genital tract and cause pelvic inflammatory disease. As many as 10 to 20 percent of women with untreated gonorrhea or chlamydia develop PID (Hook and Handsfield, 1990; Weström and Mårdh, 1984), the most common of the complications of sexually transmitted diseases.

Although the acute clinical manifestations of pelvic inflammatory disease may be quite severe, their public health significance resides primarily in their long-term sequelae. The partial or total occlusion of the fallopian tubes that can ensue from PID produces harsh and irreversible sequelae: infertility, ectopic pregnancy, chronic pelvic pain, and recurrent infection. Both gonococcal and chlamydial PID may be associated with those sequelae, but manifest differently. PIDs of chlamydial origin generally produce less severe symptoms than those of gonococcal cause, and they appear to produce more tubal damage and correspondingly higher rates of infertility and ectopic pregnancy. In part, this may be caused by the more indolent character of chlamydia, which makes women with chlamydial PID less likely to seek timely treatment than women with gonococcal PID (Hillis et al., 1993).

Rates of infertility consequent to a pelvic inflammatory disease are high, even in developed countries. In a landmark study of Swedish women treated for one episode of PID, 11.4 percent became involuntarily infertile, with the risk of infertility roughly doubling with each subsequent episode; 23.1 percent of women became infertile after two episodes of PID; and 54.3 percent became infertile after three or more episodes (Weström and Mårdh, 1990). In the absence of timely, effective treatment, which is the normative circumstance in Sub-Saharan Africa, this risk becomes even greater: according to data from the preantibiotic era, 45–75 percent of women who had suffered from PID became infertile (Weström and Mårdh, 1990). Delay in PID treatment is a critical risk factor for impaired fertility; women who wait to seek health care for more than two days after onset of symptoms have a threefold increase in risk of infertility or ectopic pregnancy compared with those who seek care promptly. This risk is highest for women with chlamydial infection: 17.8 percent of those who delayed seeking health care developed impaired fertility; none of those who sought prompt treatment became so afflicted (Hillis et al., 1993).

Ectopic pregnancy is caused by partial occlusion of the fallopian tubes, in which the damaged tube hampers the passage of the fertilized ovum into the uterus. Absent emergency care, it is frequently fatal. In Sweden, women with a history of any pelvic infection have a risk of ectopic pregnancy 6 to 10 times greater than women with no such history, and the first conception following an infection leads to ectopic pregnancy in almost 10 percent of women (Weström et al., 1992). In Africa, studies from Zimbabwe and Gabon implicate both gonorrhea and chlamydia in the development of ectopic pregnancy (De Muylder et al., 1990; Ville et al., 1991), although the Gabon study shows a stronger association between chlamydia and ectopic pregnancy, which is consistent with the pattern of association suggested by the Swedish data.

While chronic pelvic pain has neither the emotional significance of infertility nor the fatal character of ectopic pregnancy, it is the most disabling of all PID sequelae, often so insidious and severe that it interferes with daily activities. It affects 15 to 18 percent of all women who have had a pelvic inflammatory disease and is often associated with infertility (Weström, 1980). In industrialized countries, up to one-third of women who have had a single episode of PID develop recurrent infections because of inadequate treatment, increased vulnerability of damaged tubes, repeated exposure to sex partners who remain untreated, or unaltered risky behaviors (Weström and Mårdh, 1990). This risk, as is the case for all the other sequelae of PID, may be much greater in Sub-Saharan Africa simply because of the pervasive lack of access to effective care.

Adverse Pregnancy Outcomes Adverse pregnancy outcomes, which include congenital or perinatal infection, low birthweight, and fetal death, are a major public health problem in Sub-Saharan Africa, and linked to both genital discharge syndromes and genital ulcer diseases. When STDs occur during pregnancy, a mother may pass the infection to her child, either during pregnancy or at the time of delivery. Thus, not only the pregnant woman herself but her entire family is affected, so that she becomes the unwitting, critical link between horizontal and vertical transmission.

Congenital infections occur during pregnancy; perinatal infections occur around the time of birth. Either may result in transient illness, permanent disability, or neonatal death. In Sub-Saharan Africa, the most common and best-documented congenital or perinatal infections caused by STDs include *ophthalmia neonatorum*, congenital syphilis, and congenital HIV infection. Ophthalmia neonatorum, an eye infection that develops within the first month of life, is one of the most common infections of newborns related to maternal STDs, and may be caused by gonorrhea, chlamydia, or both. Easily preventable by instillation of medication in the eye at birth, untreated it may result in blindness. In a Nairobi hospital where ocular prophylaxis at birth had been discontinued, *ophthalmia neonatorum* occurred in 42 percent of infants whose mothers were infected with gonorrhea, and in 31 percent of infants whose mothers had chlamydia (Laga et al., 1986).

Congenital syphilis is a very serious condition, often debilitating when it is not fatal. Approximately one-third of women with syphilis are delivered of live infants with syphilis, who then go on to suffer the ravages of that disease; untreated, the disease can proceed to fatality (Schultz et al., 1990). HIV-infected babies have an even worse prognosis, since no good therapeutic options are yet available. In a Rwanda study, 38 percent of HIV-infected infants had died by the age of 6 months (Lepage and Van de Perre, 1988a,b).

HIV-infected mothers have a risk of transmitting HIV to their babies ranging from 13 to 45 percent, with a tendency toward higher rates in Africa (Blanche et al., 1989; Hira et al., 1989; Lallemant et al., 1994; Lepage et al., 1993; Newell, 1992; Ryder et al., 1989; St. Louis et al., 1993; Tovo et al., 1988). One reason that has been postulated for the difference in transmission rates between countries is that, compared with those from industrialized countries, African HIV-infected women are generally in poor health because of poor nutritional status and frequent infections, and thus are at greater risk of transmitting HIV to their infants (Lepage et al., 1993). HIV may be transmitted during pregnancy, during birth, or through breast milk, but the relative contribution of these different modes of transmission to infection is still unclear in most African countries. A collaborative French-American study showed that the uptake of zidovudine by HIV-infected pregnant women reduces the risk of mother-to-child transmission by approximately one-third (Connor et al., 1994). The complexity of the regimen used in this study and the cost of the drug, however, make it unlikely that this kind of therapy will become available to most of the HIV-infected women of Sub-Saharan Africa in the near future.

Low birthweight, defined as live birth below 2,500 grams, occurs because of intrauterine growth retardation, premature delivery, or both. Many factors, both infectious and noninfectious—such as diet, smoking, and hypertension—may cause low birthweight. The relative contribution of each of these factors remains to be determined, and undoubtedly varies substantially according to their local prevalence. In developing countries, up to 30 percent of infants are below 2,500 grams at birth, compared with only 2 to 10 percent of infants in industrialized countries (Barnes, 1979). Because 70 percent of mortality and morbidity during the first month of life occurs among low birthweight babies (Barnes, 1979), STDs would appear to be an important factor in child survival.

Syphilis and genital herpes appear to be associated with both intrauterine growth retardation and premature delivery, while gonorrhea, chlamydia, and trichomoniasis induce premature delivery without affecting intrauterine growth (Brunham et al., 1990a; Cotch, 1990). In a study in Nairobi, Elliot and colleagues suggested that treatment of maternal gonorrhea may reduce prematurity rates by 14 percent (Elliot et al., 1990). Studies from Kenya, Rwanda, Zaire, and Zambia have identified a significant association between HIV infection and low birthweight (Braddick et al., 1990; Bulterys et al., 1991; Hira et al., 1989; Ryder et al., 1989; Temmerman et al., 1992b), which appears to derive from intrauterine growth retardation.

Fetal death, occurring either before 20 weeks of gestation (spontaneous abortion), or at or after 20 weeks of gestation (stillbirth), also appears to be associated with several types of sexually transmitted infections. Studies from industrialized countries suggest that spontaneous abortion is more frequently associated with gonorrhea or genital herpes, with stillbirth more often linked with chlamydia or syphilis (Brunham et al., 1990a; Cooper-Poole, 1986; Mtimavalye and Belsey, 1987). Schulz and his colleagues have estimated that at least 50 percent of women with untreated syphilis may lose the fetus they are carrying (Schulz et al., 1990). In Zambia, pregnant women with untreated syphilis had a risk of bearing a stillborn child 28 times higher than pregnant women without syphilis (Watts et al., 1984). In another Zambian study, 42 percent of stillbirths were attributed to syphilis (Ratnam et al., 1982), and in Ethiopia, data suggest that 5 percent of all pregnancies are lost to that disease (Bishaw et al., 1983).

Enhanced HIV Transmission   The relationships between HIV infection and other STDs are complex, intriguing, and in large measure speculative. STDs may enhance HIV transmission either by increasing the infectivity of HIV-infected persons or by increasing the susceptibility to HIV infection of non-HIV-infected persons. Several studies, mostly from Africa, indicate that both genital ulcers and genital discharge syndromes enhance the risk of HIV transmission (Cameron et al., 1989; Laga, 1990; Laga et al., 1990; Plummer et al., 1991; Wasserheit, 1992). HIV also may alter the natural course of other STDs, including their response to treatment. In Zimbabwe and Kenya, HIV-infected persons have an increased risk of treatment failure for chancroid (Latif, 1989; MacDonald et al., 1989). All of these interactions are worrisome. If coinfection with HIV prolongs or increases the infectivity of individuals with genital ulcers, and if genital ulcers facilitate transmission of HIV infection, then at the community level the two infections have the potential to greatly amplify each other (Wasserheit, 1992).

Cervical Cancer   Cervical cancer is a major public health problem throughout the world, and it is the most common cancer in Africa (Parkin et al., 1988; see also Chapter 7). It is strongly associated with several types of human papillomavirus (HPV), the etiologic agent of genital warts (WHO, 1987) and increasingly recognized as important human carcinogens.

HIV-infected women are at increased risk for cervical dysplasia, a precursor lesion for cervical cancer (Laga et al., 1992; Schafer et al., 1991; Wright et al., 1994a). Furthermore, HIV infection may adversely alter the course and treatment of cervical dysplasia and cancer (Frutcher et al., 1992; Klein et al., 1992; Maiman et al., 1990; Rellihan et al., 1990; Schwartz et al., 1991; Wright et al., 1994b). Compared with women of unknown HIV serostatus, HIV-infected women have a ninefold greater risk of recurrent or persistent cervical intraepithelial neoplasia following loop electrosurgical excision (Wright et al., 1994b).

If detected and treated early, cervical cancer is almost always curable; in the absence of early treatment, it is almost always fatal. In Sub-Saharan Africa, many women die from cervical cancer because their disease is only diagnosed at an advanced, incurable stage.

Gender Differentials in STDs and HIV Infection

Gender is linked to biological and behavioral factors that contribute to crucial differences in the acquisition, course, and consequences of STDs. Compared with men, women are less likely to have control over the circumstances of their sexual activity. If they have sex with an infected partner, they are more likely to acquire an STD, including HIV infection; if they have an STD or HIV infection, they are less likely to seek health care; if they seek health care, they are less likely to be treated effectively, are more likely to develop complications, and, finally, frequently pay a heavier social toll for STDs, including HIV and their sequelae. These individual factors operate against a backdrop of such societal features as the low status of women and the high ratios of males to females in urban areas. These societal factors clearly influence sexual behavior and are discussed in greater detail below.

Control Over the Circumstances of Sexual Intercourse

Gender typically influences economic and social status and, in most societies, women's roles are defined primarily by their sexual and reproductive relationships with men, relationships that place severe limitations on the extent of women's control of their own sexuality (Aral, 1990). Compared with men, in most societies women also have fewer options about when, where, how, and with whom they will have sex.

Acquisition of STDs and HIV Infection and Development of Complications

Gender affects the efficiency of transmission of some STDs. Transmission of STD pathogens that produce discharge or are present in genital secretions—such as gonococci, chlamydiae, trichomonads, and HIV—appears to be more efficient from male to female than vice versa, at least partly because of the prolonged exposure to organisms when infected ejaculate is retained in the vagina. In contrast, the transmission of syphilis, chancroid, and genital herpes, all of which cause genital ulcers, differs little by gender. This may be because transmission of these STDs depends on small breaks in the genital skin that probably occur in both sexes during vigorous coitus. Sexual behaviors may also synergize with biological factors to promote STD transmission. For example, the practice of "dry sex" (use of intravaginal desiccants to increase friction during coitus) in some parts of Sub-Saharan Africa—such as Malawi, Zaire, and Zambia (Brown et al., 1992; Dallabetta et al., 1990; Nyirenda, 1992)—frequently causes breaks in the vaginal surface (Brown et al., 1992), which may enhance the risk of acquiring HIV infection and other STDs. Finally, unavailability of female-controlled barrier methods of birth control restricts women's ability to protect themselves against all STDs, including HIV infection.

Health-Seeking Behavior

Another gender-related consequence of STDs is the exacerbation of their sequelae brought about by differences in health-seeking behavior. Although in some industrialized countries women are more likely than men to seek health care and subsequently receive appropriate treatment, this is rarely the case in Sub-Saharan Africa (Ehrhardt and Wasserheit, 1991). First, women may not suspect that they have an STD. Indeed, women with STDs are more frequently asymptomatic than men: 50 to 80 percent of women infected with gonorrhea are asymptomatic (Jones and Wasserheit, 1991), compared with 20 to 40 percent of men (Rothenberg and Potterat, 1990). In addition, when STD symptoms are present in women, they are often subtle, and may resemble changes that normally occur during the menstrual cycle, such as increased vaginal discharge, lower abdominal pain, and vaginal bleeding. Finally, cultural factors may influence the way women perceive the significance of their symptoms. For example, in regions where women are circumcised, practice "dry sex," or where STDs are widespread, pain during coitus, irregular vaginal bleeding, or pelvic pain may be considered the norm.

Another major reason for gender differentials in seeking care for STDs is the female-specific, stigmatizing character of STDs, including HIV infection. Women face very strong sociocultural barriers to STD care, which are frequently fueled by the judgmental attitudes of health care providers. Finally, financial barriers for accessing care for HIV and other STDs may be stronger for women than for men, because women are frequently either of lower socioeconomic status than men or do not have independent financial resources.

Detection and Treatment of STDs

Even if they do seek health care for STDs, women are less likely than men to receive correct diagnosis and adequate treatment, for several reasons. First, most health care providers have limited expertise in STD management in women; they also share a common misconception that STDs affect only promiscuous women and prostitutes. Second, as discussed earlier, because STD signs and symptoms in women are often subtle and nonspecific, clinical diagnosis is not reliable. Third, in many Sub-Saharan African settings, laboratory tests are not available, even though it is women who would benefit most from laboratory tests because of the poor predictive value of female STD syndromes, particularly for vaginal discharge. Finally, the increased antimicrobial resistance of many pathogens to older antibiotics such as penicillin requires that new, more expensive drugs be used. Once again, women may be disproportionately affected: most sexually active women in Sub-Saharan Africa are either pregnant or breastfeeding at any given time, yet antibiotics that are effective and safe under those conditions may be neither available nor affordable.

The Social Implications of STDs and HIV Infection

Both STDs and their complications have far greater social significance for women than they do for men. Uncomplicated STDs typically cause personal embarrassment and domestic conflicts, but whoever is responsible for bringing a given infection into the relationship, it is the woman who is typically blamed and who endures the most serious consequences; these may include violence, divorce, and social ostracism. The complications of STDs, especially impaired fertility, are even more devastating. Although male infertility scientifically explains about one-third of all infertility, women are customarily blamed when a couple cannot have children. In parts of Africa, it is not uncommon for the female of an infertile couple to look for another male to make her pregnant (Rob et al., 1987), out of fear of being rejected by her husband and in-laws and becoming a social outcast. As a result, many infertile men may never become aware of their infertility. For women, childlessness, whether through infertility or poor pregnancy outcome, can be a major tragedy. Not only does it cause personal pain for the women themselves, but it becomes a paramount infirmity in a society that values women primarily for their ability to produce healthy offspring. Infertile women may be divorced by the same husbands who infected them with the STD that produced the infertility. The same is true of HIV-infected women, who are at risk of abandonment by the very men who transmitted the infection (de Bruyn, 1992). Ostracized by society, divorced women have few survival options other than prostitution, which increases STD transmission and the risk of infertility in the larger community, creating a vicious cycle of disease; misery; and, increasingly, death.

In this way, STDs and their complications affect individuals, communities, and, eventually, whole societies. In some areas, notably the so-called "infertility belt," which extends from Gabon in the west of Africa to southwestern Sudan in the east, STDs have had a dramatic impact on fertility rates. Brunham estimates in a mathematical model that a 20 percent gonorrhea prevalence in sexually active adults may produce up to a 50 percent reduction in net population growth, an estimate consistent with fertility levels actually observed in some parts of Uganda (Brunham et al., 1991). The consequences of HIV infection are even more striking. In another mathematical model, Anderson predicts that in some Sub-Saharan African countries, HIV infection may reverse demographic growth from positive to negative over a few decades (Anderson et al., 1988).

Yet another dramatic—and paradoxical—effect of STDs on society is their potential for jeopardizing family planning programs. STDs may decrease acceptance and continuation of contraceptive methods in two ways: directly, by creating the perception of a contraceptive side effect, and indirectly, by creating a fear of fertility impairment in the face of complications of STDs. Numerous studies in Bangladesh have found that the most common reason given for discontinuing a contraceptive method is the perception of a method-associated side effect (Akbar et al., 1981; Bhatia, 1982; Jain and Sivin, 1977; Rob et al., 1987). Similar findings have turned up all over the globe and can be extrapolated comfortably to other settings. Absent accurate diagnosis and effective education and therapy, it is far easier for a woman to blame a vaginal discharge on her current contraceptive method than to confront the possibility of having been infected by her husband—who is then, by definition, unfaithful. The net result is that the woman stops using her contraceptive method in the mistaken belief that it caused the unrelated infection (Wasserheit, 1989).

The indirect impact of STDs on family planning is equally important. Several authors have postulated that high levels of infertility or frequent adverse pregnancy outcomes might result in a compensatory decrease in acceptance of family planning methods (O'Reilly, 1986; Rosenberg et al., 1986). In societies that value children highly, couples are unlikely to undertake voluntary fertility regulation unless they are confident that they will be able to raise as many healthy children as they desire (Wasserheit, 1989).

STDs and HIV Infection Throughout the Female Life Span

The relative contribution of different risk factors for STDs, including HIV infection, varies with age. Increased vulnerability to STDs may be the result of biological or behavioral factors, and these may go in the same or in the opposite direction. In adolescence, for example, biological and behavioral factors act concurrently to increase dramatically the risk of HIV infection and other STDs and their complications. In later years, however, these factors may have different weights. In the adult, biological factors tend to decrease in importance and to be outweighed by behavioral factors. In the elderly, while physiological changes may facilitate the transmission of HIV and other STDs, behavioral factors tend to be protective (Ehrhardt and Wasserheit, 1991).

The striking changes that occur in cellular morphology in the vagina and cervix over the female life span have a direct effect on susceptibility to STDs and on the spectrum of infections found at each stage. During the first few weeks of life, the vagina and cervix of the newborn are lined by squamous epithelial thick cells that are relatively resistant to infection. From one month until menarche, changes in this lining increase susceptibility to STDs, especially to chlamydia and gonorrhea. Then, beginning at puberty, under hormonal influence, the cervico-vagina vault will again be covered by a thicker layer of squamous cells that are more resistant to some infections. The junction between squamous cells and the columnal cells that are the site of attachment for chlamydial and gonococcal infection is called the zone of ectopy. In the adolescent, the zone of ectopy is found on the surface of the cervix, where it is particularly susceptible to chlamydia, gonorrhea, and HIV. In young adulthood, the zone will usually migrate from the surface of the cervix to a less-exposed position in the cervical canal, reducing susceptibility to those infections (Cohen et al., 1985).

Sexuality and sexual behavior are forbidden subjects in many societies. As a result, real data on these topics are quite limited, particularly in developing countries. Most of our knowledge about sexual behavior comes from studies in industrialized countries, and it may not be applicable to Sub-Saharan Africa. In addition, sexual behavior in Sub-Saharan Africa is likely to vary a great deal across its many cultures and countries. At the same time, biological factors are more likely to be similar across cultures. This section enlarges upon the key biological and behavioral risk factors that are unique to each stage of the female life span.

Infancy, Childhood, and Adolescence

Infancy   During infancy, STDs, including HIV infection, are rarely transmitted sexually unless sexual abuse has occurred. Instead, they result from intrauterine or perinatal transmission of maternal infections. Behavioral risk factors for congenital infections therefore concern the infant's mother.

The consequences of congenital and perinatal infections associated with STDs and HIV infection include, at the extreme, blindness and other physical disabilities, mental retardation, and death. All the morbidities may have continuous, severe consequences throughout childhood, adulthood, and senescence. In addition, congenital infections affect not only the baby, but also its mother, who has to care for the sick or disabled child, perhaps for her remaining lifetime. Also, the children born to HIV-infected mothers, whether infected themselves or not, will, if they outlive their parents, become orphans, representing an extra burden for the older members of the community, often the grandmothers.

Childhood   STDs and HIV infection during childhood are relatively rare, and result almost entirely from sexual abuse. Sexual activities during childhood are exploratory and sporadic; while such sexual play between children of the same age is normative, sexual behavior between adults and children is not. Sexual abuse of children by strangers or by family members has received very little attention in Sub-Saharan Africa, and may well merit more. There are no studies of the region that would permit evaluation of the extent of emotional injury and long-term impact on the subsequent psychosexual development of sexually abused children or the magnitude of the problem. Studies from industrialized countries indicate that the extent of trauma varies and that the effects are nonspecific and may influence later sexual, emotional, or substance abuse behavior (Browne and Finkelhor, 1986). Sexual abuse of children may be more likely than rape of adult women to result in STD and HIV transmission because penetration is more likely to be traumatic in children.

Adolescence   This is the period when behavioral and biological factors combine to maximize the risk for STDs and HIV infection. As noted, during puberty and adolescence, several physiological changes occur in the female genital tract that result in a particularly high risk. In addition, adolescence is a period of life in which many women have their first sexual encounter, and it is the time when sexual behavior patterns become established. Furthermore, when the initial sexual encounter is traumatic, it may be a high-risk event for male-to-female HIV transmission (Bouvet et al., 1989). Age at sexual debut (time of first sexual intercourse) and sexual activities during adolescence follow secular trends and also vary greatly according to culture. Studies indicate that an earlier age of sexual debut is associated with higher total numbers of sex partners over a lifetime. In Ethiopia, where child marriage is practiced, half of 2,111 women surveyed had experienced their first sexual intercourse before the menarche (Duncan et al., 1990). That same early sexual activity was associated with an increased prevalence of STDs, PID, and cervical cancer later in life. The study also indicates that the younger the age at first marriage or first coitus, the shorter the duration of the marriage and the greater the likelihood of divorce (Duncan et al., 1990).

The extent of sexual assault in Sub-Saharan Africa is unknown. As in other parts of the world, rapes are rarely reported (see also Chapters 2 and 8). Instead, the incident is often settled between the families involved through compensation, in cash or goods, by the perpetrator to the family of the woman raped. There is evidence that rape is a serious problem in parts of Sub-Saharan Africa. In Kenya, when 71 teenage girls were raped during one night in the dormitory of a boarding school, a Kenyan newspaper described the incident as a common occurrence, and as sanctioned by the principal and his staff (Heise et al., 1994). There is a good chance that sexual abuse is a menace for African women throughout their lives. In South Africa, as one example, the incidence of rape appears to exceed rates in the United States, with an annual incidence of 34 rapes per 1,000 women, compared with 18 per 1,000 women in the United States (Heise et al., 1994).

Finally, the limited health knowledge and constrained health-seeking behavior of adolescents compound the impact of physiological factors on STD and HIV infection morbidity. Many adolescents are unable to recognize or to understand the significance of STD or HIV symptoms and have little or no independent access to health care, or are afraid to utilize existing services.

Adulthood In adulthood, behavioral factors dominate the risk for STDs and HIV infection and are characteristically tied to the sex partner's sexual behavior. The physiological changes that affect the risk for STDs, including HIV infection, during the adult reproductive years are related primarily to the menstrual cycle, pregnancy, and contraceptive use.

The menstrual cycle seems to play a key role in the risk of PID. Symptomatic gonococcal and chlamydial PID appear to occur more frequently during the first week of the menstrual cycle, probably because of the retrograde flow of menstrual blood from the uterus into the fallopian tubes. During pregnancy, although the lower genital tract, particularly the cervix, may be more susceptible to infections, the upper genital tract appears to be protected from infections by gestational anatomical changes.

Sex during menses has been hypothesized, although not shown, to be a risk factor for female-to-male transmission (De Vincenzi, 1994). Although there is no evidence thus far to suggest that pregnancy aggravates the course of HIV infection, several studies have documented the occurrence of serious HIV-related infections during pregnancy (Selwyn and Antoniello, 1993).

Contraceptives may play a prominent part in altering the risk of HIV and other STDs during the reproductive years, and even beyond. Barrier contraceptive methods such as condoms and diaphragms serve as a mechanical barrier to pathogens. Oral contraceptive pills seem to increase risk of cervical chlamydial infection, but appear to decrease the frequency and severity of PID. Users of intrauterine devices have increased risk of developing PID, particularly during the first four months following insertion, and this risk varies by geographic area; Africa has the highest rates of all the world's regions (Farley et al., 1992).

Behavioral risk factors for STDs include sexual and health-seeking behavior. Because men tend to have more partners and engage in riskier sexual behavior than women, women's risk for STDs, including HIV infection, is more closely related to their husbands' sexual behavior than their own. Nonsexual transmission of STD pathogens present in the blood—such as HIV, treponemes (which cause syphilis), and hepatitis B virus—may be a concern for health workers, particularly for midwives and traditional birth attendants, who are usually women and who frequently come into contact with abundant quantities of blood.

The lifelong impacts of STDs and their long-term sequelae are tremendous, and were described earlier. Obviously, the earlier in life those sequelae occur, the longer women have to bear their consequences. In addition, women may be more susceptible to such consequences, notably the psychological and social repercussions, in part because they are affected by HIV and other STDs at an earlier age than men.

Maturity and Senescence As people become older, their sexual activity often decreases as a result of physiologic changes and societal influences. During senescence, increased biological risk for STDs compensates for decreased behavioral risk.

The physiologic changes that occur in women include atrophic changes in the vagina, with thinning of the epithelium, reduced lubrication, and narrowing and shortening of the vaginal canal. A vagina that is dry can be injured more easily by penile penetration (Holmes, 1990; Mooradian and Greiff, 1990), placing a woman at greater risk for transmission of HIV infection and other STDs from an infected partner.

Sexual behavior at older ages is determined by sexual interest, which is influenced, in turn, by the hormonal environment and sociocultural factors. The level of sexual activity among older people, particularly women, varies greatly across cultures. While sexual activity is socially acceptable or desirable for older men, it may not be so for older women. In Sub-Saharan Africa, for example, the limited available evidence suggests that many women cease to be sexually active at menopause.

A different, yet major aspect of the burden of the HIV epidemic on women, including older women, is the care of the sick. Indeed, it is women who—as health care workers, community members, or family members—provide most of the care for people with chronic illnesses, including HIV infection and AIDS (Richardson, 1989).

MAGNITUDE OF THE PROBLEM

Morbidity

This section provides general information on the extent of the problem of sexually transmitted diseases, including HIV infection, in Sub-Saharan Africa and estimates the prevalence of five common STDs across the countries of the region.

There are noteworthy differences in the magnitude of the STD burden between the industrialized and the developing countries. First, sexually transmitted diseases including HIV infection are much more prevalent in most developing countries, particularly in Sub-Saharan Africa, than in the majority of industrialized countries. Second, developing countries, again particularly those in Sub-Saharan Africa, have a higher incidence of complications of STDs than industrialized countries experience, and these complications are often more severe. Third, different kinds of STDs predominate in developing and industrialized countries. For example, the proportion of STDs characterized by genital ulcers is greater in developing countries than in industrialized countries; in Sub-Saharan Africa, chancroid and syphilis account for the majority of genital ulcers, while in industrialized countries, herpes is the main cause of those lesions (Meheus et al., 1990). Finally, while in industrialized countries HIV infection is often transmitted through homosexual contact and injecting drug use, and affects predominantly males, in Sub-Saharan Africa, HIV infection is almost exclusively transmitted heterosexually and affects both women and men equally, except for substantial mother-to-child transmission.

The following statistics highlight the severity of the problem in Sub-Saharan Africa.

- STDs are among the top five reasons for clinic attendance in many Sub-Saharan African countries (Meheus, 1990). For example, STDs account for 13 percent of adult outpatient visits in Zimbabwe (Zimbabwe, 1989), and for 5 to 10 percent of outpatient visits in Zambia (Hira et al., 1992b). In some countries, PID is the most common diagnosis among women attending STD clinics. In Zimbabwe, 47 percent of women attending an STD clinic had a pelvic inflammatory disease (Latif, 1981), and in Ethiopia at least 39 percent of gynecological outpatients had signs or symptoms suggestive of PID (Perine et al., 1980). Even though many women with PID are never diagnosed and the majority are not hospitalized (Carty et al., 1972), it is one of the leading causes of gynecological admission (Brown and Cruickshank, 1976; De Muylder, 1989; Perine et al., 1980; Ratnam et al., 1980b; Zacarias and Aral, 1985).

- In many countries of Sub-Saharan Africa, where the prevalence of syphilis among pregnant women is at least 10 percent, Schulz and colleagues estimate that 5 to 8 percent of all pregnancies that last beyond 12 weeks will fail to produce a healthy infant because of congenital syphilis, or syphilis-related fetal death or infant death (Schulz et al., 1987).

- In some Sub-Saharan African countries—for example, Cameroon, Ethiopia, and Kenya—as many as 4 to 6 percent of newborn babies develop gonococcal ophthalmia, a condition that, untreated, leads to blindness (Galega et al., 1984; Lepage and Van de Perre, 1988a; Muhe and Tafari, 1986).

- In Sub-Saharan Africa, HIV infection has not only reached high levels of prevalence—overall, affecting one in 40 adults, and in certain cities as many as 30 percent of pregnant women (see Appendix, Table 11-8)—but is also rapidly spreading, particularly in urban areas and among selected subgroups, such as prostitutes (Nkowame, 1991).

- In several African cities, AIDS is the leading cause of death among young women and men.

Prevalence

Estimates of the prevalence of HIV infection and other STDs among women in Sub-Saharan Africa must be made cautiously. Although more information on STDs is available in Sub-Saharan Africa than in other parts of the developing world, the quantity, quality, and heterogeneity of data across countries and populations limit the ability to precisely define the extent of STD morbidity in the region. There is virtually no surveillance system in Sub-

Saharan Africa to assess incidence, and most available data derive from prevalence studies in family planning, antenatal, and STD clinics. For certain diseases and syndromes—gonorrhea, chlamydia, trichomoniasis, syphilis, and HIV infection—data are relatively abundant, while for others—chancroid, genital ulcers, PID, cervical cancer, adverse outcomes of pregnancy, and ectopic pregnancy—data are patchy at best.

Despite these constraints, it is possible to estimate the burden of STDs across Sub-Saharan African countries by examining five common diseases: gonorrhea, chlamydia, trichomoniasis, syphilis, and HIV infection. Prevalence data have been compiled for each disease by country, for low-risk, high-risk, and very high-risk populations. The three populations were defined as follows: (1) low-risk populations were women attending antenatal clinic or family planning clinics, or women sampled in community-based studies who are probably fairly representative of the general population; (2) high-risk populations were women attending STD clinics, or women with symptoms suggestive of STDs who were attending other clinical facilities; and (3) very high-risk populations were women engaged in prostitution. To obtain sufficient data for prevalence estimates that could be considered moderately robust, the authors reviewed studies from the past 4 years for HIV, and for the past 20 years for the other STDs.

For all STDs except HIV infection, disease-country-population-specific prevalence was estimated by taking the median value when data from more than one study were available for a given country; the assumption was that a single study represented the country prevalence in countries that had only one disease-population-specific study. For HIV[1] infection, because the number of studies varies tremendously across countries and across regions within countries, a slightly different approach was used to avoid biasing estimates toward countries or regions with the highest number of studies. To estimate the population-specific HIV prevalences by country, the authors first calculated population-specific median HIV prevalences by region within a given country, and then took the median of those medians for each country. For all five diseases, to estimate the disease-population-specific prevalences for Sub-Saharan Africa, the median of all the country-specific median prevalences was taken.

The individual study prevalences and the median country prevalences reveal that: (1) the amount of data varies greatly between countries; (2) most studies concern HIV infection; there are relatively few data on other STDs; (3) there are large variations in disease prevalence, within and among countries; and (4) prostitutes constitute a major reservoir of STDs. Furthermore, the prevalences of STDs, including HIV infection, are generally higher in Sub-Saharan Africa than in industrialized countries, even among low-risk populations. In addition, in most Sub-Saharan African countries, as in the industrialized countries, chlamydia is more prevalent than gonorrhea in populations considered at low risk (Appendix Tables 11-6, 7, and 8 and Tables 11-3 and 11-4, below).

Table 11-4 shows the median STD and HIV prevalences for Sub-Saharan Africa. Because of the heterogeneity among countries, these figures are necessarily crude, and almost meaningless when considered as absolute quantities. Nevertheless, they are useful in assessing the relative importance of "core groups" in the transmission of the five STDs in the region as a whole. Core groups are defined as groups of individuals who are highly sexually active, and thus contribute disproportionately to disease transmission in a given population (Yorke et al., 1978). Core groups usually include prostitutes, their clients, and other individuals who have multiple sex partners, such as those in the military and long-distance truck drivers. The ratio of STD prevalence in prostitutes to the STD prevalence in low-risk populations can be derived from Table 11-4, which shows diminishing rates per 100 women for HIV infection (7), gonorrhea (5.2), syphilis (2.5), chlamydia (2.3), and trichomoniasis (1). These descending values suggest that core groups in Sub-Saharan Africa play a critical role in the transmission of HIV infection and gonorrhea, but are less important in the transmission of syphilis and chlamydia, and have little influence in the transmission of trichomoniasis. The role of the core group inferred through this analysis of STD is consistent with what has been postulated elsewhere, with the exception of syphilis, which elsewhere has been highly associated with core groups. This discrepancy may be brought about by the measurement of syphilis by syphilis serology in the data being used here, a measure that indicates either a past or a current infection. In addition, while compared with the general population, core groups may have a much higher prevalence of current infectious syphilis, their prevalence of positive syphilis serology may not be significantly greater.

STD and HIV prevalence among high-risk groups is significantly correlated with STD and HIV prevalence in low-risk groups (p < 0.05), using Pearson's correlation coefficient. Data on persons attending STD clinics must be examined with caution, however, because various health services in different countries may attract very heterogeneous populations that may not be comparable across countries.

TABLE 11-3 Median STD Prevalences (median prevalence per 100 women)

Country	Low-Risk Population					High-Risk Population					Very-High-Risk Population				
	GC	CT	TV	TP	HIV	GC	CT	TV	TP	HIV	GC	CT	TV	TP	HIV
Angola					0.3				25						
Botswana				17	0						20		17	22	45
Burkina Faso				18					20	21					
Central African Republic	10			10											
Cameroon	12	9	12	10	0.9	21		7				39			7.1
Côte d'Ivoire					6.5	10						65			35
Ethiopia	9			10	4.9	19					30	6	24	37	21
Guinea Bissau					0										
Gabon	6	15		13		15	16	23		3.7					
Gambia, The	7	7	32	11	0		14							71	
Ghana	3	4				3	7								49
Kenya	7	8	11	4	8.4	23	7	11	6		28			37	75
Madagascar												18	39	25	
Malawi	5	3	26	14	20	20	5	32	25		29		27	21	
Mozambique				6	0.1										
Niger	5			0	1	15		16	4						4.9
Nigeria	5	9	21	4											6.5
Rwanda		16		7	15					72				49	
Senegal	2	8	19	7	0.2	3	8	16	14	0.1	15	16	21	23	3.4
Somalia	0	18		10							11			47	3
South Africa	10	1	36	12	0.8	11	13	31	0	6.5					16
Sudan						6		20						29	
Swaziland	3		26	12	2.3										
Tanzania	7	7	14	16	12					13	51	25		23	58
Uganda	2	7	43	5	13					59				6	
Zaïre	2	6	16	1	3.8						23	14	22	16	32
Zambia	11		39	8	18	23	13		29						
Zimbabwe	5	6	23	9	11	19		35	19	65					

NOTE: GC, gonorrhea; CT, chlamydia; TV, trichomoniasis; TP, syphilis; HIV, HIV infection type 1.
Low-risk population includes women attending antenatal or family planning clinics or women sampled in community based-studies.
High-risk population includes women attending STD clinics, or women with symptoms suggestive of STDs.
Very-high-risk population includes women engaged in prostitution. Median prevalences are calculated using data from the Appendix.

TABLE 11-4 Median STD Prevalences in Sub-Saharan Africa (per 100 women)

Population	Disease				
	Gonorrhea	Chlamydia	Trichomoniasis	Syphilis	HIV Infection
Low risk	5	8	23	10	3
High risk	15	11	20	19	17
Very high risk	26	18	23	25	21

NOTE: Low-risk population includes women visiting antenatal or family planning clinics or women sampled in community-based studies. High-risk population includes women attending STD clinics or women with symptoms suggestive of STDs. Very-high-risk population includes women engaged in prostitution. Median prevalences are calculated using data from Table 11-3.

A mapping of country prevalences (Figures 11-1, 11-2, and 11-3) reveals a clustering of diseases: highest prevalences occur in eastern and southern Africa, and in a limited region of central Africa that includes Cameroon and the Central African Republic. The pattern of gonorrhea prevalences resembles that of syphilis, although the correlation between the prevalences of these two diseases was not statistically significant. The highest prevalence of HIV infection occurs in East Africa and in the northern part of southern Africa. The very high prevalence of STDs in other regions, particularly in southern Africa, in Cameroon, and the Central African Republic, suggests that those regions have the potential for very rapid spread of HIV. Nevertheless, caution is advisable in predicting where the next wave of the HIV epidemic will strike, since there are almost no data from several large parts of Sub-Saharan Africa, notably from many countries of western Africa.

Mortality

The burden of diseases has traditionally been measured in mortality. As health interventions evolve and disease patterns shift, other indicators, such as morbidity and quality of life, must also be used to measure disease impact and to set health priorities. Indeed, measuring the burden of diseases solely by mortality may mask the extent of a problem. The sexually transmitted diseases are an excellent example: the disease burden derived from STDs is primarily the product of frequent and severe morbidity rather than mortality. Nevertheless, of the six major STD complications, four (ectopic pregnancy, adverse pregnancy outcomes, cervical cancer, and enhanced HIV transmission) are potentially fatal, and HIV infection itself has an extremely high mortality rate, and it is now a major cause of death among young adults in some regions of Africa. In Abidjan, Côte d'Ivoire, AIDS is the leading cause of death in adult men, and in a study in Rwanda, approximately 90 percent of mortality among childbearing urban women is attributed to HIV infection (De Cock et al., 1990; Linden et al., 1992).

Economic Impact

The cost attributable to a disease is the sum of direct costs (drugs, hospitalization, transportation, provider payments) and indirect costs (loss of productivity and physical, psychological, and social impacts) (Drummond et al., 1989). Indirect costs are extremely difficult to quantify, primarily because estimating physical, psychological, and social costs requires culture-specific value judgments. They are, however, crucial.

The general level of health care provided in a country corresponds largely, though not totally, to its level of economic development. In the case of STD care, for instance, laboratory tests (even inexpensive microscopic examinations) are unavailable in most Sub-Saharan African countries. It is crucial, then, to take opportunity costs into consideration, as well as the actual number of dollars spent, when estimating costs and comparing them across countries.

Although few data are available on the direct costs of STDs, the magnitude and complexity of that group of diseases, including the frequent need for hospitalization, indicates that they are very high. In addition, costs of

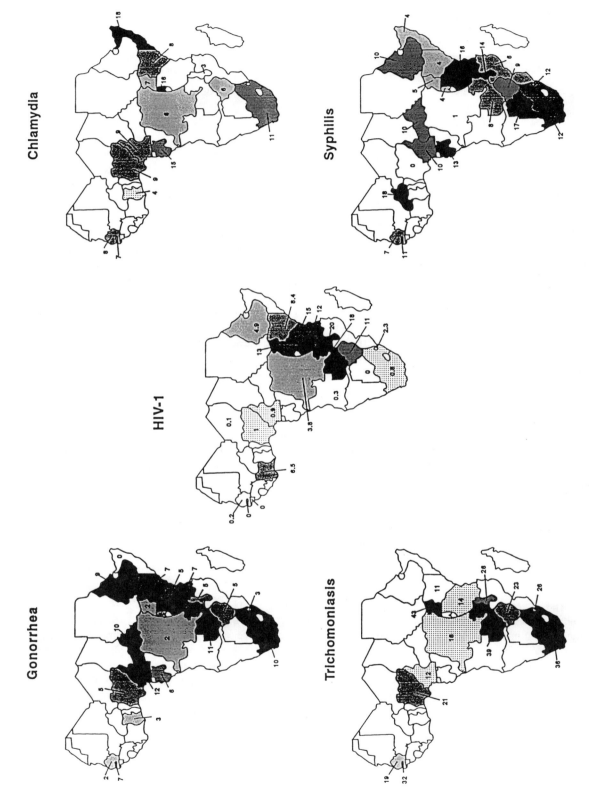

FIGURE 11-1 Disease prevalence in low-risk populations (per 100 women). The intensity of shading is proportional to disease prevalence. No shading: no data.

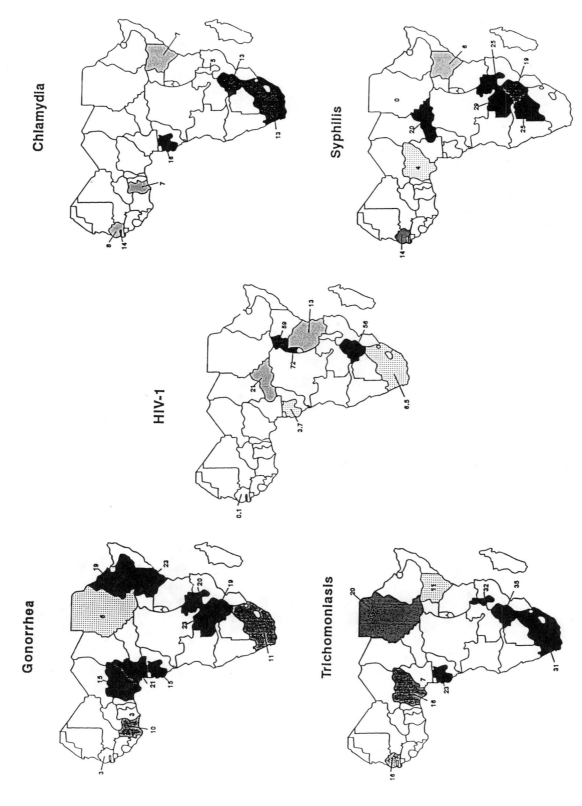

FIGURE 11-2 Disease prevalence in high-risk populations (per 100 women). The intensity of shading is proportional to disease prevalence. No shading: no data.

258

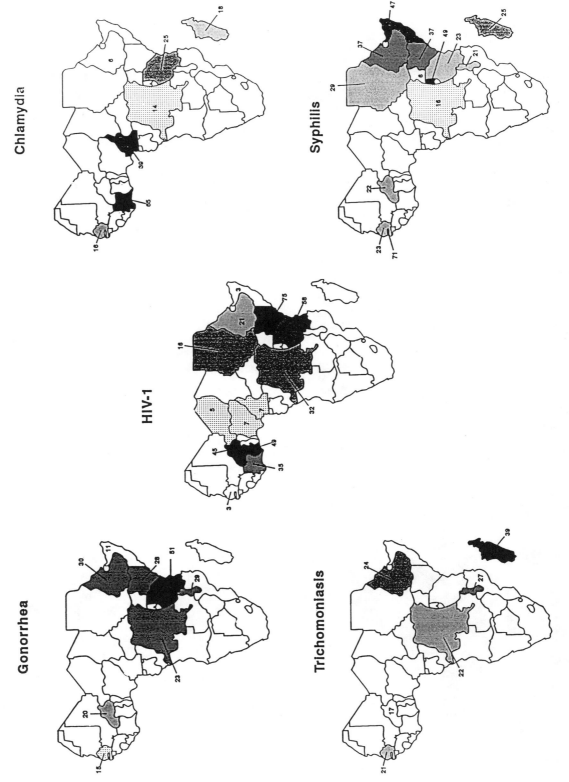

FIGURE 11-3 Disease prevalence in very-high-risk populations (per 100 women). The intensity of shading is proportional to disease prevalence. No shading: no data.

case management of STDs have markedly increased with the emergence of antimicrobial resistance and correspondingly poor response to STD treatment in HIV-infected persons. Poor countries now have to spend their scarce foreign currency to import costly antibiotics. In addition to the cost of Western medicine, people in Sub-Saharan Africa spend a considerable amount of money on traditional medicine to treat STDs and their sequelae.

The largest economic burden of STDs is not primarily the direct financial cost of treating diseases, but rather its indirect costs. Over and Piot have estimated the cost of the STD burden (including HIV infection) in healthy life-years lost per capita each year relative to other diseases in Sub-Saharan Africa. They found that in urban areas with high prevalences,[2] STDs account for up to 17 percent of productive healthy life-years lost and are second only to measles in their disease burden (Over and Piot, 1991). Because this model omits consideration of the devastating psychological and social costs of infertility in women, the total economic burden of STDs in Sub-Saharan Africa is higher. Treatment for infertility in Sub-Saharan Africa is very costly and failure rates are high, but what may appear to be an irrational expenditure of scarce resources is, instead, hard evidence of the high psychological and social costs of infertility and, by extension, the diseases that cause it.

SOCIETAL DETERMINANTS OF STDS AND HIV INFECTION

Several societal factors have been postulated as determinants in the transmission of STDs, including HIV infection: population-age composition, sex ratio, urbanization, population mobility, war and social unrest, sexual norms, women's social status, and the availability of health services (Aral, 1990; Brunham and Embree, 1990). Clearly such factors are interrelated and will change, independently and in association, in the course of socioeconomic development. The impact of each factor on STDs and HIV infection will therefore be time-dependent: the effect of one factor may be contingent on changes in the other factors.

Population-Age Composition

The population of Sub-Saharan Africa is characterized by a youthful age composition and fertility rates that are higher than in any other major region of the world (Cohen, 1993). In parts of the developing world, the marked decline in childhood mortality resulting from advances in medical sciences, childhood immunization, and improved sanitation has not been paralleled by a comparable decline in natality. This is particularly true for Sub-Saharan Africa, where birth rates have not changed since 1950 (Caldwell and Caldwell, 1990), although this figure masks considerable variation among regions and individual countries (Cohen, 1993).

The age composition of a community can influence STD and HIV rates in several ways. First, a broad-based age pyramid, dominated by young people, implies a large and increasing proportion of the population in its sexually active years. Second, all STDs are significantly age-related, with the highest STD and HIV rates occurring in young adults. Third, such a population structure may hamper the ability of the older generation to guide the younger generation's sexual norms and behaviors. Fourth, the relative scarcity of older men may increase promiscuity between a few older men and many younger women, given that sexual union between older men and younger women is almost universally accepted and practiced (Aral, 1990).

Urbanization, Sex Ratio, and Population Mobility

Rapid urbanization is a cardinal demographic feature of virtually all developing countries. In Africa, that phenomenon rests on the base of the region's urban centers, which were created during the colonial period. In many of these centers, only male workers were allowed, and the numerous waves of migration since independence have consisted mainly of young men looking for work (Larsen, 1989). Agriculture and mining have generated dormitory townships where men stay temporarily, sometimes for months, without going back to their homes, leaving wives and families in their rural villages. These cumulative processes have created a marked disequilibrium between the numbers of men and women in the region's urban settlements. In Nairobi and Harare, as just two examples, there are 50 to 80 percent more men than women. Social movement between status groups is another important factor that promotes anonymity, loosens societal structure, and, in turn, increases risky sexual behavior.

Population mobility is not solely a phenomenon brought about by urbanization and industry. In traditional societies, migration is often seasonal and is associated with herding and agriculture. In Botswana, for instance, Tswanas may have as many as four homes to accommodate seasonal migrations. In many areas, particularly in urban centers, the relative scarcity of women, combined with population mobility, poverty, and social inequities, creates an environment all too conducive to prostitution, thereby swelling the high-risk core group.

War and Social Unrest

War and social unrest not only engender geographic and social mobility, but add extreme levels of mental and physical violence. In Mozambique, between 1975 and 1989, an estimated 1.6 million people (10 percent of the population) were displaced by the frequent RENAMO (Mozambique National Resistance) attacks on rural populations (Cliff, 1991). Gersony reports that 15 percent of refugees reported systematic rape of civilian women by RENAMO combatants, and in areas controlled by RENAMO (Gersony, 1988):

> [a] function of the young girls and women is to provide sex for the combatants . . . these women are required to submit to sexual demands, in effect to be raped, on a frequent, sustained basis. . . . One of the frequent refugee complaints (verified by medical workers in some of the refugee camps) is the level of infection with venereal diseases which this practice proliferates. Severe beating is inflicted on young girls and women who resist sexual demands.

Sexual Norms, Women's Social Status, and Patterns of Sexual Behavior

Perhaps because sexuality is such a fundamental element of human life, it is complex, sensitive, and somewhat hidden, so that the gap between proscribed sexual norms and sexual practices can be quite wide (Holmes and Aral, 1991). They are undoubtedly interrelated, nevertheless, and both are influenced by the status of women.

Larsen (1989) has described two patterns of sexual behavior in Sub-Saharan Africa. Schematically, the first pattern characterizes societies of patrilineal descent, in which women tend to be socioeconomically dependent on men, and widows are inherited by their husbands' kin. In such a situation women have little control over their lives and very few sex partners, while men have sex with several women, usually prostitutes, who themselves have sex with many men. The second pattern characterizes matrilineal societies, in which women are comparatively more independent and both men and women have multiple sexual partnerships. Prevalence of HIV and other STDs tends to be higher in the patrilineal than in the matrilineal societies (Larsen, 1989).

Availability and Utilization of Health Services

Availability of health services influences the prevalence of STDs by reducing the size of the pool of infected persons through treatment. The principal impact of treatment is on the bacterial STDs, and while this may have a substantial indirect impact on the spread of HIV, any direct impact on the virus itself is lacking. In addition, unless there are routine screening programs that can identify infected individuals, and perhaps curtail risky behavior, availability of health services primarily influences diseases that are symptomatic. And, although in some industrialized countries women tend to be more likely than men to seek health care and thus receive appropriate treatment (Ehrhardt and Wasserheit, 1991), this is rarely the case in Sub-Saharan Africa. Furthermore, care for STDs appears to be an exception, for a variety of reasons.

CONCLUSIONS

STDs and HIV infection in women are among the most challenging problems facing the international health community. As Table 11-5 indicates, STDs and HIV infection can occur at any age, but the importance of both behavioral and biologic risk factors for these diseases ebbs and flows across the life span in ways that have important implications for both research and intervention. Because both of these kinds of factors peak during

TABLE 11-5 Risks of Sexually Transmitted Diseases and HIV Infection among Females in Sub-Saharan Africa by Stage of the Life Span and Type of Risk Factor

	In Utero/ Infancy	Childhood (ages 1–14)	Adolescence/Young Adulthood (ages 15–24)	Mature Adulthood (ages 25–49)	Postmenopause (age 50+)
Risk of exposure (importance of behavioral risk factors)	Low-medium	Low	High	High	Low
Risk of acquisition if exposed (importance of biologic risk factors)	High	High	High	Medium	High

NOTE: Because STDs and HIV infection can be acquired at any point during the life span, this table, unlike those in Chapters 3 to 10, presents the comparative risks of acquisition of, and exposure to, STDs and HIV infection. Also, the life span age categories defined here differ slightly from those of the other chapter tables, because they represent age groupings with similar risks of acquisition and exposure.

adolescence and young adulthood, this period constitutes the stage of highest risk in the life span of women. Both STDs and HIV infection occur most frequently in populations that are difficult to reach, and they are intertwined with sexuality and gender role, which in turn are determined by underlying socioeconomic factors. Those issues may be difficult to confront. Failure to identify and address these socioeconomic factors, however, narrows the ability to effectively prevent and control all STDs, including HIV infection. Limited data also suggest that the socioeconomic costs of HIV infection and other STDs are substantial. From a programmatic perspective, because of the impacts of STDs on reproductive health and HIV transmission, it is likely that interventions to prevent and control STDs in addition to HIV infection will synergistically promote family planning, child survival, and safe motherhood, and have a profoundly positive impact on the health of females across their entire life span.

RESEARCH NEEDS

This section highlights selected research issues of high priority in the reduction of STD/HIV morbidity among women in Sub-Saharan Africa and, in some cases, among women worldwide. Some of this research, particularly that involving basic science, may best be done in industrialized countries. Research done in developing countries must be relevant to the needs of those countries and carried out by local scientists in collaboration with local policy planners. Research involving both developing and industrialized countries should be collaborative and strongly encouraged, since it is in the common interest of both sets of nations.

Operational Research

Operational research is one of the most crucial areas of research for the improvement of public health. It concerns the translation of knowledge into action and it integrates information from a variety of disciplines: psychology, sociology, anthropology, epidemiology, clinical medicine, microbiology, and administration. Operational questions that are critical for reducing sexually transmitted diseases in women include the following:

• How can we effectively integrate STD control with other relevant programs such as AIDS prevention, family planning, and antenatal care into a comprehensive health care package that is more accessible and acceptable to women?

- What characteristics of health care systems would allow them to better serve the needs of women?
- How should counseling, testing, and partner notification for both HIV and other STDs be done in settings where resources are scarce and where such activities may lead to violence against women? In the absence of routine screening for women, the only way to identify asymptomatic women with STDs may be through their male sex partners.
- How should programs be designed to reach groups at high risk for STDs, including HIV infection, such as prostitutes, their clients, and long-distance truck drivers?
- How can traditional practitioners such as traditional birth attendants be involved in the prevention of HIV infection and other STDs?

Technology Development

Two technological issues are fundamentally important for women. The first is the development of noninvasive, simple, rapid, and affordable diagnostic tests for STDs (particularly for gonorrhea and chlamydia) that would permit the identification of women with asymptomatic infections. The second is the development of female-controlled prevention methods, such as safe intravaginal microbicidal agents, that would allow women to protect themselves against STDs, including HIV infection, and unwanted pregnancy.

Behavioral Research

The design of interventions to bring about behavioral change requires that people's behavioral patterns be understood, in this case the sexual and health-care-seeking behaviors that are the major determinants of STDs, including HIV infection. It is also important to understand reproductive decisions as another essential determinant of sexual behavior that may be influenced dramatically by the mortality associated with HIV infection. Research questions that may be relevant to understanding those behaviors and developing interventions to control HIV and other STDs include the following:

- What are the factors that determine sexual, health-seeking, and reproductive behaviors?
- What are the factors that determine women's social status?
- How does women's social status influence sexual, health-seeking, and reproductive behaviors?

Intervention trials, with comparison groups, to assist women in building the skills and self-esteem to reject unsafe sexual behavior should be developed. Special effort should be directed toward adolescent girls to help them avoid becoming infected with HIV and other STDs, recognizing the unique physiological and psychological factors that influence the spread of these diseases during adolescence.

Individual behaviors clearly are determined by societal factors. The influence of each of those factors and the interactions among them must be defined if individual behavior is to be well understood. This chapter attempted to explore, at the country level, the associations among such societal factors as urbanization, women's status, access to health services, and STD/HIV prevalence. The scarcity and poor quality of data and the lack of good indicators impeded that exploration in many cases. Methodologies for measurement of societal indicators, data collection, and data analysis that are appropriate to the sensitive context and dimensions of STDs must be developed.

Clinical Research and Epidemiology

- The clinical and epidemiological predictors of STDs in women must be refined to develop better management algorithms for asymptomatic as well as symptomatic infections.
- The relative importance of and the gender differences in HIV-associated diseases should be determined to assist in the development of simple management algorithms for opportunistic infections and neoplasms.
- The natural history of subclinical PID must be better described to improve detection.

- Both the impact of STDs, including HIV infection, on adverse pregnancy outcomes and the influence of pregnancy on the course of STDs need to be better understood to provide adequate care to women of reproductive age.
- Simple, cheap treatment regimens for HIV-infected pregnant women to reduce perinatal transmission should be developed.

NOTES

1. There are two types of HIV: HIV-1 and HIV-2. In these analyses, only HIV-1 was considered because it is more uniformly distributed across Sub-Saharan Africa.

2. High urban prevalence is defined as: HIV > 10 percent and gonorrhea > 5 percent among sexually active adults; syphilis > 10 percent among pregnant women.

REFERENCES

Adjorlolo, G. 1992. Natural history of HIV-2. Intl. Conf. AIDS 8:session 50.

Ahmed, H., K. Omar, Y. Adan, M. Guled, L. Grillner, and S. Bygdeman. 1991. Syphilis and human immunodeficiency virus seroconversion during a 6-month follow-up of female prostitutes in Mogadishu, Somalia. Intl. J. Stud. AIDS 2(2):119–123.

Aissu, T., M. C. Raviglione, J. P. Narain, et al. 1992. Monitoring HIV-associated tuberculosis in Uganda: Seroprevalence and clinical features. Intl. Conf. AIDS 8 (poster PoC 4023).

Akbar, J., J. Chakraborty, N. Jahan, et al. 1981. Dynamics of depo medroxyprogesterone acetate (DMPA) use effectiveness in the Matlab Family Planning Health Services Project. Paper presented at Bangladesh Fertility Research Programme, Seventh Annual Contributors' Conference, Dacca.

Akinsete, I., O. S. Ayelari, Y. Olurinde, and A. S. Akanmu. 1991. The pattern of HIV infection at the Lagos University Teaching Hospital (LUTH) Lagos, Nigeria, from January 1988–December 1990. Intl. Conf. AIDS 7(1):374 (abstract no. M.C. 3306).

Aladesanmi, A. F. K., G. Mumtaz, and D. C. W. Mabey. 1989. Prevalence of cervical chlamydial infection in antenatal clinic attenders in Lagos, Nigeria. Genitour. Med. 65:130.

Anderson, R. M., R. M. May, and A. R. McLean. 1988. Possible demographic consequences of AIDS in developing countries. Nature 4:1087–1093.

Aral, S. O. 1990. Sexual behavior as a risk factor for sexually transmitted disease. Pp. 185–198 in Reproductive Tract Infections: Global Impact and Priorities for Women's Reproductive Health, A. Germaine, K. K. Holmes, P. Piot, and J. Wasserheit, eds. New York: Plenum.

Arya, O., H. Nsanzumuhire, and S. Taber. 1973. Clinical, cultural, and demographic aspects of gonorrhoea in a rural community in Uganda. Bull. WHO 49:587–595.

Arya, O. P., S. R. Taber, and H. Nsanze. 1980. Gonorrhea and female infertility in rural Uganda. Am. J. Obstet. Gynecol. 138:929–932.

Asiimwe, G., G. Tembo, W. Naamara, et al. 1992. AIDS surveillance report: June 1992. Ministry of Health, AIDS Control Programme Surveillance Unit, Entebbe, Uganda. Photocopy.

Ballard, R. C., and H. Fehler. 1986. Chlamydial infections of the eye and genital tract in Southern Africa. S. Afr. Med. J. Oct.(Suppl):76–79.

Ballard, R. C., H. G. Fehler, M. O. Duncan, et al. 1981. Urethritis and associated infections in Johannesburg: the role of *Chlamydia trachomatis*. S. Afr. J. Sex. Trans. Dis. 1:24–26.

Ballard, R. C., et al. 1986. Chlamydial infections of the eye and genital tract in developing societies. Pp. 479–486 in Chlamydial Infections (Proceedings of the Sixth International Symposium on Human Chlamydial Infections), D. Oriel, et al., eds. Cambridge, U.K.: Cambridge University Press.

Barnes, T. E. C. 1979. Obstetrics in the Third World with particular reference to field research into delivery of maternal care to the community. Pp. 109–136 in Recent Advances in Obstetrics and Gynaecology, J. Stallworthy, and G. Bourne, eds. New York: Churchill Livingstone.

Barongo, L. R., J. B. Rugemalila, R. M. Gabone, et al. 1992. The epidemiology of HIV infection in adolescents of Kagera region. Intl. Conf. AIDS 8 (poster PoC 4197).

Beaujan, G., and I. Willems. 1990. Prevalence of *Chlamydia trachomatis* infection in pregnant women in Zaire. Genitour. Med. 66:124–126.

Belec, P. L., G. Gresenguet, M. C. Georges-Courbot, A. Villon, M. H. Martin, and A. J. Georges. 1989. Sero-epidemiologic study of several sexually transmitted diseases (including HIV infection) in a rural zone of the Central African Republic. Bull. Soc. Pathol. Exot. Filiales 81(4):692–698.

Bello, C. S. S., O. Y. Elegba, and J. D. Dada. 1983. Sexually transmitted diseases in northern Nigeria. Five years' experience in a university teaching hospital clinic. Br. J. Vener. Dis. 59:202–205.

Bentsi, C., C. Klufio, P. Perine, et al. 1985. Genital infections with *Chlamydia trachomatis* and *Neisseria gonorrhoeae* in Ghanaian women. Genitour. Med. 61(1):48–50.

Berger, R. E. 1990. Acute epididymitis. Pp. 641–651 in Sexually Transmitted Diseases, 2d ed., K. K. Holmes, P. A. Mårdh, P. F. Sparling, et al., eds. New York: McGraw-Hill.

Bhatia, S. 1982. Contraceptive intentions and subsequent behavior in rural Bangladesh. Stud. Fam. Plan. 13:24–31.

Bishaw, T., N. Tafari, M. Zewdie, et al. 1983. Prevention of congenital syphilis. Pp 148-153 in Proceedings of the Third African Regional Conference on Sexually Transmitted Diseases, H. Nsanze, R. H. Widy-Wirski, and R. H. Ellison, eds. Basel: Ciba Geigy.

Blanche S., C. Rouzioux, M-L. Guihart Moscato, et al. 1989. A prospective study of infants born to women seropositive for human immunodeficiency virus type 1. N. Engl. J. Med. 320:1643–1678.

Borgdorff, M. W., L. R. Barongo, C. N. Van Jaarsveld, et al. 1992. Sentinel surveillance: How representative are blood donors? Intl. Conf. AIDS 8 (poster PoC 4450).

Bottiger, B., I. B. Palme, J. L. da Costa, L. F. Dias, and G. Biberfeld. 1988. Prevalence of HIV-1 and HIV-2/HTLV-IV infections in Luanda and Cabinda, Angola. J. AIDS 1(1):8-12.

Bouvet E., I. De Vincenzi, R. Ancelle, and F. Vachon. 1989. Defloration as risk factor for heterosexual HIV transmission. Lancet i: 615.

Braddick, M. R., J. K. Kreiss, J. E. Embree, et al. 1990. Impacts of maternal HIV infection on obstetrical and early neonatal outcome. J. AIDS 4:1001–1004.

Brown, McL., and J. G. Cruickshank. 1976. Aetiological factors in pelvic inflammatory disease in urban blacks in Rhodesia. S. Afr. Med. J. 50:1342–1344.

Brown, R. C., J. E. Brown, and B. A. Okako. 1992. Vaginal inflammation in Africa. N. Engl. J. Med. 20:572.

Browne, A., and D. Finkelhor. 1986. Impact of child sexual abuse: a review of the research. Psychol. Bull. 99:66–77.

Brunham, R. C., and J. E. Embree. 1990. Sexually transmitted diseases: current and future dimensions of the problem in the Third World. Pp. 35–58 in Reproductive Tract Infections: Global Impact and Priorities for Women's Reproductive Health, A. Germaine, K. K. Holmes, P. Piot, and J. Wasserheit, eds. New York: Plenum.

Brunham, R. C., K. K. Holmes, and J. E. Embree. 1990a. Sexually transmitted diseases in pregnancy. Pp. 771–801 in Sexually Transmitted Diseases, K. K. Holmes, P. A. Mårdh, P. F. Sparling, et. al., eds. New York: McGraw-Hill.

Brunham, R., M. Laga, J. Simonsen, et al. 1990b. The prevalence of *Chlamydia trachomatis* infection among mothers of children with trachoma. Am. J. Epidemiol. 132(5):946–952.

Brunham, R. C., G. P. Garnett, J. Swinton, and R. M. Anderson. 1991. Gonococcal infection and human fertility in sub-Saharan Africa. Proc. R. Soc. London. Ser. B 246(1316):173–177.

Bulterys, M., A. Chao, A. Saah, et al. 1990. Risk factors for HIV-1 seropositivity among rural and urban pregnant women in Rwanda. Intl. Conf. AIDS 6(1):269 (abstract No. Th.C.576).

Bulterys, M., A. Chao, J. B. Kurawige, et al. 1991, Maternal HIV infection and intrauterine growth; a prospective cohort study in Butare, Rwanda. Intl. Conf. AIDS 7 (abstract WC 3234).

Burans, J. P., E. Fox, M. A. Omar, et al. 1990. HIV infection surveillance in Mogadishu, Somalia. E. Afr. Med. J. 67(7):466–472.

Burney, P. 1976. Some aspects of sexually transmitted disease in Swaziland. Brit. J. Vener. Dis. 52:412–414.

Bwayo, J. J., M. Otido, D. Oduor, et al. 1992. Regular clients of female sex workers: condom use and risk of HIV-1 infection. Intl. Conf. AIDS 8 (poster PoC 4182).

Caldwell, J. C., and P. Caldwell. 1990. High fertility in sub-Saharan Africa. Sci. Am. 262(5):118–125.

Cameron, D. W., L. J. D'Costa, G. M. Maitha, et al. 1989. Female to male transmission of human immunodeficiency virus type 1: risk factors for seroconversion in men. Lancet 2:403–407.

Carswell, J. W., et al. 1987. HIV infection in healthy persons in Uganda. AIDS 1(4):223–227.

Carty, M. J., M. Nzioki, and A. R. Verhagen. 1972. The role of gonococcus in acute pelvic inflammatory disease in Nairobi. E. Afr. Med. J. 49(5):376–379.

Chang, Y., E. Cesarman, M. S. Pessin, et al. 1994. Identification of herpes-virus-like DNA sequences in AIDS-associated Karposi's sarcoma. Science 226:1865–1869.

Chao, A., P. Habimana, M. Bulterys, et al. 1992. Oral contraceptive use, cigarette smoking, age at first sexual intercourse, and HIV infection among Rwandan women. Intl. Conf. AIDS 8 (poster PoC 4338).

Chiphangwi, J., N. G. Liomba, P. Miotti, G. Dallabetta, E. Ndovi, and A. J. Saah. 1989. Serial seroprevalence studies and estimates of incidence of HIV-1 antibody in pregnant women in Malawi. Intl. Conf. AIDS 5:1023 (abstract no. G.507).

Chiphangwi, J., G. Dallabetta, A. Saah, G. Liomba, and P. Miotti. 1990. Risk factors for HIV-1 infection in pregnant women in Malawi. Intl. Conf. AIDS 6(1):158 (abstract no. Th.C.98).

Cliff, J. 1991. The war on women in Mozambique. Health consequences of South African destabilization, economic crisis, and structural adjustment. Pp. 15–33 in Women and Health in Africa, M. Turshen, ed. Trenton, N.J.: Africa World Press.

Cohen, B. 1993. Fertility levels, differentials and trends. Pp. 8–67 in Demographic Change in Sub-Saharan Africa. Washington, D.C.: National Academy Press.

Cohen, M. S., J. R. Black, R. A. Proctor, and P. F. Sparling. 1985. Host defense and the vaginal mucosa. Scand. J. Nephrol. 86:13–22.

Connor E. M., R. S. Sperling, and R. Gelber. 1994. Reduction of maternal-infant transmission of human immunodeficiency virus type 1 with zidovudine treatment. N. Engl. J. Med. 331(18):1173–1180.

Cooper-Poole, B. 1986. Prevalence of syphilis in Mbeya, Tanzania. The validity of the VDRL as a screening test. E. Afr. Med. J. 63:646–650.

Corwin, A., J. Olson, M. Omar, A. Razaki, and D. Watts. 1991. Human immunodeficiency viral type 1 infection among prostitutes in Somalia. Intl. Conf. AIDS 7(1):306 (abstract no. M.C.3032).

Cotch, M. F. 1990. Carriage of *Trichomonas vaginalis* (Tv) is associated with adverse pregnancy outcome. Interscience Conference on Antimicrobial Agents and Chemotherapy 30:199 (abstract 681).

Dabis, F., F. Lepage, A. Serufilira, F. Nsengumuremyi, P. Msellati, and P. Van de Perre. 1989. Transmission du virus VIH-1 de la mère à l'enfant en Afrique Centrale: une étude de cohorte à Kigali, Rwanda—caractérisation épidémiologique à l'inclusion. Conférence internationale sur les implications du SIDA pour la mère et l'enfant. Paris (Résumé B11).

Dada, A. J., J. Ajayi, O. Ransome-Kuti, G. Williams, E. Abebe, A. Levin, T. Quinn, and W. Blattner. 1991. Prevalence survey of HIV-1 and HIV-2 infections in female prostitutes in Lagos State, Nigeria. Intl. Conf. AIDS 7(1):371 (abstract no. M.C.3295).

Dallabetta, G., et al. 1990. Vaginal tightening agents as risk factors for acquisition of HIV. Intl. Conf. AIDS 6(1):268 (abstract no. ThC574).

Dallabetta, G., P. Miotti, G. Liomba, et al. 1992. Evaluation of clinical and laboratory markers of cervicitis in STD patients in Malawi. Intl. Conf. AIDS 8(1):29 (abstract TuB 0510).

Damiba, A., S. Vermund, and K. Kelley. 1990. Prevalence of gonorrhoea, syphilis and trichomoniasis in prostitutes in Burkina Faso. E. Afr. Med. J. 67 (7 Suppl 2A):473–477.

D'Costa, L., F. Plummer, I. Bowmer, et al. 1985. Prostitutes are a major reservoir of sexually transmitted diseases in Nairobi, Kenya. Sex Trans. Dis. 12(2):64–67.

de Bruyn, M. 1992. Women and AIDS in developing countries. Soc. Sci. Med. 34(3):249–262.

De Clercq, A. 1982. Problèmes en obstétrique et gynécologie. Pp. 627–656 in Santé et maladies au Rwanda, A. Meheus, S. Butera, W. Eylenbosch, G. Gatera, M. Kivits, and I. Musafili, eds. Bruxelles: Administration Générale de la Coopération au Développement.

De Cock, K., B. Barrere, L. Diaby, et al. 1990. AIDS—the leading cause of adult death in the West African city of Abidjan, Ivory Coast. Science 249:793–796.

De Cock K. M., S. B. Lucas, S. Lucas, J. Agness, A. Kadio, and H. D. Gayle. 1993. Clinical research, prophylaxis, and care for HIV disease in Africa. Am. J. Public Health. 83(10):1385–1389.

Delacolette, C., K. Kihemu, C. Delacolette-Lebrun, and R. Habyambere. 1986. Prévalence et sensibilité aux antibiotiques de l'infection à *Neisseria gonorrhoeae* en milieu rural au Kivu, Zaïre. Ann. Soc. Belge Méd. Trop. 66:87–90.

Del Mistro, A., J. Chotard, A. J. Hall, et al. 1992. HIV-1 and HIV-2 seroprevalence rates in mother-child pairs living in The Gambia (West Africa). J. AIDS 5(1):19–24.

De Muylder, X. 1989. Standardised management of PID in a developing country. Genitour. Med. 65:281–283.

De Muylder, X., M. Laga, C. Tennstedt, E. Van Dyck, G. Aelbers, and P. Piot. 1990. The role of *Neisseria gonorrhea* and *Chlamydia trachomatis* in pelvic inflammatory disease and its sequelae in Zimbabwe. J. Inf. Dis. 162:501–505.

De Schampheleire, I., et al. 1990. Maladies sexuellement transmissibles dans la population féminine à Pikine, Sénégal. Ann. Soc. Belge Med. Trop. 70: 227–235.

De Schryver, A., and A. Meheus. 1989. International travel and sexually transmitted diseases. Rapp. Trim. Stat. Sanit. Mond. 42:90–99.

De Vincenzi, I. 1994. A longitudinal study of human immunodeficiency virus transmission by heterosexual partners. N. Engl. J. Med. 331:341–346.

Diaw, I., T. Siby, I. Thior, M. Traore, L. Dabo, M. Ndaw, A. Diaw, C. Langley, N. Kiviat, I. Ndoye, et. al. 1992. HIV and STD infections among newly registered prostitutes in Dakar. Intl. Conf. AIDS 8(2):C300 (abstract no. PoC 4333).

Didier, B., N. Lorenz, L. H. Ouedraogo, Y. Zina, P. Barth, and T. Rehle. 1990. KAP-study and HIV-seroprevalence among prostitutes in rural Burkina Faso. Intl. Conf. AIDS 6(1):146 (abstract no. Th.D.52).

Dietrich, M., A. A. Hoosen, J. Moodley, and S. Moodley. 1992. Urogenital tract infections in pregnancy at King Edward VIII Hospital, Durban, South Africa. Genitour. Med. 68(1):39–41.

Dosso, M., H. Faye, Y. Diakite-Harding, H. Aissi, J. Aka, and M. Duchassin. 1986. Aspects épidémiologiques et prévalence de Neisseria gonorrhea dans les infections génitales à Abidjan: analyse de 1742 prélèvements. Bull. Soc. Path. Ex. 79:130–139.

Drescher, C., T. Elkins, O. Adkeo, et al. 1988. The incidence of urogenital *Chlamydia trachomatis* infections among patients in Kumasi, Ghana. Intl. J. Gynecol. Obstet. 27:381–383.

Drummond, M. F., G. L. Stoddart, and G. W. Torrance. 1989. Methods for the Economic Evaluation of Health Care Programmes. Oxford, U.K.: Oxford University Press.

Duncan, M., G. Tibaux, A. Pelzer, et al. 1990. First coitus before menarche and risk of sexually transmitted disease. Lancet 335:338–340.

Dupont, A., D. Schrijvers, E. Delaporte, et al. 1988. Séroprévalence de la syphilis dans les populations urbaines et semi-rurales du Gabon. Bull. Soc. Path. Ex. 81:699–704.

Ebrahim, S. H., M. R. Sunkutu, and N. Mwansa. 1993. Epidemiological and clinical features of Kaposi's sarcoma in adults in Zambia. Intl. Conf. AIDS (abstract WS-B15-1).

Ehrhardt, A. A., and J. N. Wasserheit. 1991. Effects of age and gender on sexual behavior. Pp. 97–121 in Research Issues in Human Behavior and Sexually Transmitted Diseases in the AIDS Era, J. N. Wasserheit, S. O. Aral, K. K. Holmes, and P. J. Hitchcock. eds. Washington, D.C.: American Society for Microbiology.

Elliot, B., R. Brunham, M. Laga, et al. 1990. Maternal gonococcal infection as a preventable risk factor for low birthweight. J. Infect. Dis. 161:531–536.

Engels, H., A. Nyongo, M. Temmerman, W. G. V. Quint, E. Van Marck, and W. J. Eylenbosch. 1992. Cervical cancer screening and detection of genital HPV infection and chlamydial infection by PCR in different groups of Kenyan women. Ann. Soc. Belge Med. Trop. 72:53–62.

Fakeya, R. 1986. Antitreponemal antibodies among antenatal patients at the University of Ilorin Teaching Hospital. Afr. J. Sex Trans. Dis. 1:9–10.

Farley, T. M., M. J. Rosenberg, P. J. Rowe, J. H. Chen, and O. Meirkik. 1992. Intrauterine devices and pelvic inflammatory disease: an international perspective. Lancet 339:785–788.

Fassassi-Jarretou, A., A. Mabignath-Sall, B. Narraido, et al. 1991. Impacts de *Chlamydia trachomatis* sur les femmes enceintes au Gabon. Bull. Soc. Pathol. Exot. Filiales 84(5):620–626.

Feleke, W., M. Yusuf, H. Tesfay, A. Abraham, and G. Carosi. 1992. Prevalence of syphilis among pregnant women attending urban and semi-urban health centers in Ethiopia. Intl. Conf. AIDS 8(2):B148 (abstract PoB 3371).

François-Gerard, C., J. Nkurunziza, C. De Clerq, L. Stouffs, and D. Sondag. 1992. Seroprevalence of HIV, HBV and HCV in Rwanda. Intl. Conf. AIDS 8(2):C249 (abstract no. PoC 4027).

Frank, O. 1983. Infertility in Sub-Saharan Africa. Center for Policy Studies Working Paper 97. New York: The Population Council.

Friedmann, P., and D. Wright. 1977. Observations on syphilis in Addis Ababa. 2. Prevalence and natural history. Br. J. Vener. Dis. 53:276–280.

Fruchter, R., M. Maiman, E. Serur, and S. Cuthill. 1992. Cervical intraepithelial neoplasia in HIV infected women. Intl. Conf. AIDS 8(1) (abstract MoB 0057).

Galega, F., D. Heymann, and B. Nasah. 1984. *Gonococcal ophthalmia* neonatorum: the case for prophylaxis in tropical Africa. Bull. WHO 62:95–98.

Gaye-Diallo, A., F. Denis, S. Mboup, et al. 1992. Co-infections HIV/HTLV-1 in Senegal. Intl. Conf. AIDS 8 (poster PoC 4028).

Gersony, R. 1988. Summary of Mozambican refugee accounts of principally conflict-related experience in Mozambique. Washington, D.C.: Bureau for Refugee Persons, U.S. Department of State.

Geyid, A., H. S. Tesfaye, A. Abraha, et al. 1991. A study on STD pathogens in sex workers in Addis Ababa, Ethiopia. Intl. Conf. AIDS 7(2):301 (abstract No W.C. 3023).

Gichangi, P., M. Temmerman, A. Mohamed, J. Ndinya-Achola, F. Plummer, and P. Piot. 1992. Rapid increase in HIV-1 infection and syphilis between 1989 and 1991 in pregnant women in Nairobi, Kenya. Intl. Conf. AIDS 8(2):pC249 (abstract PoC 4029).

Gini, P., W. Chukudebelu, and A. Njoku-Obi. 1989. Antenatal screening for syphilis at the University of Nigeria Teaching Hospital, Enugu, Nigeria, A six-year survey. Intl. J. Gynecol. Obstet. 29(4):321–324.

Goeman, J., A. Meheus, P. Piot, et al. 1991. L'épidémiologie des maladies sexuellement transmissibles dans les pays en développement à l'ère du SIDA. Ann. Soc. Belge Med. Trop. 71: 81–113.

Green, S. D., J. K. Mokolo, M. Nganzi, A. G. Davies, I. R. Hardy, D. J. Jackson, E. B. Klee, R. A. Elton, P. D. Hargreaves, and W. A. Cutting. 1992. Seroprevalence and determinants of HIV-1 infection in pregnancy in rural Zaire. Intl. Conf. AIDS 8(2):C247 (abstract no. PoC 4016).

Gresenguet, G., L. Belec, P. M. V. Martin, et al. 1991. Séroprévalence de l'infection à VIH-1 au sein des consultants de la clinique des maladies sexuellement transmissibles de Bangui, Centrafrique. Bull. Soc. Path. Ex. 84(3):240–246.

Guiness, L., S. Sibandze, E. McGrath, and A. Cornelis. 1988. Influence on antenatal screening on perinatal mortality caused by syphilis in Swaziland. Genitour. Med. 64:294–297.

Heise, L., A. Rulkes, C. H. Watts, and A. B. Zwi. 1994. Violence against women: a neglected public health issue in less-developed countries. Soc. Sci. Med. 39(9):1165–1179.

Hellmann, N. S., P. Nsubuga, E. K. Mbidde, and S. Desmond-Hellmann. 1990. Specific heterosexual risk behaviors and HIV seropositivity in a Uganda STD clinic. Intl. Conf. AIDS 6(1):269 (abstract no. Th.C.578).

Hillis, S. D., R. Joesoef, P. A. Marchbanks, J. N. Wasserheit, W. Cates, and L. Westrom. 1993. Delayed care for pelvic inflammatory disease as a risk factor for impaired fertility. Am. J. Obstet. Gynecol. 168:1503–1509.

Hira, P. R. 1977. Observations on trichomonas vaginalis infections in Zambia. J. Hyg. Epidemiol. Microbiol. Immunol. 2:215–224.

Hira, S. 1984. Epidemiology of maternal and congenital syphilis in Lusaka and Copperbelt Provinces of Zambia. Lusaka: Republic of Zambia.

Hira, S., C. Bhat, A. Ratnam, C. Chintu, and R. Mulenga. 1982. Congenital syphilis in Lusaka. II. Incidence at birth and potential risk among hospital deliveries. E. Afr. Med. J. 59(5):306–310.

Hira, S. K., J. Kamanga, G. J. Bhat, et al. 1989. Perinatal transmission of HIV-1 in Zambia. Br. Med. J. 299:1250–1252.

Hira, S. K., et al. 1990. Syphilis intervention in pregnancy: Zambian demonstration project. Genitour. Med. 66:159–164.

Hira, S., S. Godwin, J. Kamanga, and G. Mukelabai. 1992a. Efficacy of spermicide use and condom use by HIV-discordant couples in Zambia. Intl. Conf. AIDS 8(1) (abstract no. WeC1085).

Hira, S., R. Sunkutu, and P. Perine. 1992b. Zambian National STD Control Program: The model program in Africa. Intl. Conf. AIDS 8(2):B229 (abstract No. PoB 3829).

Hitti, J., C. K. Walker, P. S. J. Nsubuga, et al. 1992. Oral contraceptive use and HIV infection. Intl. Conf. AIDS 8 (poster PoC 4309).

Holmes, K. K. 1990. Lower genital tract infections in women: cystitis, urethritis, vulvovaginitis, and cervicitis. Pp 527–545 in Sexually Transmitted Diseases, K. K. Holmes, P. A. Mårdh, P. F. Sparling, et. al., eds. New York: McGraw-Hill.

Holmes, K. K., and S. O. Aral. 1991. Behavioral interventions in developing countries. Pp. 318–344 in Research Issues in Human Behavior and Sexually Transmitted Diseases in the AIDS Era, J. N. Wasserheit, S. O. Aral, K. K. Holmes, and P. J. Hitchcock, eds. Washington D.C.: American Society for Microbiology.

Hook, E. W., and H. H. Handsfield. 1990. Gonococcal infections in the adult. Pp. 149–165 in Sexually Transmitted Diseases, 2d ed., K. K. Holmes, P. A. Mardh, P. F. Sparling, et al., eds. New York: McGraw-Hill.

Hoosen, A. A., S. M. Ross, M. J. Mulla, and M. Patel. 1981. The incidence of selected vaginal infections among pregnant urban Blacks. S. Afr. Med. J. 59:827–829.

Hopcraft, M., A. Verhagen, S. Ngigi, and A. Haga. 1973. Genital infections in developing countries: experience in a family planning clinic. Bull. WHO. 48:581–586.

Hudson, C., A. Hennis, P. Kataaha, et al. 1988. Risk factors for the spread of AIDS in rural Africa: evidence from a comparative seroepidemiological survey of AIDS, hepatitis B and syphilis in southwestern Uganda. AIDS 2(4):255–260.

Iquatt, B., and A. Sawhney. 1988. Symptomless gonorrhoea in women in Maiduguri (northeastern Nigeria). Genitour. Med. 64:349.

Ismail, S., H. Ahmed, M. Jama, et al. 1990. Syphilis, gonorrhoea and genital chlamydial infection in a Somali village. Genitour. Med. 66(2):70–75.

Jain, A. K., and I. Sivin. 1977. Life-table analysis of IUDs: problems and recommendations. Stud. Fam. Plan. 8:24–47.

Jama, H., et al. 1987. Syphilis in women of reproductive age in Mogadishu, Somalia: Serological survey. Genitour. Med. 63:326–328.

Jones, R. B., and J. N. Wasserheit. 1991. Introduction to the biology and natural history of sexually transmitted diseases. Pp. 11-37 in Research Issues in Human Behavior and Sexually Transmitted Diseases in the AIDS Era, J. N. Wasserheit, S. O. Aral, K. K. Holmes, and P. J. Hitchcock, eds. Washington D.C.: American Society for Microbiology.

Kanyama, I. 1991. Sentinel surveillance of HIV infection in Northern Zambia. Intl. Conf. AIDS 7(1):373 (abstract no. M.C.3301).

Kapiga, S., D. J. Hunter, J. F. Shao, et al. 1992. Contraceptive practice and HIV-1 infection among family planning clients in Dar es Salaam, Tanzania. Intl. Conf. AIDS 8 (poster PoC 4343).

Kaptue, L., et al. 1990. Setting up a sentinel surveillance system for HIV infection in Cameroon. Intl. Conf. AIDS 6(abstract F.C. 597).

Kaptue, L., L. Zekeng, S. Djoumessi, M. Monny-Lobe, D. Nichols, and R. Debuysscher. 1991. HIV and chlamydia infections among prostitutes in Younde, Cameroon. Genitour. Med. 67:143–145.

Karita, E., P. Van de Perre, A. Nziyumvira, W. Martinez, J. Nyiraminani, E. Fox, and J.B. Butera. 1992. HIV seroprevalence among STD patients in Kigali, Rwanda, during the four-year period 1988-1991. Intl. Conf. AIDS 8(2):C323 (abstract no. PoC 4468).

Kitabu, M. Z., G. M. Maitha, J. N. Mungai, et al. 1992. Trends and seroprevalence of HIV amongst four population groups in Nairobi in the period 1989–1991. Intl. Conf. AIDS 8 (poster PoC 4018).

Kivuvu, Mayimona, B. Malele, N. Nzila, A. Manoka, et al. 1990. Syphilis among HIV+ and HIV- prostitutes in Kinshasa: prevalence and serologic response to treatment. Fifth Intl. Conf. AIDS in Africa. Kinshasa (abstract TPC7).

Klein, R. S., A. Adachi, I. Fleming, I, G. Y. F. Ho, and R. Burk. 1992. A prospective study of genital neoplasia and human papillomovirus (HPV) in HIV-infected women (abstract). Intl. Conf. AIDS 8(1) (abstract TuB 0527).

Kreiss, J. K., and K. G. Castro. 1990. Special considerations for managing suspected human immunodeficiency virus infection and AIDS in patients from developing countries. J. Infect. Dis. 162:955–960.

Kreiss, J., D. Koech, F. Plummer, et al. 1986. AIDS virus infection in Nairobi prostitutes. N. Engl. J. Med. 314(7):414–418.

Laga, M., et al. 1988. Prophylaxis of gonococcal and chlamydial ophthalmia neonatorum: A comparison of silver nitrate and tetracycline. N. Engl. J. Med. 318: 653–657.

Laga, M. 1990. Human immunodeficiency virus infection prevention: The need for complementary STD control. Pp. 131–144 in Reproductive Tract Infections: Global Impact and Priorities for Women's Reproductive Health, A. Germaine, K. K. Holmes, P. Piot, and J. Wasserheit, eds. New York: Plenum.

Laga, M., F. Plummer, H. Nzanze, et al. 1986. Epidemiology of ophthalmia neonatorum in Kenya. Lancet 2:1145–1149.

Laga, M., N. Nzila, A. T. Manoka, et al. 1989. High prevalence and incidence of HIV and other sexually transmitted diseases (STD) among 801 Kinshasa prostitutes. Intl. Conf. AIDS 5:74 (abstract Th.A.O.21).

Laga, M., N. Nzila, A. T. Manoka, et al. 1990. Nonulcerative sexually transmitted diseases (STD) as risk factors for HIV transmission. Intl. Conf. AIDS 6(abstract ThC 97).

Laga, M., J. P. Icenogle, R. Marsella, et al. 1992. Genital papilloma virus infection and cervical dysplasia—opportunistic complications of HIV infection. Intl. J. Cancer. 50:45–48.

Lallemant M., A. Baillou, S. Lallemant-Le Coeur, et al. 1994. Maternal antibody response at delivery and perinatal transmission of human immunodeficiency virus type 1 in African women. Lancet 343:1001–1005.

Larsen, A. 1989. Social context of human immunodeficiency virus transmission in Africa: Historical and cultural bases of East and Central African sexual relations. Rev. Inf. Dis. 11:716–731.

Latif, A. 1981. Sexually transmitted disease in clinic patients in Salisbury, Zimbabwe. Br. J. Vener. Dis. 57:181–183.

Latif, A. S. 1989. Epidemiology and control of chancroid. Eighth ISSTDR (abstract 66).

Latif, A., S. Bvumbe, J. Muongerwa, E. Paraiwa, and W. Chikosi. 1984. Sexually transmitted diseases in pregnant women in Harare, Zimbabwe. Afr. J. Sex. Trans. Dis. January-March: 21–23.

Laukamm-Josten, U., D. Ocheng, B. Mwizarubi, C. Mwaijonga, R. Swai, and M. Trupin. 1992. HIV and syphilis seroprevalence and risk factors in truckstops and nearby communities in Tanzania. Intl. Conf. AIDS 8(2):C272 (abstract PoC4162).

Leclerc, A., E. Frost, M. Collet, J. Goeman, and L. Bedjabaga. 1988. Urogenital Chlamydia trachomatis in Gabon: an unrecognised epidemic. Genitour. Med. 64:308–311.

Lepage, P., and P. Van de Perre. 1988a. Clinical manifestation of AIDS in infants and children. Bailliere's Clin. Trop. Med. Commun. Dis. 3(1):89–101.

Lepage, P., and P. Van de Perre. 1988b. Strategies in the identification and control of HIV infected women in Africa. Pp. 215–255 in AIDS in Children, Adolescents, and Heterosexual Adults, A. J. Schinazi-Nahmias, ed. New York: Elsevier.

Lepage, P., P. Van de Perre, P. Msellatl, et al. 1993. Mother-to-child transmission of human immunodeficiency virus type 1 (HIV-1) and its determinants: a cohort study in Kigali, Rwanda. Am. J. Epidemiol. 137(6):589–599.

Liljestrand, J., S. Bergström, F. Nieuwenhuis, and B. Hederstedt. 1985. Syphilis in pregnant women in Mozambique. Genitour. Med. 61(6):355–358.

Linden, C. P., S. Allen, A. Serufilira, et al. 1992. Predictors of mortality among HIV-infected women in Kigali, Rwanda. Ann. Intern. Med. 116:320–328.

Luyeye, M., et al. 1990. Prevalence et facteurs de risque pour les MST chez les femmes enceintes dans les soins de santé primaires à Kinshasa. Fifth Int. Conf. AIDS in Africa. Kinshasa (abstract T.P.C.8).

Mabey, D. C., et al. 1984. Sexually transmitted diseases among randomly selected attenders at an antenatal clinic in The Gambia. Br. J. Vener. Dis. 60:331–336.

Mabey, D. 1986. Syphilis in Sub-Saharan Africa. Afr. J. Sex. Trans. Dis. 6:2(2):61–64.

Mabey, D., and H. Whittle. 1982. Genital and neonatal chlamydial infection in a trachoma endemic area. Lancet 2(93):300–301.

MacDonald, K. S., W. Cameron, L. J. D'Costa, et al. 1989. Evaluation of fleroxacin (RO-23-6240) as single-oral-dose therapy of culture-proven chancroid in Nairobi, Kenya. Antimicrob. Ag. Chemother. 33:612–614.

Maiman, M., R. G. Fruchter, E. Serur, J. C. Remy, G. Feuer, and J. Boyce. 1990. Human immunodeficiency virus infection and cervical neoplasia. Gynecol. Oncol. 38:377–382.

Mandara, N., S. Takulias, J. Kanyawana, and F. Mhalu. 1980. Asymptomatic gonorrhoea in women attending family planning clinics in Dar-es-Salaam, Tanzania: results of a pilot study. Trop. Geogr. Med. 32:329–332.

Mane, P., G. R. Gupta, and E. Weiss. 1994. Effective communication between partners: AIDS and risk reduction for women. AIDS 8 (Suppl):S325–S331.

Mann, J. M., N. Nzilambi, P. Piot, N. Bosenge, M. Kalala, H. Francis, R. C. Colebunders, P. K. Azila, J. W. Curran, and T. C. Quinn. 1988. HIV infection and associated risk factors in female prostitutes in Kinshasa, Zaire. AIDS 2(4):249–254.

Mann, J. M., D. J. M. Tarantola, and T. W. Netter, eds. 1992. AIDS in the World. Cambridge, Mass.: Harvard University Press.

Manneh, K. K., R. S. Njie, R. Sarr, et al. 1992. HIV status of antenatal women reporting for routine blood test at the Royal Victoria Hospital. Intl. Conf. AIDS 8 (poster PoC 4015).

Manoka, A., M. Laga, M. Kivuvu, et al. 1992. Syphilis among HIV+ and HIV- prostitutes in Kinshasa: Prevalence and serologic response to treatment. Intl. Conf. AIDS 6(3):102 (abstract SB27).

Martin, D. H., L. Koutsky, D. A. Eschenbach, et al. 1982. Prematurity and perinatal mortality in pregnancies complicated by maternal *Chlamydia trachomatis* infections. J. Am. Med. Assoc. 247:1585.

Mason, P. R., et al. 1983. Epidemiology and clinical diagnosis of *Trichomonas vaginalis* infection in Zimbabwe. Centr. Afr. J. Med. 29(3):53–56.

Mason, P., D. Katzenstein, T. Chimbira, and L. Mtimavalye. 1989. Vaginal flora of women admitted to hospital with signs of sepsis following normal delivery, cesarean section or abortion. The Puerperal Sepsis Study Group. Centr. Afr. J. Med. 35(3):344–351.

Mason, P., et al. 1990. Genital infections in women attending a genito-urinary clinic in Harare, Zimbabwe. Genitour. Med. 66(3):178–181.

Mason, P. R., L. Gwanzura, and F. Le Bacq. 1992. Correlation between positive syphilis serology and HIV infection in Zimbabwe. Intl. Conf. AIDS 8 (poster 4303).

Matasha, E., J. Changalucha, H. Grosskurth, et al. 1992. Commercial sexual workers intervention programme: A pilot project in northern Tanzania: operational data and intermediate results. Intl. Conf. AIDS 8(2): pD495 (abstract PoD 5639).

Mboup, L., et al. 1991. Surveillance sentinelle des infections à VIH. Bull. Epidémiol. VIH:3.

M'Boup, S. 1992. Natural history of HIV-2. Intl. Conf. AIDS 8(session 50).

Mboya, T. O. 1992. Traditional behavior and AIDS: Analysis and change through community participation. Intl. Conf. AIDS 8 (poster PoD 5697).

Mbugua, G., G. Gachihi, S. Adaw, F. Mueke, K. Mandalya, and E. Mupate. 1989. HIV seroprevalence survey among high risk females at Mombasa, Kenya. Intl. Conf. AIDS 5:1014 (abstract W.G.P.27).

Mbugua, G., L. Muthami, J. Kitama, S. Oogo, and P. Waiyaki. 1991. Rising trend of HIV infection among antenatal mothers in a Kenyan rural area. Intl. Conf. AIDS 7(2):366 (abstract W.C. 3283).

McCallum, M., et al. 1973. A survey of selected vaginal flora in Malawian women. Centr. Afr. J. Med. 19(8):176–178.

McCarthy, M. C., and A. E. El Hag. 1990. HIV-I infection in Juba, southern Sudan. Intl. Conf. AIDS 6(2):232 (abstract no. F.C.605).

McCarthy, M. C., J. P. Burans, N. T. Constantine, et al. 1989. Hepatitis B and HIV in Sudan: a serosurvey for hepatitis B and human immunodeficiency virus antibodies among sexually active heterosexuals. Am. J. Trop. Med. Hyg. 41(6):726–731.

Mefane, C., and M. Toung-Mve. 1987. Syphilis chez la femme enceinte à Libreville (Gabon). Bull. Soc. Path. Ex. 80(2):162–167.

Meheus, A. 1990. Women's health: importance of reproductive tract infections, pelvic inflammatory disease and cervical cancer. Pp. 61–91 in Reproductive Tract Infections: Global Impact and Priorities for Women's Reproductive Health, A. Germaine, K. K. Holmes, P. Piot, and J. Wasserheit, eds. New York: Plenum.

Meheus, A., W. Eylenbosch, and A. Ndibwami. 1975. Serological evidence for syphilis in different population groups in Rwanda. Trop. Geogr. Med. 27(2):165–168.

Meheus, A., F. Friedman, E. Van Dyck, and T. Guyver. 1980. Genital infections in prenatal and family planning attendants in Swaziland. E. Afr. Med. J. 57(3):212–217.

Meheus, A., K. F. Schulz, and W. Cates. 1990. Development of prevention and control programs for sexually transmitted diseases in developing countries. Pp. 1041–1046 in Sexually Transmitted Diseases, K. K. Holmes, P. A. Mårdh, P. F. Sparling, et. al., eds. New York: McGraw-Hill.

Melnick, S. L., R. Sherer, T. A. Louis, et al. 1994. Survival and disease progression according to gender of patients with HIV infection. JAMA 272(24):1915–1921.

Minkoff, H. L., C. Henderson, H. Mendez, et al. 1990. Pregnancy outcomes among mothers infected with human immunodeficiency virus and uninfected control subjects. Am. J. Obstet. Gynecol. 163:1598–1604.

Mirza, N. B., et al. 1983. Microbiology of vaginal discharge in Nairobi, Kenya. Br. J. Vener. Dis. 59:186–188.

Mlisana, K., S. Monokoane, A. Hoosen, J. Moodley, M. Adhikari, and L. Taylor 1992. Syphilis in the "unbooked" pregnant women. S. Afr. Med. J. 82(1):18–20.

Mofenson, L. M., P. Stratton, and A. Willoughby. 1992. HIV in pregnancy and effects on the fetus and infant. Year Book Obstet. Gynecol.:xiii–xlii.

Mokwa, K., V. Batter, F. Behets, et al. 1991. Prevalence of sexually transmitted diseases (STD) in childbearing women in Kinshasa, Zaire, associated with HIV infection. Intl. Conf. AIDS 7(2):358 (abstract No. W.C. 3251).

Mooradian, A. D., and V. Greiff. 1990. Sexuality in older women. Arch. Intern. Med. 150:1033–1038.

Mouden, J. C., C. Genin, J. C. Gruel, and P. Coulanges. 1988. Cyto-microbiological and serological study for the screening of sexually transmissible diseases in Malagasy multiparous women. Arch. Inst. Pasteur Madagascar 54(1):217–228.

Mtimavalye, L., and M. Belsey. 1987. Infertility and sexually transmitted diseases: major problems in maternal and child health and family planning. International Conference on Better Health for Women and Children through Family Planning, Nairobi, 5–9 October.

Muhe, L., and N. Tafari. 1986. Is there a critical time for prophylaxis against neonatal ophthalmia? Genitour. Med. 62:356–357.

Mungai, J., G. Maitha, M. Kitabu, et al. 1992. Prevalence of HIV and other STD's in three populations in Nairobi for the year 1991. Intl. Conf. AIDS 8(2):C362 (abstract PoC4714).

NACP/MOH (Ethiopia). 1992. Surveillance and research activities on HIV/AIDS: Activities accomplished so far in Ethiopia, 1984–91. Ethiopia NACP/MOH data. Photocopy.

Nasah, B., R. Nguematcha, M. Eyong, et al. 1980. Gonorrhea, trichomonas, and candida among gravid and non-gravid women in Cameroon. Intl. J. Gynecol. Obstet. 18:48.

Naucler, A., S. Anderson, P. Albino, et al. 1992. Association between HTLV-1 and HIV-2 infections in Bissau, Guinea-Bissau. AIDS 6(5):510–511.

Neequaye, A. R., J. A. A. Mingle, G. Ankra-Badu, et al. 1987. Human immune deficiency virus infections in Ghana. AIDS and Associated Cancers in Africa, Second International Symposium, Naples: 85–93.

Ndour-Sarr, A. N., D. S. Ba, T. Ndoye, A. Gueye, T. Siby, C. S. Boye, A. Child, A. Diouf, N. Mbaye, F. Kebe, et al. 1992. HIV infection in pregnant women in Dakar. Intl. Conf. AIDS 8(2):C285 (abstract no. PoC 4241).

Ndumbe, P., A. Andela, J. Nkemnkeng-Asong, E. Watonsi, and Nyambi. 1992. Prevalence of infections affecting the child among pregnant women in Yaounde, Cameroon. Med. Microbiol. Immunol. 181(3):127–130.

Newell, M. L. 1992. Risk factors for mother-to-child transmission of HIV-1. Lancet 339:1007–1012.

Nkowame, B. 1991. Prevalence and incidence of HIV infection in Africa: a review of data published in 1990. AIDS 5 (Suppl 1):S7–16.

Nkya, W. M. M. M., W. P. Howlett, C. Assenga, et al. 1987. Seroepidemiology of HIV-1 infection in the Kilimanjaro region. AIDS and Associated Cancers in Africa, Second International Symposium, Naples: 61–65.

Nkya, W. M., S. H. Gillespie, W. Howlett, J. Elford, C. Nyamuryekunge, C. Assenga, and B. Nyombi. 1991. Sexually transmitted diseases in prostitutes in Moshi and Arusha, Northern Tanzania. Intl. J. STD AIDS 2(6):432–435.

Nkya, W. M., W. P. Howlett, K. I. Klepp, B. Nyombi, and C. Assenga. 1992. HIV-cohort study of self-proclaimed prostitutes in Moshi and Arusha towns, northern Tanzania. Intl. Conf. AIDS 8(2):D496 (abstract no. PoD 5645).

Nsanze, H., S. Waigwa, N. Mirza, et al. 1982. Chlamydial infections in selected populations in Kenya. Pp. 421–424 in Chlamydial Infections, P. A. Mardh, et. al., eds. New York: Elsevier.

Nsofor, B. I., C. S. Bello, and C. G. Ekwempu. 1989. Sexually transmitted diseases among women attending a family planning clinic in Zaria, Nigeria. Intl. J. Gynaecol. Obstet. 28(4):365–367.

Nsubuga, P., F. Miremba, S. Kalibbala, et al. 1992. Reported sexual behavior and sexually transmitted infection prevalence among women attending a prenatal clinic in Kampala, Uganda. Intl. Conf. AIDS 8(2):C346 (abstract PoC4619).

Nyirenda, M. J. 1992. A study of the behavioral aspects of dry sex practice in Lusaka urban. Intl. Conf. AIDS 8(2):D461 (abstract No. PoD 5448).

O'Farrell, N., A. A. Hoosen, A. B. Kharsany, and J. van den Ende. 1989. Sexually transmitted pathogens in pregnant women in a rural South African community. Genitour. Med. 65(4):276–280.

O'Farrell, N., I. Windsor, and P. Becker. 1990. Risk factors for HIV-I amongst STD clinic attenders in Durban, South Africa. Intl. Conf. AIDS 6(2):232 (abstract no. F.C.604).

Ogbonna, C., I. Ogbonna, A. Ogbonna, and J. Anosike. 1991. Studies on the incidence of *Trichomonas vaginalis* amongst pregnant women in Jos area of Plateau State, Nigeria. Angew. Parasitol. 32(4):198–204.

Okepere, E. E., E. E. Obaseiki-Ebor, and S. M. Oyaide. 1987. Type of intra-uterine contraceptive device (IUCD) used and the incidence of symptomatic *Neisseria gonorrhoeae*. Afr. J. Sex Trans. Dis. 3:7–8.

Ole-Kingori, N., K. I. Klepp, K. S. Mnyika, et al. 1992. Population-based HIV-screening in Arusha, Tanzania: A pilot study. Intl. Conf. AIDS 8 (poster PoC 4031).

Omanga, U., F. Fendler, M. Bamba, M. Sulu, and B. Mikanga. 1989. Sero-épidémiologie de la syphilis congénitale à Kinshasa, Zaïre. Ann. Soc. Belg. Med. Trop. 69(4): 313–318.

Omer, E. E., et al. 1980. Study of sexually transmitted disease in Sudanese women. Trop. Doctor 10:99–102.

Omer, E. E., R. D. Catterall, M. H. Ali, H. A. El-Naeem, and H. H. Erwa. 1985a. Vaginal trichomoniasis at a sexually transmitted disease clinic at Khartoum. Trop. Doctor 15:170–172.

Omer, E., T. Forsey, S. Darougar, M. Ali, and H. El-Naeem. 1985b. Seroepidemiological survey of chlamydial genital infections in Khartoum, Sudan. Genitour. Med. 61:261–263.

O'Reilly, K. R. 1986. Sexual behavior, perceptions of infertility and family planning in sub-Saharan Africa. Afr. J. Sex Trans. Dis. 2:47–49.

Orubuloye I. O., J. C. Caldwell, and P. Caldwell. 1993. African women's control over their sexuality in an era of AIDS. Soc. Sci. Med.:37(7):859–872.

Osoba, A., and A. Onifade. 1987. Venereal diseases among pregnant women in Nigeria. W. Afr. Med. J. 11(1):23–25.

Ouattara, S. A., D. Diallo, M. Meite, et al. 1988. Epidémiologie des infections par les virus de l'immunodéficience humaine VIH1 et VIH2 en Côte d'Ivoire. Med. Trop. 48(4):375–379.

Ousseini, H., J. L. Pecarrere, D. Meynard, et al. 1991. Evolution de la séroprévalence des infections à VIH-1 et VIH-2 à l'Hôpital National de Niamey, Niger. Bull. Soc. Path. Ex. 84(3):235–239.

Over, M., and P. Piot. 1991. HIV infections and sexually transmitted diseases. Pp. 455–527 in Disease Control Priorities in Developing Countries, D. T. Jamison, W. H. Mosley, A. R. Measham, and J. L. Bobadilla, eds. Washington, D.C.: World Bank.

Parkin, D. M., E. Läärä, and C. S. Muir. 1988. Estimates of the worldwide frequency of sixteen major cancers in 1980. Intl. J. Cancer 41:184–197.

Perine, P. 1983. Congenital syphilis in Ethiopia. Med. J. Zambia 17(1):12–14.

Perine, P., M. Duncan, D. Krauss, et al. 1980. Pelvic inflammatory disease and puerperal sepsis in Ethiopia. Am. J. Obstet. Gynecol. 138:969–977.

Piot, P., and M. Laga. 1990. STD control in developing countries. Pp. 281–295 in Reproductive Tract Infections: Global Impact and Priorities for Women's Reproductive Health, A. Germaine, K. K. Holmes, P. Piot, and J. Wasserheit, eds. New York: Plenum.

Plummer, F., M. Laga, R. Brunham, et al. 1987. Postpartum upper genital tract infections in Nairobi, Kenya: Epidemiology, etiology, and risk factors. J. Infect. Dis. 156(1):92–98.

Plummer, F. A., D. W. Cameron, N. Simonsen, et al. 1991. Co-factors in male-female transmission of human immunodeficiency virus type 1. J. Infect. Dis. 163:233–239.

Quarcoopome, C. O. 1983. Ophthalmia neonatorum: problems of prophylaxis and treatment in Africa. WHO PBL/ON/83-1:1–4. Geneva.

Ratnam, A. V., S. Din, T. Chatterjee. 1980a. Sexually transmitted diseases in pregnant women. Med. J. Zambia 14:75–78.

Ratnam, A. V., S. N. Din, and T. K. Chatterjee. 1980b. Gonococcal infection in women with pelvic inflammatory disease in Lusaka, Zambia. Am. J. Obstet. Gynecol. 138:965–968.

Ratnam, A. V., S. Din, S. Hira, et al. 1982. Syphilis in pregnant women in Zambia. Br. J. Vener. Dis. 58:355–358.

Rellihan, M. A., D. P. Dooley, T. W. Burke, M. E. Berkland, and R. N. Longfield. 1990. Rapidly progressing cervical cancer in a patient with human immunodeficiency virus infection. Gynecol. Oncol. 36:435–438.

Retel-Laurentin, A. 1973. Fecondité et syphilis dans la région de la Volta Noire. Population 28:793–815.

Richardson D. 1989. Women and the AIDS Crisis, 2d ed. London: Pandora.

Rob, U., J. F. Phillips, J. Chakraborty, et al. 1987. The use effectiveness of the Copper-T-200 in Matlab, Bangladesh. Intl. J. Obstet. Gynecol. 25:315.

Ronald, A., and S. O. Aral. 1990. Assessment and prioritization of actions to prevent and control reproductive tract infections in the Third World. Pp. 199–225 in Reproductive Tract Infections: Global Impact and Priorities for Women's Reproductive Health, A. Germaine, K. K. Holmes, P. Piot, and J. Wasserheit, eds. New York: Plenum.

Rosenberg, M. J., K. F. Schulz, and N. Burton. 1986. Sexually transmitted diseases in Sub-Saharan Africa. Lancet 849:152–153.

Rothenberg, R. B., and J. J. Potterat. 1990. Strategies for management of sex partners. Pp. 1081–1086 in Sexually Transmitted Diseases, K. K. Holmes, P. A. Mårdh, P. F. Sparling, et. al., eds. New York: McGraw-Hill.

Rushwan, H. 1980. Etiologic factors in pelvic inflammatory disease in Sudanese women. Am. J. Obstet. Gynecol. 138:877–879.

Ryder, R. W., W. Nsa, S. E. Hassig, et al. 1989. Perinatal transmission of the human immunodeficiency virus type 1 to infants of seropositive women in Zaire. N. Engl. J. Med. 320:1637–1642.

Salehe, O., G. Riedner, Y. Hemed, H. Kazimbazi, T. Rehle, and F. von Sonnenburg. 1992. HIV infection among STD patients and correlated conditions in Mbeya, Tanzania. Int. Conf. AIDS 8(2):C362 (abstract no. PoC 4715).

Samb Noone, D., F. Van Der Veen, M. Sene, A. Thiam, L. Van De Velde, and D. Diouf. 1992. Sentinel surveillance of STDs, and its implications for AIDS control in Senegal. Int. Conf. AIDS 8(2):C299 (abstract PoC4328).

Sangare, A., G. Leonard, M. Verdier, et al. 1988. Comparison of C. trachomatis, HIV, HTLV-I. Prevalence in Ivory Coast populations. Abstract No FP33, IIIe International Conference on AIDS and Associated Cancers in Africa, Arusha, Tanzania.

Schafer, A., W. Friedmann, M. Mielke, B. Schwartlander, and M. A. Koch. 1991. The increased frequency of cervical dysplasia-neoplasia in women infected with the human immunodeficiency virus is related to the degree of immunosuppression. Am. J. Obstet. Gynecol. 164:593–599.

Schulz, K. F., W. Cates, and P. R. O'Mara. 1987. Pregnancy loss, infant death, and suffering: legacy of syphilis and gonorrhea in Africa. Genitour. Med. 63:320–325.

Schulz, K. F., J. M. Schulte, and S. M. Berman. 1990. Maternal health and child survival: Opportunities to protect both women and children from the adverse consequences of reproductive tract infections. Pp. 145–182 in Reproductive Tract Infections: Global Impact and Priorities for Women's Reproductive Health, A. Germaine, K. K. Holmes, P. Piot, and J. Wasserheit, eds. New York: Plenum.

Schrijvers, D., E. Delaporte, M. Peeters, et al. 1988. Role of sexually transmissible pathogens in transmitting HIV-1. Genitour. Med. 64:(6)395–396.

Schwartz, L. B., M. L. Carcangiu, L. Bradham, and P. E. Schwartz. 1991. Rapidly progressing squamous carcinoma of the cervix coexisting with human immunodeficiency virus infection: clinical opinion. Gynecol. Oncol. 41:255–258.

Scott, D. A., A. L. Corwin, N. T. Constantine, M. A. Omar, G. Guled, M. Yusef, C. R. Roberts, and D. M. Watts. 1991. Low prevalence of human immunodeficiency virus-1 (HIV-1), HIV-2, and human T-cell lymphotropic virus-1 infection in Somalia. Am. J. Trop. Med. Hyg. 45(6):653–659.

Selwyn, P. A., E. E. Schoenbaum, K. Davenny, et al. 1989. Prospective study of human immunodeficiency virus infection and pregnancy outcomes in intravenous drug users. J. Am. Med. Assoc. 261:1289–1294.

Selwyn, P. A., and P. Antoniello. 1993. Reproductive decision-making among women with HIV infection. Pp. 174–185 in HIV Infection in Women, M. A. Johnson and F. D. Johnstone, eds. London: Churchill Livingstone.

Sende, P., T. Abong, and G. Garrigue. 1986. *Chlamydia trachomatis*: étude de la prévalence chez la femme enceinte, la femme inféconde, et l'homme souffrant d'une uréthrite chronique. Afr. J. Sex. Trans. Dis. 2:72–74.

Senkoro, K., J. Newell, H. Grosskurth, et al. 1992. Syphilis and STD syndromes in Northern Tanzania: Prevalences, risk factors and association with the seroprevalence of HIV. Intl. Conf. AIDS 8 (poster PoC 4329).

Senyonyi, I. B. 1987. Prevalence des infections gynécologiques à *Chlamydia trachomatis* et à *Neisseria gonorrhoeae* chez 199 femmes examinées en consultation prénatales ou en consultation pour planning familial à Kigali et à Kabgayi. Rev. Med. Rwandaise 19:85–89.

Shao, J., S. Kapiga, D. Hunter, G. Lwihula, J. Mtui, and E. Mbena. 1992. Sexually transmitted diseases (STD) and HIV-1 infection among family planning clients in Dar-es-Salaam, Tanzania. Intl. Conf. AIDS 8(2):pC300 (abstract PoC 4330).

Sheller, J., N. Pedersen, and B. Kvinesdal, et. al. 1990. HIV-infection, syphilis og genitale laesioner i Maun, Botswana. Ugesk. Laeger. 152(20):1441–1443.

Sibailly, T. S., G. Adjorlolo, H. Gayle, et al. 1992. Prospective study to compare HIV-1 and HIV-2 perinatal transmission in Abidjan, Côte d'Ivoire. Intl. Conf. AIDS 8 (abstract WeC 1065).

South Africa, RSA Department of National Health and Population Development. 1991. AIDS in South Africa: Status on World AIDS Day 1991. Epidemiolog. Conf. 18(11:229–249.

South Africa, RSA Department of National Health and Population Development. 1992. Second National Survey of Women Attending Antenatal Clinics, South Africa, October/November 1991. Epidemiol. Conf. 19(5) 80–92.

St. Louis, M. E., M. Kamenga, C. Brown, et al. 1993. Risk for perinatal HIV-1 transmission according to maternal immunologic, virologic, and placental factors. JAMA 269(22): 2853–2859.

Tafari, N., D. Zewdi, B. Gebrehiwot, and T. Kebede. 1990. The simultaneous occurrence of perinatal HIV-1 and syphilis in Central Ethiopia: implications for control measures. Intl. Conf. AIDS 6(2):446 (abstract no 3176).

Tembo, G., J. Twa-Twa, G. Assimwe, et al. 1991. AIDS surveillance report: December 1991. Ministry of Health, AIDS Control Programme Surveillance Unit, Entebbe, Uganda. Photocopy.

Temmerman, M., F. Mohamed Ali, J. Ndinya-Achola, S. Moses, F. Plummer, and P. Piot. 1992a. Rapid increase of both HIV-1 infection and syphilis among pregnant women in Nairobi, Kenya. AIDS 6:1181–1185.

Temmerman, M., T. K'Oduol, F. A. Plummer, J. O. Ndinya-Achola, and P. Piot. 1992b. Maternal HIV infection as a risk factor for adverse obstetrical outcome. Intl. Conf. AIDS 8(2) pC283 (abstract PoC 4232).

Temmerman, M., E. N. Chomba, and P. Piot. 1994. HIV-1 and reproductive health in Africa. Intl. J. Obstet. 44:107–112.

Tovo, P. A., M. de Martino, G. Caramia, and the Italian Register for HIV Infection in Children. 1988. Epidemiology, clinical features, and prognostic factors of paediatric HIV infection. Lancet 2:1042–1045.

Twa-Twa, J., G. Tembo, G. Assimwe, et al. 1991. AIDS surveillance report (first and second quarter) for the year 1991. Ministry of Health, AIDS Control Programme Surveillance Unit, Entebbe, Uganda. Photocopy.

Ulin, P. R. 1992. African women and AIDS: negotiating behavioral change. Soc. Sci. Med. 34(1):63–73.

UNDP (United Nations Development Programme). 1992. Human Development Report 1992. New York: Oxford University Press.

Ursi, J., E. van Dyck, C. van Houtte, et al. 1981. Syphilis in Swaziland. A serological survey. Br. J. Vener. Dis. 57:95–99.

Van de Perre, P., N. Clumeck, M. Steens, G. Zissis, M. Carael, R. Lagasse, S. De Wit, T. Lafontaine, P. De Mol, and J. P. Butzler. 1987. Seroepidemiological study of sexually transmitted diseases and hepatitis B in African promiscuous heterosexuals in relation to HTLV-III infection. Eur. J. Epidemiol. 3(1):14–8.

van Rensburg, H., and J. Odendaal. 1992. The prevalence of potential pathogenic micro-organisms in the endocervix of pregnant women at Tygerberg Hospital. S. Afr. Med. J. 81(3):156–157.

Venter, A., J. Pettifor, F. Exposto, and M. Sefuba. 1989. Congenital syphilis—who is at risk? A prevalence study at Baragwanath Hospital, Johannesburg, 1985–1986. S. Afr. Med. J. 76(3):93–95.

Ville, Y., M. Leruez, E. Glowaczower, J. N. Roberston, and M. E. Ward. 1991. The role of *Chlamydia trachomatis* and *Neisseria gonorrhea* in the aetiology of ectopic pregnancy in Gabon. Br. J. Obstet. Gynaecol. 98(12):1260–1266.

Vink, G., and J. Moodley. 1989. Gonorrhea in black women attending a gynaecological outpatient department. S. Afr. Med. J. 58(2):901–902.

Walker, U., and W. Hofler. 1989. Prevalence of *Chlamydia trachomatis* in pregnant women and infertility cases in Abeokuta, Nigeria. Trop. Med. Parasitol.40(1):77–78.

Wasserheit, J. N. 1989. The significance and scope of reproductive tract infections among Third World women. Intl. J. Gynecol. Obstet. (Suppl) 3:145–168.

Wasserheit, J. N. 1992. Epidemiological synergy: interrelationships between human immunodeficiency virus infection and other sexually transmitted diseases. Sex. Trans. Dis. 19:61–77.

Wasserheit, J. N., and K. K. Holmes. 1990. Reproductive tract infections: Challenge for international health policy, programs, and research. Pp. 7–33 in Reproductive Tract Infections: Global Impact and Priorities for Women's Reproductive Health, A. Germaine, K. K. Holmes, P. Piot, and J. Wasserheit, eds. New York: Plenum.

Watson, P. 1985. The use of screening tests for sexually transmitted diseases in a Third World community—a feasibility study in Malawi. Eur. J. Sex. Trans. Dis. 2:63–65.

Watts, T., S. Larsen, and S. Brown. 1984. A case-control study of stillbirths at a teaching hospital in Zambia, 1979–80: Serological investigations for selected infectious agents. Bull. WHO 62:803–808.

Weissenberger, R., A. Robertson, S. Holland, et al. 1977. The incidence of gonorrhea in urban Rhodesian black women. S. Afr. Med. J. 52(28):1119–20.

Welgemoed, N., A. Mahaffey, and J. Van den Ende. 1986. Prevalence of *Neisseria gonorrhoeae* infection in patients attending an antenatal clinic. S. Afr. Med. J. 69(1):32–34.

Wessels, P. H., G. J. Viljoen, N. F. Marais, J. A. de Beer, M. Smith, and A. Gericke. 1991. The prevalence, risks, and management of *Chlamydia trachomatis* infections in fertile and infertile patients from the high socioeconomic bracket of the South African population. Fertil. Steril. 56(3):485–488.

Weström, L. 1980. Incidence, prevalence and trends of acute pelvic inflammatory disease and its consequences in industrialized countries. Am. J. Obstet. Gynecol. 138:880–892.

Weström, L., and P. A. Mårdh. 1984. Salpingitis. Pp. 615–632 in Sexually Transmitted Diseases, K. K. Holmes, P. A. Mårdh, P. F. Sparling, et al., eds. New York: McGraw-Hill.

Weström, L., and P. A. Mårdh. 1990. Acute pelvic inflammatory disease (PID). Pp. 593–613 in Sexually Transmitted Diseases, K. K. Holmes, P. A. Mårdh, P. F. Sparling, et al., eds. New York: McGraw-Hill.

Weström, L., R. Joesoef, G. Reynolds, A. Hagdu, and S. Thompson. 1992. Pelvic inflammatory disease and fertility: A cohort of 1844 women with laparoscopically verified disease and 657 control women with normal laparoscopic results. Sex. Trans. Dis. July-August:185–192.

Whiteside, A. 1991. HIV infection and AIDS in Zimbabwe: An assessment. Southern Africa Foundation for Economic Research. Economic Research Unit, University of Natal.

Whiteside, A. 1992. An evaluation of the likely impact of AIDS on the Mananga medical service subscribing companies. Draft report: 1–12. Photocopy.

Widy-Wirski, R., and J. D'Costa. 1980. Maladies transmises par voie sexuelle dans une population rurale en Centrafrique. Pp. 651-656 in Rapport Final, 13e Conférence Technique. Yaounde, Cameroon: OCEAC.

World Bank. 1992. World development indicators. Pp. 209–308 in World Development Report 1992: Development and Environment. New York: Oxford University Press.

World Bank. 1993. World Development Report 1993: Investing in Health. New York: Oxford University Press.

WHO (World Health Organization). 1987. Genital human papillomavirus infections and cancer: Memorandum from a WHO meeting. Bull. WHO 65(6):817–827.

WHO (World Health Organization). 1993. Report of a Consultation on Women and HIV/AIDS. WHO/GPA/DIR/94.1. Geneva.

WHO (World Health Organization). 1994. Women and AIDS: Agenda for Action. WHO/GPA/DIR/94.4. Geneva.

Wright, T. C., T. V. Ellerbrock, M. A. Chiasson, N. Van Devanter, and S. Xiao-Wei. 1994a. Cervical intraepithelial neoplasia in women infected with human immunodeficiency virus: prevalence, risk factors, and validity of Papanicolaou smears. Obstet Gynecol. 84:591–597.

Wright, T. C., J. Koulos, F. Schnoll, J. Swanbeck, T. V. Ellerbrock, M. A. Chiasson, and R. M. Richart. 1994b. Cervical intraepithelial neoplasia in women infected with the human immunodeficiency virus: outcome after loop electrosurgical excision. Gyn. Oncol. 55:253-258.

Yorke, J. A., H. W., Hethcote, and A. Nold. 1978. Dynamics and control of the transmission of gonorrhea. Sex. Trans. Dis. 5:51–56.

Yvert, F., J. Riou, E. Frost, and B. Ivanoff. 1984. Les infections gonococciques au Gabon (Haut-Ogooué). Pathol. Biol. 32(2):80–84.

Zacarias, F. R., and S. O. Aral. 1985. STD control in less developed countries: The time is now. Intl. J. Epidmiol. 14:505–509.

Zekeng, L., P. Barth, R. Salla, L. Kaptue, B. Schmidt-Ehry, and T. Rehle. 1990. Seroepidemiological study of sexually transmitted agents (HIV, hepatitis B virus, *T. pallidum*) among sentinel populations in the northwest and southwest provinces, Cameroon. Int. Conf. AIDS 6(2):230 (abstract FC 598).

Zekeng, L., R. Salla, L. Kaptue, et al., 1992. HIV-2 infection in Cameroon: No evidence of indigenous cases. J. AIDS 5(3):319–320.

Zimbabwe, Central Statistical Office, Ministry of Health. 1989. Annual Report. Harare.

APPENDIX

TABLE 11-6 Genital Discharge Syndrome

Country	Year	Population	N	Ref.	GC	CT	TV
Low-risk population							
Cameroon	1977	PP	296	87	14		
	1980	AN (asymptomatic)	110	180	14		15
	1980	FP (asymptomatic)	53	180	2		8
	1980	PP (asymptomatic)	296	180	10		
	1986[a]	AN		234		9	
Central African Republic	1980	AN		268	10		
Ethiopia	1973–75	PP (asymptomatic)	200	209	9		
Gabon	1981	AN	530	270	6		
	1988	PP (asymptomatic)	598	137		10	
	1987–89	AN	2,305	82		19	
Gambia, The	1982	AN	87	145	7	7	
	1982	AN (asymptomatic)	100	144	7	7	32
Ghana	1983	AN		213	3		
	1988[a]	AN (asymptomatic)	110	74		4	
Kenya	1973	FP	200	111	18		26
	1981	AN	54	188	0	6	
	1981	FP	57	188	17	4	
	1984	PP	728	131	7	23	
	1984	PP	845	212	7	21	
	1985	PP	175	99	4	17	
	1985–86	PP	2,732	127	6	9	
	1985–87	Trachoma area	168	35		4	
	1988–89	AN	549	161	3		2
	1990	AN	269	242	7		
	1990	FP		80		6	11
	1992	AN	5,674	178	10		
Malawi	1973	AN	100	162			19
	1990	AN	6,483	57	5	3	32
Nigeria	1971	AN	208	203	3		21
	1971–75	Gyn (IUD users)	282	256	5		27
	1971–75	Asymptomatic housewife	130	256	5		15
	1983–85	FP	500	196	4		
	1988	AN	80	253		11	
	1988	Infertile	20	253		15	
	1989[a]	FP	150	189	0–8		0–8
	1989[a]	No FP	50	189	6		4
	1989[a]	AN	46	6		6	
	1991[a]	AN (rural)	250	195			25
	1991[a]	AN (urban)	250	195			38
Rwanda	1987	AN + FP	199	236	5		
	1987	AN + FP	198	236		16	
Senegal	1983	AN		213	19		
	1987	AN	236	176	2		
	1990		511	93			30
Senegal	1987	AN	200	68	2	7	
	1989–92	AN	781	227	1	8	16
Somalia	1987	All village	200	115	0	18	
South Africa	1980[a]	AN	105	110	10		23
	1980[a]	AN	80	110	90		
	1981	AN (asymptomatic)	1,200	260	11		
	1983	AN		213	10		
	1986	AN	88	12		13	

TABLE 11-6 Continued

Country	Year	Population	N	Ref.	GC	CT	TV
Low-risk population							
South Africa	1986[a]	AN	231	14		1	
	1986[a]	FP	62	14		16	
	1987	AN	193	193	6	11	49
	1991[a]	AN (white, high SES)	41	261		7	
	1992[a]	AN (asymptomatic)	170	72	4	5	
	1992[a]	AN	206	249	7	11	
Swaziland	1973	OPD (all women)	179	39			29
	1973	AN	215	39			50
	1978	AN	51	167	4		23
	1978	FP	52	167	2		15
Tanzania	1978	FP (asymptomatic)	341	147	8		
	1983	AN		213	8		
	1986[a]	AN		69	6		
	1991–92	AN	2,009	237	5		14
Uganda	1971–72	Community (Ankole)	168	9	2		
	1971–72	Community (Teso)	295	9	22		
	1980	Low fertil. district	336	10	18		
	1980	High fertil. district	246	10	2		
	1992[a]	AN	450	101	1	7	43
Zaire	1985	AN	208	64	2		4
	1988	AN	101	17		9	
	1990	AN	701	142	2	6	17
	1991	AN	1,875	174	1	5	16
Zambia	1977[a]	AN	218	102			39
	1979	AN (asymptomatic)	161	216	11		
Zimbabwe	1976	AN	50	259	2		
	1976	FP	100	259	12		
	1983	AN	199	154			31
	1986–87	PP (asymptomatic)	111	155	5	6	14
High-risk population							
Cameroon	1980	AN (symptomatic)	610	180	15		21
	1980	FP (symptomatic)	81	180	21		7
	1980	PP (symptomatic)	42	180	21		2
Côte d'Ivoire	1986[a]	Symptoms		73	10		
Ethiopia	1973–75	PP (puerperal sepsis)	67	209	28		
	1973–75	PID (outpatient)	100	209	19		
	1973–75	PID (hospital)	46	209	15		
Gabon	1980–82	Symptomatic (vaginal D/C)	261	270	15		23
	1988[a]	Symptomatic (vaginal D/C)	252	137		18	
	1988[a]	Symptomatic (LAP)	265	137		14	
Gambia, The	1982	Gyn (symptomatic)	23	145		14	
Ghana	1985	Gyn	162	20	3	5	
	1985	Gyn (LAP)	40	20	0	10	
	1985	PP (hospitalized)	148	20	3		
	1985	PP (hospitalized)	39	20		8	
Kenya	1981	STD (symptomatic)	58	188	23	7	
	1982	STD (vaginal D/C)	122	171	26		34
	1982	STD (vaginal D/C)	58	171		7	
	1985	PP (preterm)	166	99	11	13	
	1992	STD		80		4	11
	1992	STD+FP	212	80			11

TABLE 11-6 Continued

Country	Year	Population	N	Ref.	GC	CT	TV
High-risk population							
Malawi	1992	STD	505	58	15		26
	1992	STD	175	58		5	
	1990	STD	255	57	25		36
Nigeria	1971–75	Gyn (symptomatic)	228	256	17		19
	1977–81	STD	435	19	13		11
	1988[a]	Gyn	120	114	15		
Senegal	1990	Gyn	250	68	4	8	
	1989–92	Gyn	795	227	2	8	16
South Africa	1980	STD	135	19	13		
	1980[a]	AN (symptomatic)	127	110	9		31
	1980[a]	Gyn	100	252	11		
	1986[a]	STD	135	14		13	
Sudan	1976	Gyn (symptomatic)	147	224	1		12
	1977	STD (symptomatic)	613	199	7		20
	1976–78	STD (vaginal D/C)	132	200	4		
	1976–78	STD (vaginal D/C)	144	200			
	1976–78	STD (vaginal D/C)	114	200			20
	1985[a]	STD	404	201	8		
	1985[a]	STD	613	199			20
Zambia	1977[a]	Gyn	518	102			31
	1979	STD (nonpregnant)	1,000	216	19		
	1979	STD (pregnant)	170	216	23		
	1979	PID (hospitalized)	100	216	46		
Zimbabwe	1976	Gyn	118	259	11		
	1979–80	STD	234	200	23		
	1982	STD (pregnant)	160	133	26		38
	1983	STD	156	154			37
	1986–87	PP (puerperal sepsis)	95	155	19	16	12
	1990[a]	STD	100	153	19	8	32
Very-high-risk population							
Burkina Faso	1990	CSW	127	59	20		17
Cameroon	1991[a]	CSW	168	122		39	
Côte d'Ivoire	1988[a]	CSW		228		65	
Ethiopia	1991[a]	CSW	282	90	30		24
	1992	CSW	46	28	30	6	
Kenya	1981	CSW (upper SES)		60	16		
	1981	CSW (middle SES)		60	28		
	1981	CSW (lower SES)		60	46		
Madagascar	1987	CSW	298	175			39
	1987	CSW	40	175		18	
Malawi	1990	CSW (STD)	274	57	29		27
Senegal	1989–92	CSW	397	227	13	17	18
	1989–92	CSW	653	70	16	14	24
Somalia	1990[a]	CSW	89	38	11		
Tanzania	1991[a]	CSW	106	185	51		
	1991[a]	CSW	47	185		25	
	1992[a]	CSW	70	156			
Zaire	1989[a]	CSW	801	130	23	14	22

NOTE: GC, gonorrhea; CT, chlamydia; TV, trichomoniasis; AN, antenatal; PP, postpartum; FP, family planning; LAP, lower abdominal pain; D/C, discharge; CSW, commercial sex worker; SES, socioeconomic status.

[a]No study date.

TABLE 11-7 Syphilis

Country	Year	Population	N	Ref.	Non-T	Trep	Non-T +Trep	GUD
Low-risk population								
Botswana	1985–87	AN	113	238			17	3
Burkina Faso	1973[a]	Village (Karba)	208	217	18			
	1973[a]	Village (Dedougo)	239	217	32			
	1973[a]	Village (Moko)	133	217	8			
Cameroon	1989–90	AN	544	184		16		
	1990[a]	AN	608	272		24		
	1990[a]	AN	900	121			10	
Central African Republic	1980	AN		268			10	
Ethiopia	1974–75	AN	2,717	208	18		17	
	1977[a]	AN	337	86	13	11	11	
	1990[a]	AN	1,719	240			7	
	1992[a]	AN	100	83			9	
Gabon	1983	AN	527	165			12	
	1984	AN	715	165			13	
	1985	AN	623	165			14	
	1986	Urban	211	77			15	
	1987	Semi-rural	277	77			9	
Gambia, The	1986[a]	AN (rural)	100	143	15	11		
	1986[a]	AN	238	143	26		13	
	1982	AN (urban)	100	144	9	1	1	
Kenya	1984	PP	1,013	131		11	4	
	1985	PP	133	99			5	
	1988–89	AN	549	161			4	
	1989–91	AN	4,883	91			4	
	1992[a]	AN	5,674	178			3	
Malawi	1985[a]	AN	182	257	18		14	
	1990	AN	6,483	57	13			7
Mozambique	1985	AN 10 districts	1,468	140	8		6	
Nigeria	1971	AN	208	203			0	
	1979–84	AN	29,083	92	3		0.4	
	1986[a]	AN		81			2	
	1989[a]	FP	150	189		15		
	1989[a]	Controls (non-FP)	50	189		12		
Rwanda	1972	AN	862	166	3			
	1972	Students	153	166	1			
	1980	AN	2,321	62	4			
	1987[a]	Asympt. blood donor	33	248		15	6	
	1989[a]	AN		54	4	4		
Senegal	1989–92	AN	781	227			6	
	1990	AN	511	93			8	
Somalia	1985–86	AN	67	117	3	3	3	
	1987	Village	200	115		23	16	
South Africa	1981	AN	1,200	260			21	
	1985–86	AN	9,071	250	3			
	1987	AN	193	193			12	
	1992[a]	AN (asymptomatic)	170	72			8	
South Africa	1992[a]	AN (unbooked)	114	172			31	
Swaziland	1978	FP	52	167	6			6
	1978	AN	51	167	14			2
	1981[a]	AN	90	247	10	33		
	1986	PP (asymptomatic)	283	96			13	
Tanzania	1983–84	AN	5,430	51	19		16	
	1991–92	AN	2,009	237			3	
	1992[a]	Community	115	136			16	

TABLE 11-7 Continued

Country	Year	Population	N	Ref.	Non-T	Trep	Non-T +Trep	GUD
Low-risk population								
Uganda	1986	Outpatients	24	112	0	8	0	
	1986	AN	1,011	43		26		
	1992[a]	AN	405	190			10	
Zaire	1988	PP	314	198			2	
	1990	AN	701	142			1	
	1991	AN	1,857	174		2	1	2
Zambia	1979–80	PP (asympt. live birth)	261	258		29	4	
	1980[a]	AN	163	215			18	
	1981	PP	464	104			7	
	1982[a]	AN	202	214	14	13	13	
	1984[a]	AN		101	13			
	1985–86	AN	5,007	103			8	
Zimbabwe	1985–87	PP (asymptomatic)	104	67		19	9	
High-risk population								
Botswana	1985–87	AN	175	238		25	16	
Central African Republic	1988[a]	Hosp	30	18			20	
Kenya	1985	PP (preterm)	157	79			6	
Malawi	1992[a]	STD	505	58			25	
Nigeria	1977–81	STD	435	19			4	
Senegal	1989–92	Gyn	796	227			14	
Sudan	1976–78	STD (vaginal D/C)	152	200	8		0	
Zambia	1979–80	PP (stillbirth)	262	258		54	29	
Zimbabwe	1982	STD (pregnant)	160	133			4	
	1990	STD	100	153	44		33	
Very-high-risk population								
Burkina Faso	1990	CSW	127	59	22			
Ethiopia	1991[a]	CSW	203	90			37	
Gambia, The	1986[a]	CSW	31	143	74	71		
Kenya	1981	CSW (upper SES)	71	60			37	2
	1981	CSW (middle SES)	51	60			31	6
	1981	CSW (lower SES)	71	60			53	6
	1985	CSW (low SES)	64	126			55	42
	1989[a]	CSW	366	161			22	
Madagascar	1987	CSW	298	175	25			
Malawi	1990	CSW (STD)	274	57	21			
Rwanda	1973	CSW	43	166	30			
	1987[a]	CSW	33	248	58	82		
Senegal	1989–92	CSW	653	70	6	31		
	1989–92	CSW	397	227			40	
Somalia	1985–86	CSW	85	117			45	
	1989	CSW	57	232			51	
	1990	CSW	155	2	69		47	
	1990[a]	CSW	89	38		28		
Sudan	1987	CSW	202	163			29	
Tanzania	1992[a]	CSW	70	156	18			16
	1991[a]	CSW	106	185	27	74		
Uganda	1986	Bar girls	36	112	46	6		
Zaire	1989[a]	CSW	801	150		28	16	7
	1990[a]	CSW	1,233	125		28	16	7

NOTE: Non-T, non-treponemal test; Trep, treponemal test; Non-T+Trep, positive non-treponemal test confirmed by treponemal test in most cases; GUD, genital ulcer disease; D/C, discharge; AN, antenatal; PP, postpartum; FP, family planning; CSW, commercial sex worker; SES, socioeconomic status.

[a]No study date.

TABLE 11-8 HIV-1 Infection

Country	Year	Population	N	Ref.	HIV-1
Low-risk population					
Angola	1986	AN (Luanda)	357	25	0.3
Botswana	1985–87	AN (Maun)	113	121	0
Cameroon	1987–90	AN (4 cities/towns)	2,417	273	0.9
Côte d'Ivoire	1992	AN (Abdidjan)	12,750	239	9.5
	1992	15–49 (Abidjan)	10,136	1	9.4
	1991	15–49 (Abidjan)	3,833	1	8.7
	1987	AN	246	204	3.6
Ethiopia	1991	AN (Diredawa)	360	179	6.9
	1991	AN (Metu)	322	179	2.8
Gambia, The	1990	AN (Banjul)	1,057	149	0.3
	1989	Vil (Gunjur)	98	65	0
	1988	Vil (Essau)	96	65	0
	1988	Vil (Kankunku)	103	65	0
	1988	Vil (Badjakunda)	105	65	0
	1988	Vil (Brikama)	109	65	0
	1989	Vil (Sibanor)	108	65	0
	1989	Vil (Diabugu)	97	65	0
	1989	Vil (Farafeni)	99	65	0
	1988	Vil (Gambisara)	98	65	0
Guinea Bissau	1989–90	AN (Bissau)	272	181	0
Kenya	1991	AN (national)	4,599	159	10.1
	1990	AN (national)	7,232	159	6.6
Malawi	1990[a]	AN	1,482	47	21.6
	1988	AN	247	48	19.0
Niger	1987–88	AN (Niamey)	1,477	205	0.1
Nigeria	1988–90	AN (Lagos)	500	5	1.0
Rwanda	1992	AN (Kigali)	128	84	31.3
	1989	AN (urban)	164	37	20.1
	1989–91	AN (Butare)	5,288	46	9.8
	1989	AN (rural)	193	37	4.2
Senegal	1990	AN (Dakar Reg)	182	157	1.2
	1990	AN (Kaolak Reg)	496	157	0.4
	1991	AN (Dakar Reg)	299	157	0.3
	1992	AN (remote areas)	781	227	0.3
	1990	AN (Ziguinchor)	825	157	0.2
	1992	AN (various areas)	2,120	88	0.2
	1991–92	AN (Dakar)	4,698	183	0.2
	1991	AN (Kaolak Reg)	240	157	0
	1991	AN (Ziguinchor)	715	157	0
	1990	AN (St Louis)	603	157	0
	1991	AN (St Louis)	418	157	0
South Africa	1991	AN (national)	17,155	157	0
	1991	AN (national)	1,576	157	0.6
Swaziland	1990	AN		266	2.3
Tanzania	1991	All 15–54 (Arusha)	148	197	12.8
	1991–92	FP (Dar es Salaam)	2,009	237	12.5
	1992	AN (Mwanza region)		24	11.6
Tanzania	1991–92	FP (Dar es Salaam)	2,285	120	11.5
	1992	Rural (10–19) Kagera	717	16	3.2
	1992	All (Mwanza town)	590	156	1.9
	1987	AN (Moshi town)	180	187	1.1
Uganda	1992	AN (Aber)	239	11	17.2
	1990–91	AN (Hoima)	346	3	13.0
	1989	AN (Jinja)		11	24.9

TABLE 11-8 Continued

Country	Year	Population	N	Ref.	HIV-1
Low-risk population					
Uganda	1992	AN (Jinja)	296	11	24.7
	1991	AN (Jinja)	300	11	22.0
	1990–91	AN (Jinja)	1,485	3	18.0
	1990	AN (Jinja)		11	15.8
	1990–91	AN (Kabale)	791	3	12.5
	1990	AN (Kampala)	628	245	36.6
	1991	AN (Kampala)	512	245	29.7
	1992	AN (Kampala)	285	11	29.5
	1992	AN (Kampala)	269	11	29.4
	1989	AN (Kampala)	2,017	245	29.0
	1991	AN (Kampala)	266	11	27.8
	1990	AN (Kampala)	426	245	27.0
	1991	AN (Kampala)	305	11	26.9
	1988	AN (Kampala)	88	245	25.0
	1989	AN (Kampala)	498	245	24.5
	1992	AN (Kilembe)	257	11	25.3
	1992	AN (Mbale)	255	11	17.3
	1991	AN (Mbale)	264	11	12.1
	1991	AN (Mbale)		241	12.0
	1990	AN (Mbale)		11	11.0
	1989	AN (Mbale)		11	9.0
	1992	AN (Mbarara)	205	11	30.2
	1991	AN (Mbarara)	217	11	24.4
	1989	AN (Mbarara)	1,017	245	21.6
	1990–91	AN (Mbarara)	1,098	3	20.6
	1991	AN (Moyo)		241	12.8
	1990	AN (Moyo)		241	11.0
	1989	AN (Moyo)		241	3.3
	1989	AN (Moyo)	615	245	3.3
	1992	AN (Mutolere)		11	5.6
	1991	AN (Mutolere)		11	4.1
	1992	AN (Palisa)	236	11	7.6
	1991	AN (Potal)	689	11	23.1
	1992	AN (Tororo)	222	11	13.1
	1991	AN (Tororo)	257	11	12.8
	1990	AN (Tororo)		11	4.1
Zaire	1988–91	AN (Kimpese)	9,129	194	3.8
Zambia	1991[a]	AN (Solwezi—periurban)		119	30.0
	1991[a]	AN (Kabompo—rural)		119	20.0
	1991[a]	AN (Mukinge—rural)		119	16.0
	1991[a]	AN (Mwinilunga—rural)		119	9.0
Zimbabwe	1989	AN (Mash. W)	295	267	20.0
	1989	AN (Mat. N)	289	267	11.1
	1989	AN (Midlands)	298	267	7.7
High-risk population					
Central African					
Republic	1989	STD (Bangui)	76	95	21.0
Gabon	1988	STD (Southeast)	734	231	3.7
Rwanda	1990	STD (Kigali)		123	75.0
	1989	STD (Kigali)		123	74.0
	1988	STD (Kigali)		123	70.0
	1991	STD (Kigali)		123	69.0
Senegal	1992	Gyn (remote areas)	795	227	0.1

Continued

TABLE 11-8   Continued

Country	Year	Population	N	Ref.	HIV-1
High-risk population					
South Africa	1990[a]	STD (Durban)	937	194	3.2
	1991	STD (J'burg Black)	1,626	223	9.8
Tanzania	1991–92	STD (Mbeya)	299	226	48.8
	1992	STD (urban,w/syph)		235	21.0
	1992	STD (urban,w/out syph)		235	14.0
	1992	STD (north,w/syph)		235	9.5
	1992	STD (north,w/out syph)		235	8.9
	1992	STD (rural,w/syph)		235	4.5
	1992	STD (rural,w/out syph)		235	3.0
Uganda	1990[a]	STD (Kampala)	96	98	60.5
	1989–91	STD (Kampala, 20–29)		107	59.0
	1989–91	STD (Kampala, 30–39)		107	55.0
	1989–91	STD (Kampala, 10–19)		107	45.0
	1989–91	STD (Kampala, 40–49)		107	40.0
	1989–91	STD (Kampala, 50+)		107	20.0
Zimbabwe	1991	STD (Karoi)	72	152	65.3
Very-high-risk population					
Burkina Faso	1990[a]	CSW (rural)	38	88	44.7
Cameroon	1988	CSW (Younde)	168	122	7.1
Côte d'Ivoire	1987	CSW	210	204	35.3
Ethiopia	1990	Bar girls (Adis)	858	179	42.0
	1989	Bar girls (Adis)	966	179	22.0
	1989	CSW (Adaitu)	110	179	41.8
	1988	CSW (Adaitu)	116	179	32.8
	1990	CSW (Adis)	1,225	179	54.2
	1989	CSW (Adis)	2,663	179	24.3
	1988	CSW (Adis)	330	179	19.4
	1988	CSW (Arbaminch)	255	179	8.2
	1989	CSW (Asmara)	379	179	5.8
	1988	CSW (Asmara)	389	179	2.3
	1988	CSW (Asseb)	352	179	31.5
	1988	CSW (Assela)	326	179	12.9
	1988	CSW (Awasa)	260	179	15.4
	1991	CSW (Baherdar)	366	179	69.4
	1990	CSW (Baherdar)	362	179	55.0
	1989	CSW (Baherdar)	353	179	48.2
Ethiopia	1988	CSW (Baherdar)	324	179	35.8
	1988	CSW (Bobi)	213	179	12.2
	1988	CSW (Dessie)	312	179	38.1
	1990	CSW (Diredawa)	366	179	48.1
	1989	CSW (Diredawa)	361	179	30.5
	1988	CSW (Diredawa)	361	179	18.0
	1988	CSW (Gewane)	119	179	30.3
	1988	CSW (Gonder)	367	179	14.7
	1988	CSW (Jimma)	309	179	9.7
	1988	CSW (Keren)	361	179	2.5
	1988	CSW (Massawa)	318	179	1.3
	1988	CSW (Mekele)	363	179	24.2
	1988	CSW (Meteka)	79	179	17.9
	1990	CSW (Metu)	165	179	36.4
	1989	CSW (Metu)	240	179	12.5
	1988	CSW (Metu)	262	179	5.3
	1988	CSW (Moyale)	99	179	16.2

TABLE 11-8 Continued

Country	Year	Population	N	Ref.	HIV-1
Very-high-risk population					
Ethiopia	1991	CSW (Nazareth)	328	179	65.6
	1990	CSW (Nazareth)	315	179	52.4
	1989	CSW (Nazareth)	354	179	31.1
	1988	CSW (Nazareth)	333	179	19.5
	1989	CSW (Nekemt)	294	179	31.3
	1988	CSW (Nekemt)	274	179	15.3
	1988	CSW (Shashemene)	325	179	19.4
Ghana	1986–87	CSW (return from Côte d'Ivoire)	151	182	49.0
Kenya	1991	CSW (Nairobi)	490	40	85.9
	1991	CSW (Nairobi)	524	124	75.2
	1990	CSW (Nairobi)	981	124	73.8
	1989	CSW (Nairobi)	656	124	67.2
Niger	1987–89	CSW (Niamey)	610	205	4.9
Nigeria	1990	CSW (Lagos)	546	55	10.3
	1988–90	CSW (Lagos)	117	5	2.6
Senegal	1985–92	CSW (Dakar)	1,364	158	4.7
	1990	CSW (Dakar)	471	157	4.5
	1991	CSW (Dakar)	665	157	4.4
	1989–91	CSW (Dakar,Regis)	653	96	4.4
	1985–92	CSW (Dakar,Regis)	2,216	158	4.3
	1991	CSW (Kaolack)	113	157	11.5
	1990	CSW (Kaolack)	106	157	4.7
	1990	CSW (St Louis)	74	157	2.7
	1991	CSW (St Louis)	69	157	0
	1992	CSW (various area)	1,342	88	2.4
	1991	CSW (Ziguinchor)	138	157	1.4
	1990	CSW (Ziguinchor)	194	157	0.5
	1992	CSW (remote)	397	227	13.8
Somalia	1990	CSW (Mogad, Merca, Ch)	303	52	3.0
Sudan	1989	CSW (Juba)	50	164	16.0
Tanzania	1987–89	CSW (Moshi—Arusha)	212	186	72.2
	1987	CSW (Kili)	52	187	57.7
	1992	CSW (Niwanza town)	103	156	39.8
Zaire	1988	CSW (Kin)	801	130	37.2
	1988[a]	CSW (Kin)	377	148	26.8

[a]No study date.

NOTE: AN, antenatal; FP, family planning; Vil, village; w/syph, with syphilis; w/out syph, without syphilis; CSW, commercial sex worker.

Appendix A

Demographic Overview and State of the Data

From a demographic standpoint, a study of the mortality and morbidity of females in Sub-Saharan Africa is a difficult task. The lack of data on cause-specific mortality and morbidity, particularly data disaggregated by gender, is a recurrent theme throughout this report. Although African countries have made considerable advances in expanding their demographic data bases, data of the kind needed for this book are scanty. Data are almost nonexistent for females of certain age groups, and for both males and females for a number of diseases and conditions. The data that do exist are from scattered sources, most of which are subject to underreporting or other sources of bias. In general, researchers are just beginning to construct a composite picture of mortality and morbidity of females over the course of their lifetime in Sub-Saharan Africa. This composite picture combines information from varying sources of data, but still suffers from large gaps; in addition, details of specific regional and local variations are rarely available.

This appendix reviews the nature of the evidence on female mortality and morbidity in Sub-Saharan Africa, while recognizing the limited sources and reliability of the available data. It presents current levels and trends in female mortality and morbidity and highlights gaps in the information. In view of the scarcity of available data, the appendix is also prescriptive, suggesting areas that require more data for a better understanding of female health.

DATA ON FEMALE MORTALITY AND MORBIDITY ACROSS THE LIFE SPAN

Data on Mortality

Sources and Measures

Demographers have long incorporated a life span perspective in data collection and analysis through either cohort measures or measures based on stable populations that reflect the fertility or mortality experience of a birth cohort as it ages. Most common is the use of a synthetic cohort, where fertility or mortality is expressed as the level that would be experienced by a cohort of males or females living through the age-specific rates prevailing at a given time. The key to this approach is the availability of age-specific rates. Life expectancy at birth is a measure that summarizes mortality experience throughout the life span.

Age-specific rates are traditionally based on vital registration data, providing numbers of deaths by age, sex, and cause of death; and on census data, providing age and sex-specific "denominator" data. Vital registration data in Africa are scanty, however. Sub-Saharan Africa lacks vital registration systems (with the exception of Mauritius and South Africa) that even approach the United Nations standards for completeness.

Another traditional source of information on mortality and morbidity is based on the health care services, but this information is of limited use in Sub-Saharan Africa. One reason for this is that the majority of deaths occur outside the health care system. Another is that health care service information is usually restricted to inpatients in tertiary facilities, and there are substantial selection biases among the populations that use these health services, reflecting, for example, differentials in access to health services according to age, gender, and geography or a higher level of risk among those utilizing the services. Access may be lower, for instance, in young teenage groups or in rural areas (Graham, 1991; Timaeus, 1991d). Only a small proportion of women at risk in Sub-Saharan Africa have access to hospitals (Graham, 1991). Much of the health care provided to the African population is through smaller, community-based primary health care services (Ewbank, 1988), and evidence suggests that deaths among patients in contact with these facilities tend to be omitted in health service statistics because of incomplete recordkeeping (Graham, 1991).

Since the 1960s, demographic data have improved substantially. Censuses and surveys, described below, have filled some of the statistical needs traditionally met through vital registration data. Most important to the current level of knowledge about African mortality, however, has been the development of survey instruments and methodologies to measure mortality through specific retrospective questions asked of a mother or other family member about births and deaths, which can be included in a census or survey. These questions, described below, result in estimates of mortality over a broad age group. Indicators most often used are the probability of survival from birth to exact age 5, and the conditional probability of survival from age 15 to age 50. The estimates thus reflect "partial lifetime" mortality over a substantial age period. The mortality measures refer to the time period over which the deaths occurred, although greater weight is generally given to the information from more recent deaths. Expert matching of these estimates with model schedules of mortality, developed on the basis of mortality experience over a broad range of countries and time periods, can be used to estimate life expectancy at birth.

The above methodology is most developed for the estimation of mortality among infants and children, which includes the majority of deaths in a developing country. Estimates are based on a mother's retrospective reporting of her fertility history, or a question on the number of children ever born and the number of children surviving to the time of the survey (UN, 1983). These measures also provide limited information on mortality over time. Information on survival between birth and age 5 within the two to three years immediately prior to the survey is generally considered the most accurate. Limitations of the method include probable understatement of birth and death events recalled from the past, inclusion of fostered and adopted children, and decreasing accuracy of reporting as overall numbers of births and childhood deaths decline. Whether there is a selective underreporting of female versus male deaths through use of these measures is uncertain.

Procedures to estimate adult mortality are still being developed and refined, spurred on by more recent recognition that child and adult mortality are not as closely associated as had been thought; thus, traditional methods of estimating adult mortality based on child mortality are no longer considered accurate. The most direct approach—to ask about deaths in a household in a fixed previous time period—has not proved very useful in developing countries, because it requires large sample sizes to yield sufficient numbers of observations. Indirect methods have been more successful. These methods include, for example, the widowhood and orphanhood methods (Timaeus, 1991a,b,c; UN, 1983) and the sisterhood method (Graham et al., 1988, 1989). Such methods are based on questions that ask the respondent about survival of close relatives. Estimates are converted to survival probabilities across an age span, often ages 15–60, based on assumptions about past age patterns and trends of fertility and mortality. Widowhood questions have not been as widely used in Africa as orphanhood questions, because the former require a greater number of respondents to obtain accurate estimates. Sisterhood methods are fairly recent developments and, as such, are still being evaluated, but early field trials are encouraging (Graham, 1991; Trussell and Rodriguez, 1990). Orphanhood questions may underestimate mortality for theoretical reasons, as well as because of adoption, where respondents may refer to surviving stepparents or foster parents, rather than to early mortality of the biological parents. The impact of the adoption effect is possibly greater on reporting about mothers than about fathers, which may underlie the relatively steep declines noted in female compared with male adult mortality (Timaeus, 1991d). Mortality estimates may also be biased by other reporting errors, such as age misstatements or omissions.

During the 1960s, several of the English-speaking countries initiated efforts in census data collection, and a major impetus was provided by the African Census Program in the 1970s, when 22 countries undertook census activities. A majority of Sub-Saharan African countries also undertook censuses in a 1980s round (de Graft-Johnson, 1988). Many of these efforts, however, did not include the kinds of indirect mortality measures described above, which would allow for robust estimates of mortality.

A number of Sub-Saharan African countries have conducted national and subnational household demographic surveys under internationally sponsored programs in an attempt to gather reliable demographic data—for example, the World Fertility Surveys (WFS), Contraceptive Prevalence Surveys (CPS), Demographic and Health Surveys (DHS), and a socioeconomic survey, the Living Standards Measurement Studies (LSMS). Demographic Health Surveys have now been conducted in 25 countries in Sub-Saharan Africa. These surveys have provided the bulk of the information that allows for more accurate assessment of mortality rates.

In addition to these efforts, a limited number of small-scale community studies have been conducted in various sites of Sub-Saharan Africa that provide fairly high-quality information on mortality and selected aspects of morbidity. Such studies have been conducted in Kenya (Machakos), The Gambia (Keneba), Ghana (Danfa), Nigeria (Malumfashi), Senegal (Niakhar, Bandafassi, Mlomp), and Burkino Faso (Kongoussi) among other sites (Feachem et al., 1991; Gbenyon and Locoh, 1989). These studies generally utilize population-based surveillance systems or multiround surveys. Such frequent contacts with a household over a number of years substantially improve the accuracy of data collection, but the intensive effort required limits the total number of households that can be surveyed.

Even with these useful additions, however, the availability and quality of survey data on mortality in the region, particularly by gender, are limited, and they differ according to the age category and disease examined. In part, the information collected reflects the focus of concern in the region. For example, high fertility levels and high infant and child mortality levels—compared with the rest of the world—have long been predominant causes of concern in Sub-Saharan Africa. It is not surprising, therefore, that the WFS concentrated on women in the reproductive ages at the time of the survey, and thus provided substantial data primarily on marital fertility and infant and child mortality. The DHS, in turn, has an expanded focus on health-related behaviors related to child mortality, nutrition, and morbidity, but provides little or no information on adult mortality. The longitudinal surveys mentioned above have focused on specific diseases such as malaria, measles, or schistosomiasis, or on malnutrition, and their fairly small size requires years of surveillance before reliable adult mortality information is acquired.

Based on these sources, a partial picture of mortality and cause of death in Sub-Saharan Africa can be constructed, but significant gaps in the life span remain. For example, because of low mortality rates in the ages between 5 and 15 years, even in developing countries, virtually nothing is known about health conditions in these ages for either males or females. The focus on reproductive-age women has provided little information on health conditions related to chronic and degenerative disease. The relative infrequency of a maternal death compared with child death has posed a serious obstacle to collection of accurate information on maternal deaths in a survey format.

For cause of death, data on children are more complete than those for adolescents and adults. One reason for this is that it is easier to collect data on child mortality through surveys, given the large proportion of children in the population, their high mortality rates, and the characteristic clinical presentation of many childhood diseases. By far the largest proportion of infant and childhood deaths in Africa, for example, is caused by about a half-dozen infectious and parasitic diseases, including measles, diarrhea, respiratory infections, and malaria. These are acute conditions with relatively short durations that are relatively easy to diagnose, even by lay observers. Adult deaths, in contrast, tend to be caused more often by chronic diseases with more obscure clinical manifestations and, as a result, are more difficult to diagnose accurately. Thus, data on cause of death in the older age categories are generally less complete and accurate.

In many studies, causes of death are assigned on the basis of retrospective reports from untrained observers, usually members of the deceased's family. These "verbal autopsy" methods are only reliable for the easily recognized causes that form a large proportion of all deaths in a given age group (Ewbank and Gribble, 1993). There have not been any evaluations of these methods for estimating causes of adult mortality. It is unlikely, however, that these methods will prove reliable for most causes of death among adults, especially if attempts are made to disaggregate cardiovascular disease and cancers. A possible exception to this is the diagnosis of "maternal causes" related to pregnancy and childbirth.

As data sources in Sub-Saharan Africa expand, the variation in mortality levels, trends, and causes of death among countries is becoming more evident. As a result, the traditional composite picture of mortality in the region no longer holds.

Gender Differences in Mortality

There are few data available for Sub-Saharan Africa that permit age-specific comparisons of mortality rates by gender for anything less than very wide age groupings. Therefore, comparisons from Europe and North Africa are presented here because they may be broadly informative.

Henry (1989) reviewed the European historical evidence on gender differentials in mortality. Most of the life tables he examined showed higher rates in females than in males aged 25 to 44 years in populations where fertility rates were higher than average. This excess is largely explainable through maternal mortality. At younger ages, the picture is less clear. Excess female mortality was common in some or all age groups between 5 and 19 years of age in most European countries at some point in the nineteenth century. This pattern of excess mortality in female children and adolescents, however, is not as pronounced in life tables after the nineteenth century. The reasons for this shift remain unexplained.

Figures A-1 and A-2 demonstrate the gender differentials in mortality over age 1 in Algeria and Tunisia around 1970 and in the mid-1980s. In 1968–1969, there was excess mortality among females in Tunisia at ages 1–4 and 25–44 years. By 1984, there was only a small amount of excess female mortality at ages 10–14 years. In Algeria, there was excess female mortality at ages 1–24 years in 1970, but by 1988 there was only slight excess among female children at ages 1–4 and adult females aged 25–29 years. The excess mortality among females, where it exists, is often largest proportionally during the childbearing years. Mortality rates at these ages, however, are relatively low in all populations. Excess female mortality among infants and children is often less proportionally, but it can be large in absolute terms because of the relatively high mortality rates under age 5.

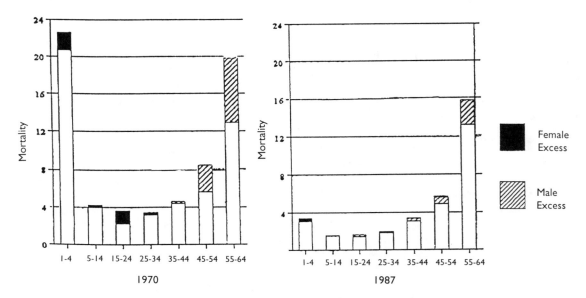

FIGURE A-1   Sex differentials in mortality by age, Algeria, 1970 and 1987. SOURCE: Tabutin, 1992, p. 204.

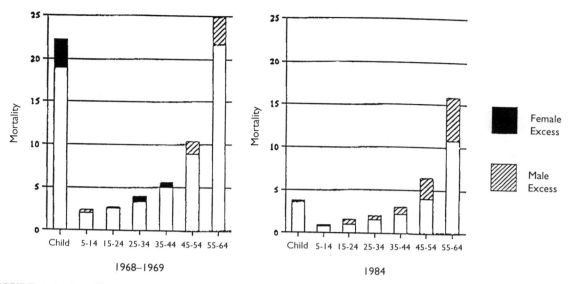

FIGURE A-2 Sex differentials in mortality by age, Tunisia, 1968–1969 and 1984. SOURCE: Tabutin, 1992, p. 205.

The data on gender differences in mortality by age in Sub-Saharan Africa are available for only very broad age groupings, and these indicate that mortality differences are small, and in most cases favor girls (Rustein, 1984; Timaeus, 1993). Less is known about gender differentials in adolescent and adult mortality, although aggregate estimates for the ages 15 to 60 years suggest that the favorable mortality experience in the female child continues through adulthood. These limited findings, coupled with the evidence from Europe and North Africa cited above, suggest that if there is significant excess female mortality in Sub-Saharan Africa, it is likely concentrated in the reproductive years.

Levels of Mortality

Table A-1 presents estimates of mortality under age 5 for countries in Sub-Saharan Africa and for North Africa. The estimates in Sub-Saharan Africa range from 47 deaths before age 5 per 1,000 live births (females in Botswana) to 281 per 1,000 (males in Mali). These estimates for Sub-Saharan Africa, with the exception of those for Togo, do not demonstrate the excess female child mortality observed for Egypt and Tunisia. If child mortality is broken down into specific age groups, however, significant differences are shown in the level of female advantage by age. Among infants, particularly among neonates, where death is largely determined by birthweight and congenital conditions, males are reported to have higher mortality rates than females, as is observed throughout the world. At ages above 1, however, where mortality is much more likely from infectious and parasitic disease, the levels are far more equal. Females, however, still enjoy a slight advantage in most Sub-Saharan countries (Gbenyon and Locoh, 1989).

Table A-2 presents estimates of adult survival for countries of Africa. Despite efforts to pull together all available data, these estimates are somewhat out of date, and describe only about 40 percent of Sub-Saharan Africa's population, excluding some major countries such as Nigeria, Ethiopia, and Zaire. The estimates are judged to be of very low to fair reliability, because they are based primarily on retrospective questions about adult deaths in censuses and surveys, and are subject to underreporting of deaths and to reporting biases, and often demonstrate inconsistency between sources when more than one source is available.

The estimates in the table demonstrate a wide range in levels of survival, although among sources judged to be of fair reliability, the data indicate that approximately 75 percent of 15-year-olds can expect to reach their 60th birthday under the levels of mortality that prevailed in the 1970s and 1980s. In selected countries, the data indicate

TABLE A-1 Summary of Infant and Child Mortality Differences by Gender, African Countries, World Fertility Surveys and Demographic and Health Surveys

Region/Country	Year	Males	Females	Male Excess
Sub-Saharan Africa				
Benin	1981	240	215	25
Botswana	1988	65	47	18
Burundi	1987	190	181	9
Cameroon	1978	139	121	18
Côte d'Ivoire	1980	219	184	35
Ghana	1979	139	121	18
Ghana	1988	160	147	13
Kenya	1978	158	145	13
Kenya	1989	96	85	11
Lesotho	1977	188	169	20
Liberia	1986	242	216	26
Mali	1987	281	277	4
Mauritania	1981	192	185	7
Namibia[a]	1992	94	89	5
Nigeria[a]	1981	170	156	14
Nigeria[a]	1990	200	182	19
Senegal	1978	278	265	13
Senegal	1986	215	202	13
Sudan	1989	140	130	10
Tanzania[a]	1991	160	147	14
Togo	1988	156	162	−5
Uganda	1988	197	179	18
Zambia[a]	1992	188	168	20
Zimbabwe	1988	93	81	12
North Africa				
Egypt	1980	208	222	−14
Egypt	1988	129	135	−5
Morocco	1980	153	148	5
Morocco	1987	118	117	1
Tunisia	1978	119	120	−2
Tunisia	1988	76	74	2

[a]Recent DHS country report data.

SOURCE: Calculated from Hill, 1991, and recent DHS country reports.

that less than 60 percent survive to their 60th year, a substantial differential from the above, but the quality of data for these countries is judged to be fairly low.

The data indicate somewhat more favorable levels of survival in adult women compared with adult men for most countries in the region. Only Mali and Malawi have estimates that suggest a female excess in the proportion dying between ages 15 and 60. As a comparison, estimates for the North African countries of Tunisia and Algeria for specific time periods in the 1960s through the 1980s do reveal excess female mortality at some ages. Nevertheless, overall mortality at ages 15 to 60 is higher for males in both countries at all time periods. Since mortality rises rapidly with age after age 40, any excess female mortality under age 40 may be counterbalanced in aggregate mortality measures by excess male mortality at ages 40–60, where the mortality rates are higher.

Socioeconomic Differences There is substantial evidence that factors such as education and, to a lesser extent, occupation and income have a potent influence on child mortality. Much less is known, however, about the

TABLE A-2 Survivorship from Age 15 to Age 60 by Sex, 1970s and 1980s

Region and Country	Date	$_{45}P_{15}$ Males	Females	Both Sexes	Reliability	Source
Western						
Benin	1978	749	779	764	Very low	Orphanhood
Côte d' Ivoire	1978–1979	646	741	694	Fair	Multiround survey
The Gambia	1978	773	812	793	Fair	Intercensal orphanhood
Ghana	1982	778	880	830	Low	Orphanhood since marriage
Liberia	1970–1971	550	584	567	Fair	Multiround survey
Mali	1986	579	541	560	Low	Recent deaths and orphanhood
Mauritania	1980	782	823	803	Fair	Orphanhood and recent deaths
Senegal	1978	652	710	682	Fair	Multiround surveys
Sierra Leone	1974	466	510	488	Very low	Orphanhood
Togo	1981	704	760	733	Very low	Recent deaths
Middle						
Cameroon	1976	644	666	654	Low	Recent deaths and orphanhood
Congo	1984	656	703	680	Very low	Recent deaths and orphanhood
Eastern						
Burundi	1981	622	699	661	Low	Orphanhood since marriage
Kenya	1974	714	769	742	Fair	Intercensal orphanhood
Madagascar	1974–1975	487	551	518	Very low	Recent deaths
Malawi	1977	741	706	723	Low	Intersurvey orphanhood
Rwanda	1978	584	629	607	Low	Recent deaths
Tanzania	1988	656	675	666	Very low	Recent deaths and orphanhood
Zimbabwe	1978	801	863	833	Very low	Orphanhood
Southern						
Botswana	1980	555	732	646	Low	Recent deaths
Lesotho	1976	503	749	627	Fair	Recent deaths and orphanhood
South Africa	1985	638	766	702	Fair	Vital registration
Swaziland	1981	561	761	663	Fair	Intercensal orphanhood
Northern						
Sudan (northern)	1975	695	768	732	Fair	Orphanhood and widowhood

SOURCES: Data from Benin (Benin, n.d.); Côte d' Ivoire (Ahonzo et al., 1984); The Gambia (Blacker and Mukiza-Gapere, 1988); Ghana and Senegal (Timæus, 1991d); Liberia, Madagascar, and Rwanda (Waltisperger and Rabetsitonta, 1988); Mali (Mali, 1980 and provisional 1987 census tables); Mauritania (Timæus, 1987); Sierra Leone (Okoye, 1980); Togo (Togo, 1985); Cameroon (Cameroon, 1978, 1983); Congo (Congo, 1978, 1987); Burundi (Timæus, 1991c); Kenya (Mukiza-Gapere, 1989); Malawi (Timæus, 1991b); northern Sudan (Sudan, 1982); Tanzania (Tanzania, 1982 and provisional 1988 census tables); Zimbabwe (Zimbabwe, 1985); Botswana (Botswana, 1972, 1983); Lesotho (Timæus, 1984); South Africa (South Africa, 1988); Swaziland (Swaziland, 1980 and unpublished 1986 census tables).

Reprinted from Timæus, 1993, p.222, in Foote et al., 1993.

relationship of socioeconomic factors to differentials in adult mortality. Timaeus (1993) cites data suggesting that adult female life expectancy in the Sub-Saharan African region in the mid-1970s was related to GNP per capita and secondary-school enrollment, although he notes that neither index alone is strongly predictive of adult survivorship.

Urban-Rural Differences Data suggest that adult mortality is lower in urban Africa than in rural Africa. This observed differential is larger in countries with high mortality rates, and this may indicate that the survival advantage of urban areas decreases as overall mortality declines. The generally lower mortality rates observed in urban Africa must, however, conceal pockets of poverty and high mortality among urban dwellers. In general, national and rural adult mortality estimates vary more among Sub-Saharan African countries than those of urban mortality (Timaeus, 1993). There are no available data on urban-rural differences in mortality disaggregated by gender.

Trends in Mortality over Time

Several studies have documented improvement in child mortality levels in Sub-Saharan Africa over the decades since World War II (see, for example, Hill, 1991; Hill and Pebley, 1989; Hill and Yazbeck, 1994). Sub-Saharan Africa has higher overall levels of child mortality than other regions, but shows similar absolute declines in these rates over time. Hill (1991) notes that in many African countries, during the 1950s, 30 to 40 percent of children died by the age of 5, and in only a few countries did less than 22 percent die. By the 1970s, few countries lost more than 27 percent, and many lost less than 22 percent of children under age 5. A breakdown of these figures by gender is not available.

Figure A-3 demonstrates the improvement in the life expectancy of adult females in a set of 15 mainland Sub-Saharan African countries (Timaeus, 1993). A comparison by region demonstrates that all western and middle African countries included in Figure A-3 experienced a rapid decline in adult female mortality for the time periods examined. Four countries—the two southern states for which data are available (Lesotho and Swaziland), northern Sudan, and Kenya—demonstrated only small gains in adult female survivorship in the 1960s and 1970s. These are also the four countries that had the lowest estimated mortality rates for females in the early 1960s. The other eastern African countries included in Figure A-3 had more rapid declines in female mortality (Timaeus, 1993). Although the methods of data collection and calculation underlying these estimates are subject to error, these data indicate a strikingly consistent improvement in female survivorship in the 1970s. Whether this trend has continued to date, and at what pace, is uncertain.

Cause-Specific Mortality Across the Life Span

Although sparse overall, much more evidence has accumulated on cause of death among children than among adults. This information is primarily available from population surveillance systems, hospital records, and vital registration. Although profiles of cause of death for the region as a whole have been published (for example, World Bank, 1993), these profiles are carefully constructed from the few small-scale studies that have been done in this region. The number of deaths in such studies is usually small, and the estimates are subject to many kinds of error and bias, so their results must be interpreted with caution.

Childhood Studies of cause of death among children culled from approximately 12 study sites in Sub-Saharan Africa are reviewed in two sources (Ewbank and Gribble, 1993; Feachem and Jamison, 1991). Infant and child mortality are dominated by a set of causes including acute respiratory infection (ARI), diarrhea, and measles, and in several areas, malaria. Low birthweight, tetanus, and birth trauma are important causes associated with neonatal mortality. Thus, the childhood mortality experience in Sub-Saharan Africa is similar to that in other countries in the predominance of ARI and diarrhea. What is unique to Africa, however, is the impact of malaria and measles. As noted earlier, gender differentials among all causes of death generally reveal a small advantage for female over male children. Malaria and measles are exceptions, however: fairly high-quality evidence from longitudinal studies indicates that young females have a greater likelihood than males of dying from either malaria or measles

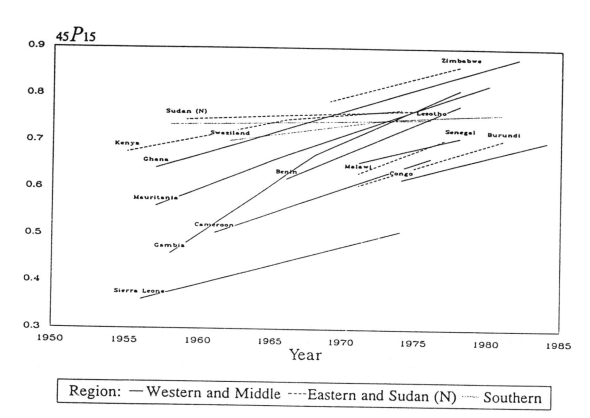

FIGURE A-3 Trends in female survivorship from age 15 to age 60. SOURCES: Data from Benin (Benin, n.d.); Côte d'Ivoire (Ahonzo et al., 1984); The Gambia (Blacker and Mukiza-Gapere, 1988); Ghana and Senegal (Timaeus, 1991c); Liberia, Madagascar and Rwanda (Waltisperger and Rabetsitonta, 1988); Mali (Mali, 1980, and provisional 1987 census tables); Mauritania (Timaeus, 1987); Sierra Leone (Okoye, 1980); Togo (Togo, 1985); Cameroon (Cameroon, 1978, 1983); Congo (Congo, 1978, 1987); Burundi (Timaeus, 1991a); Kenya (Mukiza-Gapere, 1989); Malawi (Timaeus, 1991b); northern Sudan (Sudan, 1982); Tanzania, (Tanzania, 1982, and provisional 1988 census tables); Zimbabwe (Zimbabwe, 1985); Botswana (Botswana, 1972, 1983); Lesotho (Timaeus, 1984); South Africa (South Africa, 1988); Swaziland (Swaziland, 1980, and unpublished 1986 census tables). Reprinted from Timaeus, 1993, p. 231, in Foote et al., 1993.

(see, for example, Chapter 10, and Fargues and Nassour, 1988). Causes for this differential are still being investigated. Much of the information on cause of death is from small-scale community studies; although they provide high-quality information, they yield little information on the representativeness of the findings. Thus, further work to identify the causes of death among children over a wider geographic area would be useful.

Adulthood Timaeus (1993) presents cause-specific data for adults within broad age groups from four small studies in Cape Verde, Mali, western Sierra Leone, and South Africa. For females, the risk of death in the age group 15–44 from communicable and reproductive diseases ranges from 13 to 72 per 1,000, the highest risk being in western Sierra Leone. Risk from communicable and reproductive disease is about half to two-thirds the level of risk from noncommunicable disease (except in Sierra Leone, where they are equal). For both sexes, cardiovascular disease is the leading cause of death within the age group 45–64, followed by neoplasm and digestive disease. The risk of death from injury is fairly small compared with the other major categories, but varies from 5 to 26 per 1,000 across the four sites. Data suggest that gender differentials in cause-specific mortality are generally small, particularly in the age group 15–44 years and for noncommunicable diseases, because among younger adults, higher mortality among males from injury and digestive disease is offset by deaths from maternal causes among females. It should be noted, however, that this information is , again, not representative of Sub-Saharan Africa. The widely varying profiles across sites suggest that much further work on identifying causes of death among adults is necessary to obtain a composite picture that inspires any degree of confidence.

Mortal Conditions of Special Note   Two major causes of female mortality in Sub-Saharan Africa deserve special note because of their profound adverse impact on mortality trends, not only for females themselves, but also for the many others around them who depend on their care. These two causes are maternal mortality and HIV/AIDS. As documented in Chapter 4, maternal mortality rates in Africa are higher than anywhere else in the world. In Sub-Saharan Africa, 150,000 women a year die of maternal causes, about one every 3.5 minutes. If, on average, a woman in Africa has six children during her lifetime (World Bank, 1992), and women who die in their reproductive years leave an average of two or more children (Herz and Measham, 1987), such mortality would leave nearly a million children motherless each year.

Evidence presented in Chapter 4 indicates significant variability in maternal mortality ratios among countries of Sub-Saharan Africa, with a high of 2,900 deaths per 100,000 live births in Mali and a low of 77 deaths per 100,000 live births in Zimbabwe. Five of the 33 countries for which data are available have ratios of over 1,000 deaths per 100,000 live births, over a hundred times the mortality ratio in the United States (Rosenfield, 1989), and only 12 have ratios under 200 deaths per 100,000 live births.

Within countries, certain categories of females are at greater risk than others. A very early first birth increases a woman's risk of dying from pregnancy-related causes. Women ages 15–19 face a 20 to 200 percent greater risk of pregnancy-related death than older women, and the younger the adolescent, the higher the risk (WHO, 1989). In Nigeria, for example, women under 15 were found to be 4 to 8 times more likely to die of pregnancy-related conditions than those 15–19 (Harrison and Rossiter, 1985); data from Ethiopia indicated that teenage women were twice as likely to die from pregnancy-related conditions than were women ages 20–24 (UN, 1989). In sum, pregnant adolescents have a higher likelihood of pregnancy-related complications and consequent risk of pregnancy-related mortality than women further along in their reproductive years; the risk rises again toward the end of those years.

Unlike maternal mortality, analyses of adult mortality, based on retrospective questions about adult survival, do not yet capture the growing role of HIV/AIDS in the mortality profile of Sub-Saharan Africa because of its long period from infection to death and its rapidly increasing incidence over the past decade. HIV may show an increasingly adverse effect on women in Sub-Saharan Africa because of its long incubation period, the rapid heterosexual spread of the virus, and the characteristics of the existing social structure in Sub-Saharan Africa, which may exacerbate the vulnerability of females to infection by HIV (see Chapters 2 and 11). Among young females, these problems may be even more important. Seroprevalence studies among STD clinic patients generally show higher overall HIV seroprevalence rates among men than among women, but this is far from universal. Rates are often higher among younger women (ages 15 to 34 years), and seroprevalence rates are rapidly increasing (CIR, 1993a,b; 1994a,b). The increase in seroprevalence rates is mirrored by a concomitant rise in HIV-related mortality. In a recent study in Rwanda, for example, approximately 90 percent of mortality among childbearing urban women was attributed to HIV infection (Linden et al., 1992).

Data on Morbidity

Sources and Quality

Data on morbidity in Sub-Saharan Africa are considerably scarcer and less accurate than those on mortality. Gender-specific morbidity data are available mainly from a few small-scale surveillance projects or from surveys conducted by nonmedical personnel trained to identify diseases with common and easily recognized symptoms.

As with mortality data, the quality of data on morbidity depend on the disease and age category examined. Estimates of the prevalence of observable and clinically distinct illnesses, such as a number of tropical infectious diseases or the childhood diseases, are more reliable than those for diseases that may require laboratory confirmation, such as malaria, or have less specific symptoms or subtle signs, such as most of the chronic diseases and mental disorders. Estimates of the prevalence or incidence of the diseases in this last category are derived primarily from reviews of hospital-based case series (see Chapter 7), which are highly selective in nature and probably vastly underestimate the true magnitude of disease and disability in the population. This underestimation may have a particularly severe affect for females in Sub-Saharan Africa, because their pattern of accessing and utilizing medical care is generally limited (see Chapter 2).

Estimates of Morbidity

Because available mortality data suggest that females in the region have generally lower death rates than males at any given age—except for the reproductive ages, when women experience excessive mortality from pregnancy and childbirth—efforts to study or address female morbidity across the life span have been limited. Yet a number of studies have demonstrated that although female life expectancy usually exceeds that of males, females more frequently report suffering from chronic diseases that limit their productivity. Analysis of the LSMS for Ghana and Côte d'Ivoire showed, for example, that females had higher rates of self-reported morbidity and substantially higher rates of hospitalization than males (Murray et al., 1992). A prospective study of illness in Kenya also found higher rates of morbidity among females than among males. Murray and colleagues (1992) reported that over the study period 1984–1985, men were ill 20 percent of days, and women 33 to 50 percent of days. Men experienced reduced activity 4 percent of days, while women experienced reduced activity 9 to 13 percent of days.

Disability-Adjusted Life Years

In 1993, the journal *Lancet* wrote, "Every so often an important piece of new thinking about international public health appears. *Investing in Health*, from the World Bank, is such a document" (Lancet, 1993). One of the more important contributions of the *1993 World Development Report* (*WDR*) was the estimate developed to measure the burden of disease in populations, that of the "disability-adjusted life year" (DALY) (World Bank, 1993).

It is broadly agreed that the DALYs presented in the *World Development Report*, particularly those for Sub-Saharan Africa, are subject to limitations, given the availability and quality of the epidemiologic data and the sensitivity of the underlying assumptions.[1] DALY estimates, for example, were not available disaggregated by regions within Sub-Saharan Africa. Data available to derive estimates for Africa, in particular, were by necessity based on little more data than is described here. The chapters in this report, therefore, with one exception, use original data for comparisons rather than DALY estimates. The DALY construct, however, is strongly supported by the committee presenting this report, because it provides a global comparative means for estimating the lifetime burden of disease and disability and, as such, for better understanding how disease determinants and their outcomes influence health across the human life span and across continents. The contribution of the *WDR* in this respect is novel and important, and attempts to improve the estimation of DALYs and to identify other measures of lifetime disease burden are encouraged.

Understanding Mortality and Morbidity Across the Life Span

Demographic data collection in the past has yielded substantial information regarding infant and child mortality in Sub-Saharan Africa, and more recently it has begun to yield aggregate information about the probability of survival across the middle of the life span, ages 15 to 60. Morbidity data collection, however, with its focus on specific diseases, has not yet encompassed a life span perspective, except perhaps in early childhood, when the combined effect of infectious and parasitic disease and nutritional status have been examined together. Thus, a composite picture of disease and disability by stages of the life span remains limited to only pieces of the puzzle.

Available data indicate that males suffer more of a health disadvantage at infancy than females, but that by childhood ages, health risks are more equal. If there is an overall female disadvantage at this stage of the life span, it is very small.

A majority of health concerns in Africa begin to surface during the early school years, adolescence, and the teen years. Information on STDs and HIV, early pregnancy, and safe abortion, which have a lifelong impact on the health of females, is becoming more available, but a comprehensive and representative picture remains elusive. In the early adolescent and middle teen years, deleterious lifestyle behaviors begin and take hold, and many of these, such as cigarette smoking (see Chapter 7), are known to adversely affect adult health status. Information that characterizes this process and documents the adoption and prevalence of these behaviors in females in Sub-Saharan Africa, as in males, is not yet being systematically collected.

In the adult reproductive years, little is known about how diseases and disease determinants interact, or how they cumulatively or perhaps synergistically influence health status during the later adult years. Estimates of the proportion of female deaths attributable to maternal conditions compared with other health conditions, for example, often rely on a simple indicator of deaths within certain age groups (for example, the years of fertility), and these estimates vary widely among sites and data sources. The relationship among these diseases is thus poorly defined and reveals little about the relationship of reproductive health with overall female health (see Chapter 4). More recent emphasis on adult mortality is now producing estimates on aggregate risk of death during adulthood. Little is known, however, about major causes of death among older females or males in Sub-Saharan Africa that are known to predominate among adults in other regions of the world. Cancer registries are not well developed, and little information is available on either incidence or prevalence of cardiovascular diseases, chronic obstructive pulmonary diseases, or other noncommunicable diseases believed to affect women in the region (see Chapter 7).

Mortality rates, both cause-specific and in the aggregate, are imperfect indicators of morbidity, and data on morbidity for most age groups, as indicated above, remain limited. Information on the prevalence of disease determinants (risk factors) or on disease cofactors is also absent.

To achieve a life span perspective, the relationship among diseases, disabilities, and disease determinants at different ages must be better understood, both for females and for males. At this stage, basic representative information on mortality by cause and morbidity prevalence by age group for defined populations is still a necessity. Health service statistics will probably not yield this kind of information over time, given the selective nature of the populations utilizing health services and the uncertainty of available denominator data for comparisons. It is, therefore, more realistic to assume that data from demographic and epidemiologic surveys and studies will fill these gaps.

As noted above, morbidity information, currently collected on a disease-specific basis, cannot yield the information needed for a life span perspective. DALYs have partially circumvented this problem by incorporating dimensions of disability into an aggregate measure; the feasibility of measuring disability in a setting such as Sub-Saharan Africa, however, is an open question. Furthermore, the extent to which the DALY construct can be adapted to adequately reflect health conditions prevalent in developing countries, where the epidemiological transition is at a much earlier stage, is a question that deserves further attention. It is thus clear that further work in both the conceptual and methodological arenas is required for a life span perspective for males and females to come to maturity.

CONCLUSIONS

Although African countries have made considerable advances in expanding their demographic data bases, a composite picture of female (and male) health across the stages of the life span is limited to only pieces of the puzzle. The data that exist are rarely disaggregated by gender and are from scattered sources, most of which are subject to underreporting or other sources of bias. While past demographic data collection has provided substantial information on infant and child *mortality*, and current efforts have begun to yield aggregate information about the probability of survival across the middle of the life span, ages 15 to 60; *morbidity* data collection, with its past focus on specific disease conditions, has not yet encompassed a life span perspective. Further understanding of the interrelationships among diseases and disabilities and their longer-term sequelae—coupled with advances in the conceptual and methodologic means of data collection and analysis—will be required for a better understanding of health status and disease risk across the life span.

RESEARCH NEEDS

To obtain the kinds of data that will permit a better understanding of the relationship among diseases, disabilities, and disease determinants across the female (and male) life span, the following is recommended:

• The continuation and expansion of internationally sponsored surveys to collect information on cause-specific mortality and morbidity is strongly encouraged. These surveys should ensure that all data collected are disaggregated by gender and age, and that methods of data collection and analysis are standardized to the extent possible across surveys to ensure consistent data quality and to permit valid comparisons of findings across regions, populations, and time.

• Data on causes and prevalence of disabilities should also be collected, because they will allow for more accurate estimates of disease burdens in specific populations.

• Survey efforts should focus, to the extent possible, on the tracking of defined cohorts of individuals over time, since such prospective data can provide not only reliable measures of disease incidence and mortality, but also the best picture of how diseases, disabilities, and future disease determinants interact to influence health over the life span. The use of such "population laboratories" in the past has provided important contributions to understanding mortality and morbidity dynamics in Sub-Saharan Africa, but the quality of these studies has been uneven. Careful weighing of the costs and benefits of the information to be gained in such surveys will be needed, and survey construction, data collection, and analysis should be more closely coordinated across surveys to maximize survey cost-effectiveness and the comparability and generalizability of survey results.

• Possible use of sentinel disease surveillance systems as a cost-effective means to identify and monitor changing patterns in mortality and morbidity in populations in stable catchment areas should be investigated. Data from such sources would need to be interpreted with care given the selection biases inherent in the populations tracked, but these data would ideally be supplemented with information from other, more representative, data sources, such as national or subnational household surveys.

• Development and refinement of health indexes that provide a useful means for evaluating the impact of disease and disability across the life span, such as the DALY, should be strongly encouraged. Efforts toward this end should consider the broad range of health measures used to estimate disease burden (such as DALYs), quality of life (QALYs, for example), and other health indexes currently used for the purposes of resource evaluation and allocation.

NOTE

1. To an extent, the committee shared this view and, as such, decided not to include DALYs in its report. The committee's decision, however, does not reflect a rejection of the methods or approach used by the World Bank to calculate DALYs, but rather a concern about the quality of the supporting evidentiary base for the Sub-Saharan African region.

REFERENCES

Ahonzo, E., B. Barrere, and P. Kopylov. 1984. Population de la Cote d'Ivoire. Abijan: Ministere de l'Economie et des Fiances.

Benin. No date. Enquete sur la Fecondite au Benin. Cotonou: Bureau Central de Recensement.

Blacker, J. G. C., and J. Mukiza-Gapere. 1988. The indirect measurement of adult mortality in Africa: Results and prospects. In African Population Conference, Dakar, 1988, Vol. 2. Liege: International Union for the Scientific Study of Population.

Botswana. 1972. Report on the Population Census, 1971. Gaborone: Central Statistics Office.

Botswana. 1983. 1981 Population and Housing Census: Administrative/Technical Report and National Statistical Tables. Gaborone: The Government Printer.

Cameroon. 1978. Recensement General de la Population et de l'Habitat d'Avril 1976, Tome 2. Yaounde: Direction de la Statistique et de la Compatibilite Nationale.

Cameroon. 1983. Enquete Nationale sur la Fecondite du Cameroun, 1978, Rapport Principal. Yaounde: Direction de la Statistique et de la Compatibilite Nationale.

CIR (Center for International Research, U.S. Bureau of the Census). 1993a. Trends and Patterns of HIV/AIDS Infection in Selected Developing Countries. Research Note No. 10. Washington, D.C.: U.S. Bureau of the Census.

CIR (Center for International Research, U.S. Bureau of the Census). 1993b. Trends and Patterns of HIV/AIDS Infection in Selected Developing Countries. Research Note No. 12. Washington, D.C.: U.S. Bureau of the Census.

CIR (Center for International Research, U.S. Bureau of the Census). 1994a. Recent HIV Seroprevalence Levels by Country: June 1994. Research Note No. 13. Washington, D.C.: U.S. Bureau of the Census.

CIR (Center for International Research, U.S. Bureau of the Census). 1994b. Trends and Patterns of HIV/AIDS Infection in Selected Developing Countries. Research Note No. 14. Washington, D.C.: U.S. Bureau of the Census.

Congo. 1978. Recensement General de la Population du Congo, 1974, Tome 4. Brazzaville: Centre National de la Statistique et des Etudes Economiques.

Congo. 1987. Recensement General de la Population et de l'Habitat de 1984, Tome 3. Brazzaville: Bureau Central de Recensement.

de Graft-Johnson, K. T. 1988. Demographic data collection in Africa. Pp. 13–28 in E. van de Walle, P. O. Ohadike and M. D. Saka-Diakanda, eds., The State of African Demography. Liege: International Union for the Scientific Study of Population.

DeCock, K. M., B. Barrere, L. Diaby, et al. 1990. AIDS—The leading cause of adult death in the West African City of Abidjan, Ivory Coast. Science 249:793–796.

Essex, M., S. Mboup, P. J. Kanki, M. R. Kalengayi, and P. J. Brewer. 1994. AIDS in Africa. New York: Raven.

Ewbank, D. C. 1988. Health in Africa. Pp. 85–102 in E. van de Walle, P. O. Ohadike, and M. D. Saka-Diakanda, eds., The State of African Demography. Liege: International Union for the Scientific Study of Population.

Ewbank, D. C., and J. N. Gribble, eds. 1993. Effects of Health Programs on Childhood Mortality in Sub-Saharan Africa. Working Group on the Effects of Child Survival and General Health Programs on Mortality, Committee on Population. Washington, D.C.: National Academy Press.

Fargues, P., and O. Nassour. 1988. Douze Ans de Mortalite Urbaine au Sahel. INED Travaux et Documents 123. Paris: Presses Universitaires de France.

Feachem, R. G., and D. T. Jamison, eds. 1991. Disease and Mortality in Sub-Saharan Africa. New York: Oxford University Press for The World Bank.

Feachem, R. G., D. T. Jamison, and E. R. Bos. 1991. Changing patterns of disease and mortality in Sub-Saharan Africa. Pp. 3–27 in R. G. Feachem and D. T. Jamison, eds., Disease and Mortality in Sub-Saharan Africa. New York: Oxford University Press for The World Bank.

Foote, K. A., K. H. Hill, and L. G. Martin. 1993. Demographic Change in Sub-Saharan Africa. Washington, D.C.: National Academy Press.

Gbenyon, K., and T. Locoh. 1989. Les Differences de Moralite entre garcon et filles [The Difference in Mortality Between Males and Females] in Mortalit et Societe en Afrique, G. Pison, E. van de Walle, and M. Sala-Diakanda, eds., Mortalite et Societe en Afriques au Sud du Sahara. Paris: INED.

Graham, W. J. 1991. Maternal mortality: Levels, trends, and data deficiencies. Pp. 101–116 in R. G. Feachem and D. T. Jamison, eds., Disease and Mortality in Sub-Saharan Africa. New York: Oxford University Press for The World Bank.

Graham, W., W. Brass, and R. W. Snow. 1988. Estimating maternal mortality in developing countries. Lancet 1: 416–417.

Graham. W., W. Brass, and R. W. Snow. 1989. Estimating maternal mortality: The sisterhood method. Stud. Fam. Plan. 20(3):125–135.

Harrison, K. A., and C. E. Rossiter. 1985. Maternal mortality. Br. J. Obstet. Gyn. (Suppl. 5):110–115.

Henry, L. 1989. Men's and women's mortality in the past. Population (English Selection) 1:177–201.

Herz, B., and A. R. Measham. 1987. The Safe Motherhood Initiative: Proposals for Action. World Bank Discussion Paper 9. Washington, D.C.: World Bank.

Hill, A. 1991. Infant and child mortality: Levels, trends, and data deficiencies. Pp. 37–74 in R. G. Feachem and D. T. Jamison, eds., Disease and Mortality in Sub-Saharan Africa. New York: Oxford University Press for The World Bank.

Hill, K., and A. R. Pebley. 1989. Child mortality in the developing world. Pop. Devel. Rev. 15(4):657–688.

Hill, K., and A. Yazbeck. 1994. Trends in Child Mortality, 1960–90: Estimates for 84 Developing Countries. Background Paper Number 6 for World Development Report, 1993: Investing in Health. New York: Oxford University Press.

Lancet. 1993. Editorial. World Bank's cure for donor fatigue. Lancet 342(8863):63–64.

Linden, C. P., S. Allen, A. Serufilira, et al. 1992. Predictors of mortality among HIV-infected women in Kigali, Rwanda. Ann. Intern. Med. 116:320–328.

Mali. 1980. Recensement General de la Population, Decembre 1976. Resultats Definitifs, Tome 1. Bamako: Bureau Central de Recensement.

Mukiza-Gapere, J. H. G. 1989. Biases and errors in the orphanhood method of estimating adult mortality: An empirical examination. Ph.D. thesis, University of London. Photocopy.

Murray, C. J. L., G. Yang, and X. Qiao. 1992. Adult mortality: levels, patterns, and causes. Pp. 23–111 in R. G. Feachem, T. Kjellstrom, C. J. L. Murray, M. Over, and M. A. Phillips, eds., The Health of Adults in the Developing World. New York: Oxford University Press for The World bank.

Okoye, C. S. 1980. Mortality Levels and Differentials in Sierra Leone, Vol. 2. Freetown: Central Statistics Office.

Rosenfield, A. 1989. Maternal mortality in developing countries: an ongoing but neglected epidemic. J. Am. Med. Soc. 262(3):376–379.

Rustein, S. O. 1984. Infant and Child Mortality Levels, Trends and Demographic Differentials. WFS Comparative Studies, 43. Voorburg, Netherlands: International Statistical Institute, Central Bureau of Statistics.

Rutenberg, N., and J. Sullivan. 1991. Direct and indirect estimates of maternal mortality from the sisterhood method. Pp. 1669–1696 in Proceedings, Demographic and Health Surveys World Conference, August 5–7, 1991, Vol. 3. Baltimore, Md.: Macro International.

South Africa. 1988. South African Statistics, 1988. Pretoria: Central Statistical Service.

Sudan. 1982. The Sudan Fertility Survey, 1979: Princiap Report, Vol. 1. Khartoum: Department of Statistics.

Swaziland. 1980. Report the 1976 Swaziland Population Census. Vol. 2. Mbabane: Central Statistical Office.

Tabutin, D. 1992. Excess female mortality in Northern Africa since 1965: a description. Population (English Selection) 4:187–207.

Tanzania. 1982. 1978 Population Census, Vol. 5. Dar es Salaam: Bureau of Statistics.

Timaeus, I. M. 1984. Mortality in Lesotho: A Study of Levels, Trends and Differentials Based on Retrospective Survey Data. WFS Scientific Report 59. Voorburg, Netherlands: International Statistical Institute, Central Bureau of Statistics.

Timaeus, I. M. 1987. Adult mortality in Mauritania. In Evaluation de l'Enquete Nationale Mauritanieanne sur la Fecondite. WFS Scientific Report 83. Voorburg, Netherlands: International Statistical Institute.

Timaeus, I. M. 1991a. Estimation of adult mortality from orphanhood before and since marriage. Pop. Stud. 45(3):455–472.

Timaeus, I. M. 1991b. Estimation of mortality from orphanhood in adulthood. Demography 28(2):213–227.

Timaeus, I. M. 1991c. Measurement of adult mortality in less developed countries: A comparative review. Pop. Index 57:522–568.

Timaeus, I. M. 1991d. Adult mortality: Levels, trends, and data sources. Pp. 87–100 in R. G. Feachem and D. T. Jamison, eds., Disease and Mortality in Sub-Saharan Africa. New York: Oxford University Press for The World Bank.

Timaeus, I. M. 1993. Adult mortality. Pp. 218–255 in K. A. Foote, K. H. Hill, and L. G. Martin, Demographic Change in Sub-Saharan Africa. Washington, D.C.: National Academy Press.

Togo. 1985. Recensement General de la Population et de l'Habitat, 9–22 Novembre, 1981, Tome 4. Lome: Bureau Central de Recensement.

Trussell, J., and M. Rodriguez. 1990. A note on the sisterhood estimator of maternal mortality. Stud. Fam. Plan. 21(6): 344–346.

UN (United Nations, Department of International Economic and Social Affairs). 1983. Indirect Techniques for Demographic Estimation, E.83.XIII.2. New York.

UN (United Nations). 1989. Adolescent Reproductive Behavior: Evidence from Developing Countries, Vol. 11. UN Population Studies No 109/Add.1. New York.

Waltisperger, D., and T. Rabetsitonta. 1988. Un bilan de trente ans de mesures directes de la mortalite adulte en Afrique. In African Population Conference, Dakar, 1988, Tome 2. Liege: International Union for the Scientific Study of Population.

World Bank. 1992. Better Health in Africa. World Bank, Africa Technical Department (AFTPN). (Draft unpublished tabulations, August 25). Washington, D.C.

World Bank. 1993. World Development Report 1993: Investing in Health. New York: Oxford University Press.

WHO (World Health Organization). 1989. The Health of Youth, Facts for Action. Youth and Sexually Transmitted Diseases. A42/Technical Discussions/10. Geneva.

Zimbabwe. 1985. Main Demographic Features of the Population of Zimbabwe. Harare: Central Statistics Office.

Index